Stress at Work

WILEY SERIES ON
STUDIES IN OCCUPATIONAL STRESS

Series Editors

Professor Cary Cooper
Department of Management Sciences,
University of Manchester Institute
of Science and Technology

Professor S. Kasl
Department of Epidemiology,
School of Medicine,
Yale University

Stress at Work
Edited by Cary Cooper and Roy Payne

Further titles in preparation

Stress at Work

Edited by

Cary L. Cooper

*University of Manchester
Institute of Science and Technology*

and

Roy Payne

*Medical Research Council
Social and Applied Psychology Unit
University of Sheffield*

JOHN WILEY & SONS

Chichester · New York · Brisbane · Toronto

Library of Congress Cataloging in Publication Data:
Main entry under title:

Stress at work.

Includes Index.
1. Work—Psychological aspects—Addresses, essays, lectures. 2. Stress (Psychology)—Addresses, essays, lectures. 3. Stress (Physiology)—Addresses, essays, lectures. I. Cooper, Cary L. II. Payne, Roy.
HF5548.8.S74   158.7   77-9626

ISBN 0 471 99547 9

Photosetting by Thomson Press (India) Limited, New Delhi, and printed in Great Britain by The Pitman Press, Bath, Avon.

Contributors

H. R. BEECH — *Head of the Psychology Department, Withington Hospital (University of Manchester Medical School Hospital), England.*

HAROLD BRIDGER — *Senior Consultant, Tavistock Institute of Human Relations, England.*

CARY L. COOPER — *Professor of Management Educational Methods, University of Manchester, Institute of Science and Technology, England.*

ALBERT ELLIS — *Director, Institute for Advanced Study in Rational Psychotherapy, New York, USA.*

CHARLES HANDY — *Master of St. George's College, Windsor Castle, England, and visiting Professor of Management Development, London Graduate School of Business Studies, England.*

R. VAN HARRISON — *Research Fellow, Institute for Social Research, The University of Michigan, USA.*

RAGNAR JOHANSEN — *Senior Research Fellow, Work Research Institute, Oslo, Norway.*

STANISLAV V. KASL — *Professor of Epidemiology, School of Medicine, Yale University, USA.*

JUDI MARSHALL — *Research Fellow, Department of Management Sciences, University of Manchester Institute of Science and Technology, England.*

ANTHONY J. MCMICHAEL — *Senior Research Scientist, Commonwealth Scientific and Industrial Research Organization, Adelaide, Australia.*

ROY PAYNE

Senior Research Fellow, MRC Social and Applied Psychology Unit, University of Sheffield, England.

E. CHRISTOPHER POULTON

Assistant Director, MRC Applied Psychology Unit, University of Cambridge, England.

Editorial Foreword to the Series

This book, *Stress at Work*, is the first book in the series of *Studies in Occupational Stress*. The main objective of this series of books is to bring together the leading international psychologists and occupational health researchers to report on their work on various aspects of occupational stress and health. It will start with this edited volume by some of the most distinguished academics outlining the main areas of research, conceptualization, prevention, and treatment of stress at work. The series will then be followed by a number of books on original research and theory in each of the areas described in the initial volume, such as Blue Collar Stressors, White Collar Stressors, The Interface Between the Work Environment and the Family, Individual Differences in Stress Reactions, The Person–Environment Fit Model, Behavioural Modification and Stress Reduction, Stress and the Socio-Technical Environment, The Stressful Effects of Retirement and Unemployment and many other topics of interest in understanding stress in the workplace.

We hope these books will appeal to a broad spectrum of readers—to academic researchers and postgraduate students in applied and occupational psychology and sociology, occupational medicine, management, personnel, etc.—and to practitioners working in industry, the occupational medical field, mental health specialists, social workers, personnel officers, and other interested in the health of the individual worker.

Contents

Introduction

If 'stress', or more accurately 'strain', can be said to arise from overstimulation then the bombardment we have suffered from books, magazines, television, and radio about the stressfulness of modern society must in itself have contributed to the condition. We have been shocked by 'Future Shock' (Toffler), aggravated by 'A' Types (Friedman and Rosenman), transported by Transcendental Meditation, bemused by biorhythms, and amused yet horrified by Joseph Heller's comment that 'Something Happened'. And, as Heller eloquently points out, much of whatever it is that caused something to happen, happened at work. The present volume explores what we know about stress at work on the basis of research as opposed to imaginative insight. Fact turns out to be just as interesting and perhaps more complex than even the best fiction.

We have tried to guide the reader through this complexity by dividing the book into parts, each of which concentrates on one aspect of the processes involved in stress. Two chapters do not fit neatly into this design. They are the first, by Kasl, and the last, by Payne. Their role, not surprisingly, is to begin and almost to end, since we editors have added a concluding comment. Kasl's chapter provides a comprehensive review of epidemiological studies of mental and physical health at work. It provides a context for all the other chapters as well as summarizing much of what is currently known. The chapter on epistemological issues by Payne raises the question of how future studies of stress might contribute to our knowledge in a more effective way than has been achieved by much of the previous work.

With these exceptions the design of the book follows a simple model of the stress process by concentrating on the stressors; the person stressed; the interaction between the stressors and the person; and finally what can be done to arrest the pathological consequences of physical and psychological strain.

The part on stressors in the person's environment (Part II) has three chapters and starts with an extensive review of the stressors commonly found in blue collar jobs. Christopher Poulton provides a brief review of current knowledge about the effects of lighting, noise, vibration, motion sickness, heat, cold, wind, atmospheric pollution, radiation, changes in atmospheric pressure, shiftwork, and loss of sleep. The more social psychological stressors in blue collar jobs are dealt with by Kasl. The stressors in managerial jobs are reviewed by Cooper and Marshall who concentrate on six areas: factors intrinsic to managerial jobs such as overload/underload; stressors arising from roles as defined or not defined by different organizations; strain arising from social relationships at work; careers and the expectations arising from them; the influence of the organization's structure and climate and its role in causing or alleviating strain; a 'catch-all' area looks at sources of stress arising outside the work situation, such as marriage and the effects of moving house and/or job. A final section deals with the moderating influences of personality and behavioural characteristics.

A more detailed examination of the effects of extra-organizational stressors is presented by Handy who concentrates on the relationship between work life and home life. As the title of his chapter conveys, he is particularly concerned with what causes the home life to be a help or a hindrance to work life.

Part III is concerned with the individual person and the part that individual differences in personality and behaviour play in the overall stress process. Beech turns his attention to another process—the learning process—and explores how individuals learn to be stressed and how they can be encouraged to 'unlearn' to reduce their feelings of strain.

Van Harrison's chapter has links with both Parts II and III of the book and reviews the present state of knowledge about the person–environment fit model which specifically focuses on the nature of the relationship between the person's personality, needs, abilities, etc., and the capacity of the environment to make appropriate use of them.

A more applied orientation to stress at work is contained in Part V which has three chapters. The first one is by Albert Ellis and this offers practical advice about what the individual can do to alleviate his stress whether it arises from work or not. A major argument of Ellis is that we ourselves are creators of both stressors and reactions to stressors and explores the intriguing role of the '*must*urbatory' process. Johansen's chapter describes what can be done to design work environments to produce a healthier social and psychological situation. It draws on studies done on merchant ships, but the problems encountered and the principles generated from solving them have relevance to a wide range of jobs and organizations. Harold Bridger's chapter extends our interests in dealing with stress to wider issues about the roles of culture and community in shaping the values which guide how we view and cope with stress. It integrates well with the other two chapters in the section because it deals with the individual and the organization and how they influence and are influenced by cultural values. The chapter also investigates the oft-neglected fact that stress has a positive as well as a negative effect on human development.

This outline of the book inevitably oversimplifies. Recommendations for dealing with stress are contained in many of the chapters and they are by no means the sole province of Part V. Individual differences crop up in many chapters. Most chapters in the first five parts contain comments and criticisms of methodological issues; they are not confined to the last part. With this proviso this introduction and the index should provide sufficient guidance for the busy reader to make a choice as to where to begin, but as with most books the beginning is a good place.

PART I

Stress at Work in Perspective

Chapter 1

Epidemiological Contributions to the Study of Work Stress

Stanislav V. Kasl

Yale University School of Medicine

Introduction

Ideally, this chapter should (1) identify the essence of epidemiologic methods, (2) define stress and identify stressful aspects of the work environment, and (3) review evidence on the health consequences of such stresses in studies using epidemiologic methods. Unfortunately, this ideal agenda is unworkable and naive. The first two points would undoubtedly lead to statements and postures which would vacillate between vague generalities and more precise positions—which would also be too idiosyncratic, controversial, and narrow. And the third point, if adhered to rather strictly, might leave very few studies to review.

Consequently, I have adopted a more pragmatic approach. The first priority in this review will be on the nature of the empirical evidence and the degree to which it permits inferences about the effects of some aspects of the work environment on worker health and well-being. Only secondarily will I be also concerned with such issues as defining epidemiologic methods or conceptualizing stress at work. That is, these issues are not invoked in order to accept or reject a particular study as appropriate for this review; instead, they will be raised whenever they are relevant, such as in methodological critiques or in interpretation and integration of empirical findings.

The approximate boundaries of this review can be indicated by listing the outcome variables with which I shall be primarily (but not exclusively) concerned: indicators of cardiovascular health, diverse indicators of mental health, and indices of job satisfaction. The decision to emphasize these three areas was again a pragmatic one (i.e. that's where the bulk of the evidence is which deals with health and well-being) and should not be given any greater significance than that. For example, indices of job satisfaction are included here because they tend to be sensitive to differences in work environment and not because their role in the dynamics of workers' mental health has been definitively explicated.

The scope of this review can also be approximately indicated by noting what aspects of the 'independent variable', work environment, are included or excluded. In general, I am *not* concerned with what is traditionally called the physical and chemical work environment. This is the area usually covered by standard occupational health textbooks (e.g. Mayers, 1969) and is the province of such disciplines as industrial toxicology, environmental physiology, and ergonomics (e.g. Brouha, 1967; Hamilton and Hardy, 1974). This is only an imprecise statement of exclusions intended to help the reader think of some obvious examples: chemicals which irritate the skin, carcinogens in the air which are inhaled, extremes of heat and cold, muscular activity and optimal work–rest cycles, and so on. However, since almost any aspect of the physical (and perhaps many aspects of the chemical) environment can be appraised and responded to at the psychological level, it is difficult to be precise about what exactly is irrelevant to this review. Industrial noise is a good example. Kryter (1972) has concluded that harmful effects of noise *per se* (noise as a physical stimulus) have not been demonstrated because it is likely that the harmful effects which have been suggested are due to the psychological meaning of the stimulus, not its physical properties; for example, noise on the job may mean threat of bodily harm from machinery and it is perhaps this threat which has long term consequences. Along similar lines, a laboratory study (Reim *et al.*, 1971) showed that perceived ability to control noise wiped out the adverse effects of unpredictable high-intensity noise on task performance, even though none of the subjects ever actually used the dummy switch designated for turning off the noise.

In short, we must be constantly on the lookout for an interplay between the physical setting of work and the physical task demands, and the psychological appraisal and reaction to these. For example, machine paced work requiring constant attention may be intrinsically arousing and thus elevate adrenaline levels (Frankenhauser and Gardell, 1976). But assembly line, machine paced work in an automobile factory is also a failure of the modest aspirations to find a blue collar job off the assembly line (Chinoy, 1955). And it is for this reason that Kornhauser (1965) believes that his finding of adverse mental health effects of machine pacing only among middle-aged workers ought to be interpreted as the effect of the symbolic meaning of pacing (i.e. failure), rather than as an effect of pacing itself. Given such complexities, it is no wonder that disciplines such as ergonomics are broadening their boundaries and are becoming more interdisciplinary (e.g. Shephard, 1974).

Stress at work in a limited perspective

Investigators and scholars are wont to conclude that the particular social problem they are studying or reviewing is vastly important and greatly neglected. While I do not wish to be so perverse as to argue the opposite about the social problem at hand, stress at work, nevertheless I think that one should briefly note the context of this issue: its relation to other work related problems and the relation of work role to other social roles.

I believe that it is reasonable to argue that there are three work related problems which currently draw much of the attention of policy makers, scientists, and the informed public: quality of working life (e.g. Davis and Cherns, 1975; *Work in America*, 1973; O'Toole, 1974a), unemployment (e.g. Brenner, 1973), and physical and chemical health hazards (e.g. Stellman and Daum, 1973). Stress at work as a *perceived* problem is not in competition with these three and scientists at NIOSH evidently feel that it needs some publicity in order to increase its salience (Margolis *et al.*, 1974). A recent NIOSH Research Report reviewing problems in occupational safety and health (Sleight and Cook, 1974) does have a section on 'lifestress'; however, it deals with effects of non-occupational 'stresses' (such as divorce or life changes) on work behaviour (such as accidents or absences).

The very influential report, *Work in America* (1973), does have a very small section on occupational stress. However, clearly its major and central theme—and the debate and controversy thereby precipitated (see, for example, O'Toole (1974b) and several other articles in the November 1974, issue of *J. Occup. Med.*)—concerns the prevalence of dull, routine, and meaningless jobs and the extent and significance of the resultant job dissatisfaction. Surely, the vernacular use of the term 'stress' or its most common meaning to social scientists as a 'demand which taxes the adaptive resources' (Editorial, 1975), are such as to preclude applying the term to these jobs. As we shall see below (in a later section on conceptualization of 'stress'), some uses of 'stress' include under-stimulation or under-utilization of abilities, and thus the term could be applied to the blue collar jobs which are of central concern to the *Work in America* report. However, at this point I simply wish to note that in terms of current perceptions and commonly used labels, stress at work does not appear to have as high salience as other work related problems and issues.

The other issue I wish to raise briefly concerns the relative importance of the work role and work connected problems, compared to other roles and other sources of satisfaction and dissatisfaction. While the relevant literature is not without controversy and ambiguities in interpreting findings (Gechman, 1974; Kahn, 1972, 1974a; O'Toole, 1974b; Strauss, 1974a), nevertheless a highly suggestive picture can be drawn pointing to a lower importance of the work role than the claim, on intuitive and theoretical grounds (e.g. Erikson, 1956; Friedman and Havinghurst, 1954; Miller, 1963; Tausky and Piedmont, 1967/1968), that work is a central life activity.

In several national surveys of hopes and fears of US adults (Cantril and Roll, 1971), 'good job, congenial work' are mentioned by no more than 6% to 9% of respondents, and 'unemployment' by 10% to 14%. In contrast, issues of good (ill) health and better (lower) standard of living are consistently the two most frequently listed hopes and fears, with up to 40% of respondents listing them. Highly similar findings are reported by Campbell *et al.* (1976): about 38% of a national sample of respondents rate 'an interesting job' as 'extremely important', in contrast to 70% for 'being in good health', 74% for 'a happy marriage', 67% for 'a good family life', and 62% for 'a good country to live in'. And several studies which have examined the relative contribution of job satisfaction to overall well-being and happiness (Campbell *et al.*, 1976;

Wessman, 1956; Wilson, 1967) conclude that family life and spare-time activities are clearly more important.

Studies of retirement also offer suggestive data. The results of a Harris poll (Harris, 1965) revealed that respondents (especially the younger ones) desire to retire at an earlier age than they actually expect to retire. A later study, using both a national sample and a sample of older (≥ 60) automobile workers (Barfield and Morgan, 1969), clearly showed that financial considerations are of paramount importance in plans for early retirement and that any attachment to the 'work ethic' plays a small role. When given the opportunity to retire early, one third of the workers did so and another third were planning to do so. Among those already retired (Harris, 1965), 39% indicated that retirement failed to fulfil their expectations, but less than a quarter of these dissatisfied retirees gave 'miss work' as the reason. In another study of retirees (Loether, 1965), the question 'What do you miss most about not working?' was answered by 68% of respondents with either 'nothing at all' or 'my work associates'.

Other studies of 'meaning of work' (Dubin, 1956; Gechman, 1974; Kahn, 1974a; Morse and Weiss, 1955; Orzack, 1959; Taylor, 1968) suggest that, even though some 73% to 80% of employed men would apparently continue working in the hypothetical event of an adequate inheritance, only some 9% gave the reason 'because I enjoy work' and another 10% felt that work contributed to their health or self-respect. If they did not work, only 9% would have missed doing something worthwhile. Results with another methodology, in which the respondent is presented with a number of alternative activities and is asked which one he would miss most, suggest that only about 25% of industrial workers are 'job-oriented', that is, they choose the alternative 'a day's work'. This is close to the results of a national time use study (Robinson and Converse, 1972) in which some 25% of respondents picked work related activities as the most satisfying among 'yesterday's' activities.

Overall, it would appear that lower skilled industrial workers have a rather tenuous attachment to the work role. They would continue working in the absence of financial needs, not because of any intrinsic satisfaction in work, but because society has not provided any meaningful alternatives. Blue collar workers still 'accept the necessity of work but expect little fulfillment from their specific job' (Strauss, 1974a, p. 54). Much of the theoretical writing on meaning of work in our society, Sayles and Strauss (1966) suggest, is applicable only to workers who do highly skilled and creative work.

The relevance of methods of occupational epidemiology and some illustrative findings

The textbook definition of epidemiology is 'the study of the distribution and determinants of states of health in human populations' (MacMahon and Pugh, 1970; Mausner and Bahn, 1974; Susser, 1973). It has a broad ecological orientation and concepts such as agent–host–environment, or person–place–time are central to it. It is applicable to clinical trials (Feinstein, 1968) and to health services planning, administration, and evaluation (White and Henderson, 1976). The new *Handbook of Evaluation Research* (Struening and Guttentag, 1975), compiled for social scientists, has a couple of chapters by epidemiologists in it (J. C. Cassel, M. Susser) and in general, the whole field of social epidemiology (e.g. Hinkle *et al.*, 1976; Bahnson, 1974, and the six accompanying articles in the November 1974 issue of the *Amer. J. Pub. Hlth*) represents a merging of social science and epidemiological methods. Overall, one is forced to conclude that one can neither set precise boundaries on 'epidemiologic methods', nor identify methodological approaches unique to epidemiology and not shared by some other discipline, such as social psychology, sociology, or demorgraphy. Clearly, there are differences in content, in language (retrospective cohort study), in ways of analysing data (life table methods), in special methodological concerns (limitations of hospital charts), and so on. But epidemiology, as well as the social sciences, share many problems (methods of causal analysis, strengths and weaknesses of non-experimental and quasi-experimental designs, inferences from ecological analyses, etc.) and what is good epidemiology is also good sociology or good social psychology. If any epidemiologist frets about sampling fractions and response rates, while an experimental social psychologist collars a few proverbial sophomore volunteers for his laboratory study—that's a difference in execution and standards, but not in principles.

Perhaps the most common way in which social scientists underestimate the breath of epidemiology is to equate *descriptive* epidemiology (study of distribution) with *all* of epidemiology, and ignore analytical epidemiology (study of determinants) as well as the other variants, such as clinical and social epidemiology. Stated simply, this misperception implies, for example, that an epidemiologist studies differences in morbidity or mortality by occupations, but that it takes a number of another discipline to find out why such differences exist.

The above comments notwithstanding, simple descriptive occupational epidemiology does, of course, exist and it *may* provide useful leads in the study of occupational stresses. For example, analysis of mortality due to arteriosclerotic heart disease among white US males aged 20–64 by occupations (Guralnick, 1963) leads to the observation that certain occupational groups (e.g. college presidents–professors–instructors; teachers) have rates lower than expected while other groups (e.g. lawyers and judges; physicians and surgeons; pharmacists; insurance agents and brokers; real estate agents and brokers) have considerably higher rates than expected. Since these differences are reasonably large (about two to one), but involve groups rather comparable on social status, level of physical activity, physical hazards in the work environment, and so on, it is not unreasonable to ask whether differential job 'stresses' might not be involved. The mortality differences between teachers and physicians have been observed in several countries (King, 1970); moreover, it has also been noted that general practitioners have rates of incidence of myocardial infarction (and mortality from it) twice as high as do other types of physicians

(Morris *et al.*, 1952). These data cry for a closer look at the work setting of the physicians, but as yet we only have impressionistic, informal reports (e.g. Ellard, 1974; Maddison, 1974).

Occupational differences in suicide rates have also attracted attention. For example, policemen, sheriffs, and marshals have at least twice as high rates as do teachers, lawyers, and judges (Guralnick, 1963). Among professional groups such as physicians and psychologists, women have higher suicide rates than men, even though the reverse is true in the general population (Mausner and Steppacher, 1973). Among physicians, the specialities with above average suicide rates include dentistry, psychiatry, ophthalmology, and anaesthesiology, while pediatricians, pathologists, and surgeons tend to have low rates; another interesting contrast involves optometrists whose suicide rate is about one tenth of the rate of the ophthalmologists' (Daubs, 1973).

Other suggestive reports involve the higher rates of peptic ulcer among foremen (Pflanz, 1971; Susser, 1967), and the curtailed longevity among train dispatchers before the advent of electronic equipment (McCord, 1948).

Descriptive occupational epidemiology can seldom offer definitive causal interpretations. However, it is certainly within the scope of its methodology to offer more refined analyses which may refine the causal interpretation. For example, the higher rates of coronary heart disease among drivers of double-decker London buses than among the conductors were interpreted as a function of amount of physical activity at work (Morris *et al.*, 1953). However, analyses of uniforms given out at the beginning of employment revealed a greater frequency of obesity among the drivers (Morris *et al.*, 1956), thus suggesting a self-selecting factor and throwing in doubt the original interpretation. Rosenman and Friedman (1958) further pointed out that the probable greater occupation 'stress' among the bus drivers was another tenable interpretation. And in support of this interpretation, they offered re-analyses which revealed that in the peripheral areas of London (with their lower density of traffic) the bus drivers had rates of coronary heart disease which were actually somewhat lower than for the conductors, and that the originally observed excess among the drivers applied only to the central city.

The more refined analyses of the suicide rates for optometrists and ophthalmologists (Daubs, 1973) are also illuminating, since they reveal that the much higher rates among the latter are due to the very high rates among refracting ophthalmologists; the ophthalmic surgeons have rates quite comparable to other surgeons. But since the refracting ophthalmologists do the same work as the optometrists (albeit, with their M.D. they are 'overqualified' and are doing work considered boring), the interpretation of the differential suicide rates now turns away from the occupational environment (which is similar for both groups), and points suggestively in another direction, perhaps a self-selection factor (depression?) which predisposed the ophthalmologists both towards less prestigeful and rewarding professional activity as well as towards suicide.

Health differences by occupational groups cannot be simply interpreted by *a posteriori* intuitive judgements about the stressfulness of various occupations, since later evidence may not quite support intuition. For example, are the high rates of coronary heart disease mortality among policemen, sheriffs, and marshals (Guralnick, 1963) due to occupational 'stress'? Independent evidence (Kroes *et al.*, 1974; Margolis, 1973) reveals that the most frequently mentioned 'stresses' deal with administrative issues and contacts with the court system; direct, life threatening events are mentioned much less frequently. Well, unless we invoke the notion of defensiveness and distortion in policemen's reports, this would make the policemen's job more like many clerical jobs than the way our TV-fed intuition would demand. Along similar lines, a study of RAF operational fighter pilots (Aitken, 1969) revealed that the four most frequently mentioned instances of 'personal worry and or emotional stress during the previous year' involved housing, wife, finances, and children, while concerns over flying or death were a bit farther down the list. Air traffic controlling is another occupation which has received a lot of attention because the job appears (intuitively) stressful, and because it seems to be associated with greater prevalence of hypertension, peptic ulcers, and diabetes (Cobb and Rose, 1973). Nevertheless, two studies (Singer and Rutenfranz, 1971; R. C. Smith, 1973) both reveal that the most frequently disliked aspects of the job involve administration, quality of management, pay, night shift work (which has very little air traffic), and that so-called 'stress' (high mental load, great responsibility) is either mentioned infrequently or is actually listed among the liked aspects of the job.

The above comments are not intended to suggest that we must accept the job occupants' report at face value and conclude that the jobs are not as stressful as (or stressful in the way) we may have thought on intuitive grounds. Other possibilities exist such as that the reports involve conscious or unconscious defensive distortion or that the reports are usually obtained after long term adaptation to the job environment has taken place. Even more complicated speculation might involve the notion that by some independent, 'objective' criteria such jobs are truly dangerous and stressful, and that it is the inadequate conscious perception of this situation which has health consequences, since a more accurate conscious assessment of the situation might permit better coping. However, we should also not be hasty in rejecting the validity of these reports. Two studies which measured stress response at the biochemical level have provided highly suggestive data on the circumstances of an unexpected *lack* of arousal. In one study (Rubin, 1974), the levels of serum cortisol were assessed on pilots and radar intercept officers on jet fighter bombers landing on aircraft carriers. Apparently, one could hardly find a more demanding and dangerous task than this. Results revealed elevated levels only among the pilots; the radar officers, though equally exposed to the danger, are not involved in piloting the plane and did not show higher levels. In a study of 17-OHCS levels in a combat situation (Bourne *et al.*, 1968), on the day of anticipated attack the officer and the radio operator showed an increase in corticosteroid levels, while the enlisted men showed a decrease. Yet, presumably the soldiers are at least in as great a danger during battle as are the officer and the radio operator. Both sets of results would seem to suggest that 'stress' (as reflected in the elevated levels) was not associated with the general danger of the situation, but with the more specific tasks which required a good deal of attention (arousal?) but which were not performed by all.

If it is true that facile *a posteriori* judgements of stressfulness should not be routinely invoked to 'explain' morbidity or mortality differences by occupations, then the converse is true as well: intuitive judgements regarding occupational stress will not necessarily be rewarded with subsequent differences in health outcomes. For example, in a study of white, male employees at Cape Kennedy, the *a priori* designation of some men as being under stress because of their 'intimate and vital role in launching the space vehicle for a moon landing' (Reynolds, 1974, p. 35), and other men as controls because their jobs were not associated with any responsibility for the launch, failed to reveal any reliable differences between the two groups in several cardiovascular health indicators and a symptom checklist of mental health (Reynolds, 1974; Warheit, 1974). Another example is an early study of blood pressure among prisoners (Alvarez and Stanley, 1930): the clear expectation of the authors was to find elevated levels among the prisoners and thereby to document the stressfulness of the prison setting. However, the actual finding was one of normal levels among prisoners and significantly higher levels among the prison guards: within various age groupings, the mean systolic blood pressure of the guards was 10–15 mm Hg higher than for the prisoners.

A number of reports have appeared over the years which discuss the application of epidemiologic methods to the study of occupational health issues (e.g. Bernacki, 1975; Gaffney, 1973; Proceedings, 1962) and the various relevant methodological problems and pitfalls (e.g. Enterline, 1976; McMichael, 1976). The typical paradigm is generally reasonably simple: establish differences in morbidity or mortality by occupations and place of work, and then search for environmental agents in the work place, the exposure to which might explain these differences. The actual execution of such studies, of course, may run into many problems: (1) self-selection into occupations (e.g. social class or personality differences); (2) company selection procedures, such as those exemplified by health screening into a particular job; (3) health reasons (initiated by company or the individuals) for job mobility, leaving the company, and retirement; (4) determining and measuring actual exposure; (5) various inadequacies in personnel records and company data; (6) possible biases in follow-up of subjects. And, of course, there are always possible confounding variables which may complicate interpretations in specific studies. For example, a recent report (Sterling and Weinkman, 1976) reveals some strong differences in smoking characteristics by occupations: white, male, blue collar workers are much more likely to be cigarette smokers than are white men belonging to the technical–professional–managerial grouping. Because of the broad health consequences of cigarette smoking, these differences are a potential source of serious bias if ignored. Another type of an illustration of possible confounding is the finding (Barnard and Duncan, 1975) that certain emotional stimuli (sounding of the alarm, riding the fire truck) are associated with greatly elevated levels of heart rate among fire fighters; however, since fire fighters are invariably also exposed to pollutants such as carbon monoxide, the singling out of 'emotional stress' in trying to explain any changes in cardiovascular health would be seriously amiss.

It seems to me that even though social scientists studying stress at work would learn a good deal from this particular area of occupational epidemiology, nevertheless the basic paradigm of establishing health differences and then tracing them to exposure to some environmental agent is probably too simple to be a methodological guide to the study of work stress and mental health outcomes. Consider the following contrast. Angiosarcoma of the liver is so extremely rare that just three or four cases are enough to alert health officials and start a search for agents (Creech and Johnson, 1974). The disease and its natural history are such that many traditional problems are minimized: diagnosis, distinguishing illness from illness behaviour (Kasl and Cobb, 1966), availability and effectiveness of treatment, latency between exposure and onset and death, multiple risk factors, and so on. Moreover, the search for agents produced a quick convergence on polyvinyl chloride as the probable cause. Corroborating information came in quickly from many manufacturing places around the world. Finally—and this is something not available to the social scientists examining work stress and mental health—short term laboratory studies on animals provided further confirmatory evidence. In short, a tight little package and a scientific success story.

Now consider another study, entitled 'Job stress and psychiatric illness in the U.S. Navy' (Schuckit and Gunderson, 1973). The authors identified through case files all Navy men hospitalized with a psychiatric diagnosis in the years 1966–1968, and then computed rates of 'first' (in the Navy) psychiatric hospitalization by occupation. Jobs which had high and low rates were designated as high and low 'risk' jobs, respectively. Independent assessments of 'severity of working conditions' failed to show any association with the high–low 'risk' classification. Job satisfaction data on a separate sample produced some ambiguous results, showing both more boredom and more overall job satisfaction on the high 'risk' jobs. In general, the jobs with higher rates tended to be more routine and those with lower rates, more technical. Data on characteristics of individuals revealed men in high 'risk' jobs to be older, of lower education, of lower social class of origin, more likely to be divorced or single, and so on. Since these are all characteristics the men brought with them to the jobs, and since these characteristics have been found in innumerable studies to be associated with higher rates of treated (and untreated) mental illness, the conclusion is quite compelling that this approach failed to reveal anything about job stresses—in fact, failed to be a study of job stresses. (The authors are reasonably cautious in interpreting their results, but the title of their article certainly has more marquee value than scientific scruple.)

Some issues in conceptualizing and measuring stress at work

Lazarus (1971) has noted that defining stress and related concepts makes for dull reading. Yet even this modest insight seems to be contradicted by the enormous number of publications which are apparently concerned with the concept of stress. This non-empirical literature tends to fall into several types of efforts to pin down the concept: (1) enumeration of environmental conditions which are to be considered stressful, using either concrete instances (e.g. Landy and Trumbo, 1976; Weitz, 1970) or more general theoretical concepts (e.g. Engel, 1962; Gross, 1970; McGrath, 1976); (2) restating the concept by using some other word, generally also from the vernacular, which is no more precise but perhaps less general: (a) stress as strenuous effort ... to maintain essential functions ... at a required level (Ruff and Korchin, 1967), (b) stress as 'information' interpreted as threat of loss or injury (Lipowski, 1975), (c) stress as frustration and threat which cannot be reduced (Bonner, 1967), or (d) stress as unpredictability of the future (Groen and Bastiaans, 1975); (3) defining it in terms of some 'essential' characteristics, such as: (a) unavailability of adequate responses, which has important consequences (Sells, 1970), (b) situations which are new, intense, rapidly changing, unexpected (Appley and Trumbull, 1967), or (c) in terms of motives involved in specific situations such as achievement (Pepitone, 1967); (4) attempting greater conceptual precision in order to enhance the usefulness of the term in future efforts of hypothesis testing and theory building: here, McGrath's (1970a) definition of stress as 'a *(perceived)* substantial *imbalance* between *demand* and response *capability,* under conditions where failure to meet demand has important (perceived) consequences' (p. 20) seems to have had the widest acceptance (e.g. Editorial, 1975; Lazarus, 1971). It is also the definition with the closest tie-in to the increasingly popular 'person–environment fit' formulation (e.g. Berger, 1969; Dawis *et al.,* 1964; French, 1974; French *et al.,* 1974; Lofquist and Dawis, 1969; Veroff and Feld, 1970).

Of course, there are also observers of the scene: (1) who conclude that the term is useful for no more than designating a broad area of study, a rubric for related problems (McLean, 1974), or (2) who offer a reasoned argument that the term is altogether useless and should be abandoned (Hinkle, 1973).

One of the most telling criticisms of this literature is the comment that each of these formulations is in some sense tied to a certain field of study and cannot be easily extended to all levels of human functioning (Scott and Howard, 1970). It is therefore interesting to note that most of the stress formulations specifically dealing with the work setting are of the enumeration type. For example, Landy and Trumbo (1976) have the following intuitive list of stresses: job insecurity, excessive competition, hazardous working conditions, task demands, long or unusual working hours. Gross (1970) lists three broad classes: (1) due to organizational careers (not losing job, career advancement, disengagement), (2) due to task (routinization of work, task difficulty), and (3) due to organizational structure. And McGrath (1976) has a list of six sources of stress: task, role, behaviour setting, physical environment, social environment, and characteristics which the person brings with him to the job.

The above listing of work stresses from the three illustrative sources suggests that 'stress at work' has not achieved any kind of a closure, either in the sense of concept clarification or as delineation of boundaries. However, as we shall see from the studies reviewed in subsequent sections, two major versions of 'stress at work' are implicit or explicit in most of the work: (1) the narrower version, as excess of environmental demands over the capability to meet them (other applicable, related terms are overload, overstimulation), and (2) the broader version, as inadequate person–environment fit, which includes not only the narrower version above but also the relation of needs in the person to sources of satisfaction in the work environment to meet such needs (other applicable, related terms include under-utilization, under-load, under-stimulation).

However, there is one convergence of theoretical formulations of stress, and this concerns the incorporation of the idiographic, subjective approach in stress formulations. Stated most simply, this approach formalizes the presumed wisdom of the saying 'one man's meat is another man's poison'. (For a characteristic formulation, see Gardner and Taylor (1975, p. 140): 'stress is an individual phenomenon, is subjective in nature, and can occur in anyone who feels that he or she is under pressure'.) For example, in the McGrath (1970a) formulation, the notion of imbalance between environmental demands and response capability is an idiographic one: specific demands on a particular individual and how they relate to his particular capability to meet them. But, more importantly, the emphasis is on *perceived* demands, *perceived* capability, and *perceived* consequences if demands are not met. The intellectual antecedent of this approach is—at least in part—the distinction in Lewinian theory between the life space and the foreign hull (see Cartwright (1959) and his discussion of the problem of the 'boundary zone'). Moreover, the approach gives full recognition to the importance of the process of cognitive appraisal in stress, emphasized by such writers as Lazarus (1966). Unfortunately, this convergence of theoretical formulations has led to a *self-serving methodological trap which has tended to trivialize a good deal of the research on work stress* or role stress: the measurement of the 'independent' variable (e.g. role ambiguity, role conflict, qualitative overload, etc.) and the measurement of the 'dependent' variable (role strain, distress, dissatisfaction) are sometimes so close operationally that they appear to be simply two similar measures of a single concept. For example, Lyons (1971) reports a correlation of—0.59 between 'role clarity' and an index of job tension among staff registered nurses. Yet since the latter index has many items regarding being bothered by unclear responsibility, unclear evaluation by supervisor, unclear expectations by others, etc., the correlation between the two scales becomes about as illuminating as correlating 'How often do you have a headache?' type of item with 'How often are you bothered by headaches?' form of item. Similarly, what is the meaning of an association between high qualitative overload and low self-esteem among university professors (Mueller, 1965), when the former (perceiving one's skills and abilities as not being good enough to meet job demands) and the latter (being dissatisfied with oneself and one's skills and abilities) both derive from one and the same perception of oneself?

What is the way out of this triviality trap? Certainly, an exclusive reliance on 'objective' measures ('objective' in the sense that the data are not supplied by the self-same respondent who is also describing his distress, strain or dissatisfaction; 'objective' can be either reports of others or factual data about company structure, machinery, job tasks, etc.) for assessing the independent variable, stress at work, would violate the spirit of most anybody's notion of stress. Objective and perceptual measures tend to be poorly correlated (Kahn *et al.*, 1964; Kasl, 1973; Payne and Pugh, 1976) and very rarely produce comparable associations (in magnitude) with the typical outcome measures. But since it is almost always of interest to know: (1) how outcome variables relate to objective measures of the work environment, and (2) the extent to which perceptual measures are anchored in objective data, one suggestion would be to use both sets of variables in a research design, whenever possible. Another suggestion is to make extensive use of the strategy of searching for possible modifying effects of various characteristics of the person on the association between the independent and dependent variables. For example, Kahn (1974b) found that the modest association between 'objective' role conflict (the sum of pressures to change behaviour, as reported by the role senders who had formal influence on the respondent) and experienced role conflict was really an amalgamation of a strong association among men high on anxiety-proneness and a total lack of association among men low on anxiety-proneness; similarly, the weak overall association between 'objective' role conflict and reported job tension was hiding a stronger association among flexible men and an absence of an association among rigid men. Such explication of an overall association via the influence of individual characteristics and individual differences is fully in the spirit of the idiographic, subjective formulation of stress, even though an objective measure of the work environment is actually being used. Finally, one might also suggest that even in a study where the self-report of the subjects is the only source of data, some steps towards reducing the triviality of findings can be taken if the investigator makes a strenuous effort to operationalize two conceptually distinct variables as differently and independently as possible. For example, Johnson and Stinson (1975) measured 'person–role conflict' by direct enquiry into the extent to which the subject's job entailed tasks which he felt should not be part of the job. This measure thus seems to tap a basic complaint about one's job (carrying out disliked activities) and, not surprisingly, it correlated -0.65 with overall job satisfaction among military officers and civil service personnel. Possibly, a more appropriate and more distinct operationalization of the conflict variable would have been to assess the behavioural demands (along a number of dimensions) which stem (1) from the work environment and (2) from the self (due to values and needs and aspirations, perhaps), and then compute some compound discrepancy or conflict measure.

Before closing this section, I wish to comment briefly on one approach to stress which has gained enormous popularity in recent years: social change and life events. Many of the workers in the area of 'stress and disease' (e.g. Cassel, 1974; Groen, 1971; Kagan, 1971) have zeroed in on social and cultural change in their attempts to understand a variety of illnesses. And just about anybody (it would seem) who is interested in stress and has some spare room in their questionnaire or interview schedule is using some kind of a life events list in their study—in spite of an accumulating, well-thought-through, and well-deserved criticism of the methodology (e.g. Dohrenwend and Dohrenwend, 1974; Rabkin and Struening, 1976). However, much of this literature on social change and life events is not applicable to the concerns of this review because: (1) studies of stress at work mostly examine some stable aspects of the work environment for its effects, while studies of social change seldom zero in on the work setting; (2) the results of studies using the list of life events methodology seldom permit the isolation of effects due to life events involving only work. And in those instances in which this is possible, the causal interpretation of the findings is not clear. For example, what does it mean that more depressed patients seeking treatment than matched community controls, report events involving work (particularly 'start new type of work' and 'change in work conditions') for the 6 months prior to interview (Paykel *et al.*, 1969)? Is there a recall and reporting bias? Is there a factor which may predispose towards both depression and changes at work? Do the events clearly antedate onset of depression, or only onset of helpseeking? What exactly are the changes at work which are involved: are they economic, in supervision, in new task demands, in prestige and esteem of work and job, and so on? These are, of course, obvious questions.

Because of the great prominence of the social change and life events literature, in the review below we shall be particularly on the lookout for studies which specifically examine health effects of change in the work setting.

Stress at work and indicators of cardiovascular health

There is no integrated programme of research in which stress at work and cardiovascular health are systematically studied and where new studies build on the results of earlier ones (for beginnings of concern with this issue, see J. S. House, 1974b, and Orth-Gomer, 1974). Instead, the studies to be examined in this section are truly a mixed bag, in the sense of variety of methodologies, settings, conceptualizations, and inadequacies. The overall picture is quite suggestive, but there are many gaps and very few individual studies are above methodological criticism or offer an unambiguous interpretation. And it should be no surprise to find that these studies deal almost exclusively with white males.

Overall, there does not appear to be a consistent linear gradient in coronary heart disease (CHD) mortality and morbidity due to socio-economic status (or its major components) for US white males (Antonovsky, 1968; Guralnick, 1963; Jenkins, 1971; Kitagawa and Hauser, 1973; Lehman, 1967; Marks, 1967; National Center for Health Statistics, 1965). To be sure, there are some inconsistencies due to methods: for example, ecological analyses of CHD mortality by areas tend to reveal some excess in the poorest areas (Comstock, 1971; Kitagawa and Hauser, 1973); occupational gradients in total communities do not always agree with results from a single industrial setting (Lehman, 1967); and incidence and prevalence studies do not always yield the same results (e.g. Cassel, 1971). But overall, the generalization regarding an absence of a consistent linear gradient is quite defensible. Moreover, major risk factors such as serum cholesterol and blood pressure also did not reveal a clearcut social class gradient in a national sample (National Center for Health Statistics, 1966 and 1967), though a modest inverse gradient between level of education and blood pressure should not be ignored. And cigarette smoking, as we have noted earlier, appears to be more common in the lower status blue collar occupations (Sterling and Weinkman, 1976).

More promising leads with socio-economic indicators have been obtained by investigators who constructed various derived indices of concepts generally labelled 'social mobility' and 'status incongruity' (e.g. Jenkins, 1971; Smith, 1967). While I shall briefly examine the evidence which only bears on the occupational setting, it should be recognized that: (1) various aspects of socio-cultural mobility are intercorrelated (e.g. geographical and occupational mobility) and (2) the evidence linking these concepts to CHD is very broad, e.g. geographical mobility (Syme et al., 1964), excess of wife's educational attainment over husband's (Shekelle et al., 1969), discrepancy in parental religion (Lehr et al., 1973), or place of one's residence in relation to rate of urbanization (Tyroler and Cassel, 1964). And, incidentally, there is a good deal of methodological controversy regarding the adequacy of data analysis in the status incongruity studies, particularly the extent to which main status effects have been removed before one searches for interaction-incongruity (e.g. Horan and Gray, 1974; Shekelle, 1976).

There is some evidence that the relationship between educational attainment and occupational status is associated with CHD morbidity (Bruhn et al., 1968; Christenson and Hinkle, 1961; Hinkle et al., 1966 and 1968; Wan, 1971); specifically, men with relatively low education compared to their occupational status appear to be at greater risk. (Other findings, such as higher CHD rates among those with lower education (Lehr et al., 1973) also fit in since they involved relatively high occupational categories.) The most tempting interpretation is that such a combination represents a work situation in which the job demands (high occupational status) exceed the skills and training of the employee (low education), leading to work pressures and overload. However, this is too hasty an interpretation, since Hinkle and his collaborators have clearly shown that the men without college education who go on to attain high occupational status in the Bell system are different from the college-educated men on so many diverse variables (smoking, social background, non-work activities) that the college-no-college distinction picks up broad differences in early-established life styles rather than a narrower status congruity-incongruity distinction. We need additional analyses to see whether the lower rates of CHD among the higher levels of management (Lee and Schneider, 1958; Pell and d'Alonzo, 1963) hold primarily for those with college education, and whether the role of confounding variables (which may antedate the work situation) can be partialled out.

The data on occupational mobility are also suggestive without being conclusive. The two studies of Syme (Syme *et al.*, 1964 and 1965) carried out in North Dakota and California showed that cases with CHD had experienced more occupational changes and had been fewer years in their principal occupation than matched controls. However, Wardwell and Bahnson (1973) failed to replicate these findings in Connecticut. Lehman *et al.* (1967) analysed 30-year data on a cohort of 1160 men working in the Bell system and found no differences on any one of their many indices of mobility (number of promotions, of changes in job assignment, of job titles held, of demotions, of intra-company location changes, and so on) between three age–education matched groups of men: deceased from CHD, deceased from another cause, and survivors. On the other hand, Jenkins *et al.* (1966) found that men with a 'silent' myocardial infarction were more likely to have received a job promotion within the previous three years than age–occupation matched controls. Findings from the Evans County study (Kaplan *et al.*, 1971) revealed that for upper and middle class subjects, inter- and intra-generational mobility was associated with lower CHD rates than was lack of mobility; on the other hand, lower class subjects showed lowest CHD rates if they were stable and higher rates if they were mobile. Wardwell *et al.* (1968) reported consistent data in that CHD rates were more adversely affected by intergenerational mobility (either up or down) of lower social class men than of middle or upper class men. However, complex interactions with religious status were also noted.

Obviously, the mobility data are confusing and apparently inconsistent. They demand that we begin digging below the surface of socio-demographic variables and formulate both richer hypotheses and more probing study designs, since all we know right now is that adverse health effects *may sometimes* be observed. For example, to what extent are consequences of mobility modified by various company policies of concern and support ('Ma' Bell?), by the distinction between intra- and inter-company moves, by associated residential and geographical moves, by changes in co-workers, etc.? Approached from another viewpoint, we need to ask: what exactly are the changes precipitated by a particular occupational move being studied? For example, are there some occupations (e.g. university professors in non-administrative slots) in which promotion precipitates a minimum of change in job content, while there are other settings (e.g. a scientist in research and development moving into sales and management) in which the change in job demands is quite drastic? What are some of the individual difference variables which may interact with the effects of occupational mobility? For example, Jenkins *et al.* (1966) noted that recent promotion was associated with CHD particularly among men with the characteristic of 'high sense of time urgency'.

Several reviewers (e.g. House, 1974b; Jenkins, 1971; Zohman, 1973) have noted that working excessive hours and/or holding down more than one full-time job may be associated with CHD morbidity and mortality. The supporting evidence (Bruhn *et al.*, 1968; Buell and Breslow, 1960; Russek and Zohman, 1958; Theorell and Rahe, 1972) is reasonably good, particularly as it relates to younger men. However it is not quite clear what is involved. For example, Theorell and Rahe (1972) found that cases with CHD had worked more hours overtime, but controls had spent more time doing work at home (i.e. taking their work home). Bruhn *et al.* (1968) found no differences in overtime work, only in having more than one job. And the mortality analysis (Buell and Breslow, 1960) revealed a gradient primarily among younger, light workers, but not among workers doing either sedentary, or medium-to-heavy work (farmers and farm workers were excluded altogether).

The above studies lead to consideration of another body of evidence which shows a rather remarkable agreement. Reports of being tired on awakening, of being exhausted at the end of a day, or of not being able to relax, have been found associated with CHD, both in prospective studies (Paffenbarger *et al.*, 1966; Thomas and Greenstreet, 1973) and case-control retrospective studies (Russek, 1965; Wardwell *et al.*, 1968). Moreover, these and similar reports (e.g. feelings of being overburdened) appear to be associated with higher cholesterol levels (Brooks and Mueller, 1966; Chapman *et al.*, 1966), though not in all studies (Caplan *et al.*, 1975; Schar *et al.*, 1973). However, do these results indicate that work environments which produce a sense of exhaustion or lead to inability to relax after work put the individual at greater risk for CHD? I do not believe so. The two prospective studies obtained their data when their subjects were at *school* and *before* they had begun their work careers, which would suggest that these reports tap a generalized predisposition or characteristic which the person brings with him into the work situation. This interpretation is also supported by the Wardwell *et al.* (1968) data where 'trouble relaxing after a hard day' was strongly associated with father's occupational level (antecedent variable) but not with respondent's own occupational level (concurrent variable). If this interpretation is correct, then we have a difficult problem since we do not know whether this predisposition relates to CHD irrespective of the work setting (i.e. work setting is irrelevant), or if it interacts with particular work settings (i.e. if particular job demands and responsibilities 'activate' this predisposition and thus bring about the increased risk). And, of course, a study design in which only subjective reports from the subjects are available will not be able to disentangle the two possibilities.

There is also a fair amount of suggestive evidence that job dissatisfaction and various types of complaints about work may be associated with CHD or CHD risk factors (Groen and Drory, 1967; House, 1972 and 1974a; Jenkins,

1971; Medalie et al., 1973; Sales and House, 1971; Theorell and Rahe, 1972; Wolf, 1971). This evidence involves a variety of methodologies: prospective and case-control studies, total community samples, interviews with first degree relatives of deceased, and ecological correlations between satisfaction data and standardized mortality ratios for various occupational groups. There is even some evidence that work satisfaction may make a modest contribution to overall longevity (Palmore, 1969). In short, one is convinced that there is something here but, again, it is hard to be more precise. First, other studies have failed to obtain an association between work satisfaction–complaints and CHD or CHD risk factors (Caplan, 1971; Caplan et al., 1975; Mueller, 1965; Schar et al., 1973; Wardwell and Bahnson, 1973). Second, the association may hold only for some subgroups. For example, House (1972, 1974a) found no overall association between job satisfaction and CHD risk (smoking, obesity, blood pressure, glucose, cholesterol); however, among older men in white collar occupations, the predicted association between higher dissatisfaction and higher CHD risk was found, while among younger men the reverse was true (unexpected). Third, it is not always clear what is involved. For example, the prospective study of angina pectoris (Medalie et al., 1973) found that men who reported problems with co-workers and supervisors (being 'hurt' by them or not being appreciated) were at greater risk for subsequent angina. Does this say anything about the work environment or is this just a reflection of a general neuroticism, which is known to relate prospectively to angina (Ostfeld et al., 1964)? Along the same lines, Wardwell and Bahnson (1973) suggest that cases who have had a myocardial infarction are high on 'somatization', a generalized tendency to translate conflict and affect into bodily symptoms, including reports that work affects their sleep, digestion, and so on.

There is an increasingly popular formulation which asserts that jobs or organizational roles which are associated with overload, excessive demands, and many responsibilities represent settings of high CHD risk. This formulation (e.g. Sales, 1969) is, in some sense, an attempt to provide a more focused interpretation of some of the data just reviewed. However, there is additional evidence which bears on this hypothesis which I shall now briefly consider: (1) some suggestive data on CHD differences by occupations, and (2) more specific attempts to assess overload, demands, and responsibilities and relate them to indices of cardiovascular health.

As I have noted earlier, the CHD mortality differences by occupations (Guralnick, 1963) are by themselves mostly an invitation to speculate. Somewhat more interpretable data come from the following illustrative studies. Russek (1962) reported that those specialities within medicine, dentistry, and law which were rated by experts as more 'stressful' (unspecified) had higher rates of CHD, as determined from mailed questionnaires. However, a later report (Russek, 1965) revealed a positive association between stressfulness and cigarette smoking; analyses within smoking categories revealed a much more tenuous relationship between stressfulness and CHD rates.

Moreover, a later attempt at replication in a study of lawyers (Friedman and Hellerstein, 1968) provided only minimal support—there was no overall gradient but the least stressful speciality, non-trial patent law, did have the lowest rates; prestige ratings of the law schools where the respondents were trained complicated the picture. Studies of CHD prevalence among monks (Barrow *et al.*, 1961; Caffrey, 1969) revealed lower rates among Trappist monks (who live in relative seclusion) than among Benedictine monks (who conduct seminaries, colleges, prep schools, and parishes). Since diet differences and different cholesterol levels are also involved, it is interesting to note that within each order the priests (who have more responsibilities) had higher rates than the brothers. However, another study (Groen *et al.*, 1962) did not find CHD differences between Trappist and Benedictine monks. In a study of NASA personnel (French and Caplan, 1970), prevalence rates of CHD among managers were significantly higher than among scientists and engineers; as a group, the managers had also higher levels of role conflict, subjective quantitative overload, and amount of responsibility.

Studies of CHD risk factors yield such illustrative findings as: (1) cholesterol levels go up and blood coagulation is accelerated among tax accountants as tax deadline approaches and workload goes up (Friedman *et al.*, 1958); both return to normal some 2 months after deadline. However, it is interesting to note that while the mean intra-person difference in cholesterol levels between periods of 'objective' stress and periods of normal work load was about 17 mg/100 ml, the mean intra-person difference between highest and lowest levels of subjective stress (of any kind, based on a diary) was 42 mg/100 ml. (2) Air traffic controllers have a much greater incidence and prevalence of hypertension than do second class airmen (Cobb and Rose, 1973); moreover, working in a high-density traffic area is associated with more hypertension than working in low-density traffic. (3) In a community sample (House, 1972), men who report more job pressures (including role conflict, responsibility, work overload) have higher CHD risk, especially middle-aged and older men.

Unfortunately, this picture is incomplete unless we also cite some of the evidence which does not fit easily. (1) Men in higher levels of management frequently have lower rates of CHD (e.g. Lee and Schneider, 1958; Pell and d'Alonzo, 1963); possibly, in these settings work load and responsibility go down with higher levels of management, but this is not a readily acceptable proposition without further data. (2) A large study of a number of occupations (Caplan *et al.*, 1975) revealed blood pressure levels among air traffic controllers no higher than among such groups as machine paced assemblers, electronic technicians, and supervisors; controllers at small and large airports were not significantly different. (3) Employers responsible for launching the space vehicle for moon landing and working under severe deadline pressure were no different from controls (without any responsibility for the launch) on prevalence of EKG abnormalities (Reynolds, 1974); levels and changes in cholesterol, blood pressure, and glucose also failed to differentiate the two groups. (4) Cases with myocardial infarction reported fewer responsibilities at work and less supervising of others than did matched controls (Theorell and Rahe, 1972).

The complexity of the possible relationships linking overload, excessive demands, and many responsibilities to cardiovascular health is illustrated by the programme of research conducted at the Institute for Social Research, The University of Michigan (Caplan, 1971; Caplan, Cobb, and French, 1975; Caplan et al., 1975; Cobb, 1974; French, 1974; French and Caplan, 1970 and 1972). One aspect of the complexity is that more finely differentiated variables (conceptually and operationally) lead to differential associations: (1) quantitative overload may be related primarily to CHD risk (smoking, cholesterol, heart rate) while qualitative overload may have primarily mental health consequences (low self-esteem); (2) amount of responsibility for other people and their work may be positively associated with blood pressure, while amount of responsibility for 'things' (e.g. research equipment) may be negatively associated with blood pressure. Another aspect of the complexity is the interaction between job demands and organizational setting: NASA administrators tended to have lower blood pressure in relation to the extent to which their organizational unit involved mostly administration, and higher blood pressure to the extent that it involved scientific–engineering work (French and Caplan, 1970). Complex associations are also obtained when the role of the social environment (particularly social support) is taken into consideration. French (1974) summarizes some of the NASA study data which tend to show that the association between job stresses (e.g. work load, role ambiguity) and physiological outcomes (blood pressure, serum glucose and cortisol) is positive among men with poor interpersonal relations (with co-workers, subordinates, and supervisors), and absent or negative among men with good interpersonal relations; however, psychological outcomes do not reveal this differentiation. Caplan, Cobb, and French (1975) showed that the proportion of cigarette smokers who had quit smoking was considerably greater among men who reported lower job stress (e.g. work load, time pressure, responsibility for persons and things); however, this association held only among men who were low on social support (from peers, supervisors, and subordinates).

The complexity of these findings is underscored by the volume *Job Demands and Worker Health* (Caplan et al., 1975) which only presents 'main effects and occupational differences'. Given these first level analyses, the results here are quite disappointing; for example, 'no measure of stress, personality or psychological strain correlates convincingly with cholesterol' (p. 81); the same was true of blood pressure. Clearly, we must await more complex analyses to see any linkages between the physiological data and indices of job stress.

It is difficult to see how I can deal with the topic of stress at work and cardiovascular health and not at least touch on the whole literature on 'Type A Coronary-Prone Behaviour Pattern' (Friedman, 1969; Friedman and Rosenman, 1974). However, I will do so only briefly because I believe that as yet the available evidence does not in any clear way implicate the work environment. This is because of a basic paradox in the work of Friedman, Rosenman, and their collaborators: even though Type A behaviour (characterized by such attributes as hard-driving effort, striving for achievement, competitiveness, aggressiveness, haste, impatience, restlessness, alertness, and hurried motor movements (Jenkins *et al.*, 1971) is clearly conceptualized as the result of a predisposition stimulated by appropriate environmental challenges (as Friedman and Rosenman (1974) state, 'an environmental challenge must always serve as the fuse for this' behaviour pattern), the actual work has treated it as a stable personality characteristic which by itself is an adequate predictor of CHD. In their early work, there is a complete confounding of Type A classification and occupational variables: (1) Type A men were selected from engineering, paper manufacturing, newspaper organization, TV stations, etc., while Type B (absence of A) men were selected from a municipal government employees' union, professional embalmers, and accounting firms (Friedman and Rosenman, 1959); (2) among women classified Type A, 97% were working and 67% were classified as executives, while among Type B women, only 35% were working and less than 1% were classified as executive (Rosenman and Friedman, 1961).

I believe the evidence justifies the following conclusions: (1) Type A behaviour is an established risk factor for CHD, with a relative risk of about 2·0; this was obtained in a prospective study and the increased risk is independent of other established risk factors (Rosenman *et al.*, 1975; Brand *et al.*, 1976). (2) Among men with a single previous CHD event, Type A behaviour increases the risk for recurrence of CHD, independent of other risk factors (Jenkins *et al.*, 1976). (3) The dichotomous, clinical judgement of Friedman–Rosenman predicts CHD better than a self-report measure, the Jenkins Activity Scale (Jenkins *et al.*, 1974); the loss in predictive power is about what one would expect from calculating the error of misclassification due to using the self-report test instead of the clinical judgement (Jenkins *et al.*, 1971). (4) Factor-analysis of the self-report test has yielded three factors (hard-driving, job involvement, and speed and impatience), but there are many other items which do not load on any of these three factors (Zyzanski and Jenkins, 1970). Moreover, the three factors are useless in predicting new CHD or recurrence (Jenkins *et al.*, 1974 and 1976), since only the total scale score predicts. On the Job Involvement factor, men who go on to develop CHD are, against expectation, slightly (non-significantly) lower than men who remain healthy.

For several reasons, I do not feel that this evidence, however impressive from the viewpoint of establishing a psychosocial risk factor for CHD, tells us how the work environment is implicated. The basic evidence comes from a male sample which is only 10% blue collar, with most of the remainder in middle and upper levels of managerial and technical–scientific work (Rosenman *et al.*, 1964). Consequently, we do not know if Type A behaviour is a risk factor for blue collar workers, or how it varies as a risk factor across different occupational and work settings. Nor do we know how the extent of Type

A behaviour may vary across different work settings and what components of it might be the most sensitive to such settings. The factor called Job Involvement would appear to be the one most closely tied to the occupational setting, the one most likely to represent the interplay of a predisposition and a situational stimulus. However, as we have seen, it does nothing whatever to predict CHD.

In short, I believe that we are dealing with an incompletely explicated construct. From the perspective of the concerns of this review we need to decompose this risk factor into three components: (1) the relevant personality predisposition, (2) the demands of a particular work setting, and (3) the behaviour and reaction which are precipitated when these demands 'activate' the predisposition. At least, at the minimum, we need to know a lot more about the occupational specificity and generality of Type A behaviour as a risk factor.

I should like to close this section by reminding the reader that, no matter how bewildered he/she is by this array of findings, were one to also consider other issues of a methodological or substantive nature the picture would only get worse. For example, there is fairly good evidence that the psychosocial etiology of myocardial infarction is different from that for angina pectoris (Jenkins, 1971) and that it may not always be wise to just discuss CHD in general. Results of prospective and retrospective studies need to be evaluated separately, since the illness may have many consequences, only some of which have been described (Jenkins, 1971; Lebovits et al., 1967); the same comments apply to studies of morbidity (survivors) versus mortality (non-survivors). Self-reports of CHD may produce spurious associations not found if diagnosis is based on clinical examinations; for example, Reeder et al. (1973) found such an association with their Psychosomatic Stress Index, but it vanished when the index was correlated with abnormal EKG. And the handling of confounding and interacting variables is of such varying adequacy across studies that summarizing findings becomes a very imprecise process.

Several years ago, Matsumoto (1970) sought to 'explain' the low CHD rates in Japan by hypothesizing that certain differences between Japanese and American society might be responsible. Prominent among these was his description of the work role and of the typical occupational career of a Japanese worker. It would appear that the firm one works for, the work setting, and one's co-workers truly become an extended family, which has enormous stability over time and provides an unchanging order. Work and other activities, such as leisure, become intimately intertwined and possibly a blurring of social roles takes place. I mention this essay not to evoke nostalgia in the Western reader, but only because it points dramatically to a certain class of 'social support' variables which are worth investigating. The promise of this approach is evident in the already discussed results from NASA (French, 1974) and in the observation (Cassel, 1963) that shiftworkers with a constant set of co-workers had considerably lower cholesterol levels than those whose co-workers were ever-changing. Even though the studies of work and cardio-vascular health do not add up to an impressive body of convergent evidence, the broad hypothesis involving socio-cultural change–mobility–incongruity remains dominant. Perhaps the broad socio-emotional context (and its stability) of the work setting has been inadequately explored.

Stress at work and indicators of mental health and well-being

There are several reasons why this section must be organized differently from the previous one on cardiovascular health: (1) the relevant empirical evidence suggesting links from various aspects of the work environment to mental health and well-being is enormous; (2) the danger of overlap with other (independently written) chapters in this volume is much greater; and (3) there exist a number of recent reviews of this large literature (e.g. Kahn, 1972; Kasl, 1973 and 1974; Locke, 1976; Porter and Steers, 1973; Robinson et al., 1969; Strauss, 1974a; Vroom, 1969) and one needs to build upon them instead of just re-examining the same evidence. However, since I have already noted that (1) 'epidemiologic methods' does not translate into a uniquely defined body of methods, and (2) 'stress at work' does not point to an agreed-upon set of conditions in the work environment, I am left with no boundaries and no obvious guidelines for organizing this section. What I intend to do, then, is to present an overview, which shall consist of some general propositions, a discussion of the limitation of current evidence, and some remarks regarding future research.

The most general dimension of the work environment, prestige or status level of a job, is clearly associated with higher job satisfaction and with better mental health (Gurin et al., 1960; Kahn, 1972; Kornhauser, 1965; Langner and Michael, 1963; Quinn et al., 1971; Robinson et al., 1969; Vroom, 1964 and 1969). Among the components of job satisfaction, those which deal with self-esteem, self-actualization, autonomy and pay are more closely related to job level than are job satisfaction components dealing with work conditions and relations with co-workers or supervisor (Argyris, 1964; Blauner, 1964; Kasl and French, 1962; Porter, 1962; Quinn et al., 1971). This general agreement in evidence, however, should not blind us to the fact that correlations between job level and job satisfaction or symptomatology are rather weak, seldom greater than 0·30.

The job satisfaction literature in relation to specific aspects of the work environment permits the following summary statement (Alderfer, 1969; Blauner, 1960; Caplan, 1971; Caplan et al., 1975; Indik, 1963; Kahn, 1972; Mott et al., 1965; Porter and Lawler, 1965; Quinn et al., 1971; Vroom 1964 and 1969; Zander and Quinn, 1962). Low job satisfaction is related to: (1) Conditions at work: presence of health and safety hazards, and unpleasant work conditions, such as fast paced and physically demanding work; long hours of work (if this is forced on the worker); afternoon and night shifts; unclear tasks; lack of control over work, such as pacing. (2) Work itself (job *content)*: lack of use of skills and abilities; highly fractionated repetitive task involving few different operations. (3) *The work group*: no opportunity to interact with co-workers; work groups which are large and lack cohesiveness; non-acceptance by co-workers. (4) *Supervision*: no participation in decision making; inability to provide feedback to supervisor; lack of recognition for good performance; supervisors who are not considerate or understanding. (5) *The organization*: large organization with a 'flat' organizational structure (relatively few levels in the organization); having a staff position (versus a line position); discrimination in hiring. (6) *Wages and promotion*: low financial rewards or perceived inequity in wages; lack of promotional opportunities.

The literature which links diverse aspects of mental health to specific aspects of the work environment will be summarized in a comparable way to emphasize the many similarities in results (Caplan, 1971; Caplan *et al.*, 1975; Kahn and Quinn, 1970; Kahn *et al.*, 1964; Kornhauser, 1965; Mott *et al.*, 1965; Neel, 1955; Quinn *et al.*, 1971; Zander and Quinn, 1962). *Poor* mental health is related to: (1) *Conditions at work*: exposure to health and safety hazards, and unpleasant work conditions; necessity to work fast and to expend a lot of physical effort; excessive and inconvenient hours. (2) *Work itself*: lack of use of skills and abilities; perception of job as uninteresting; repetitious work, especially on a constantly moving assembly line; role overload, both qualitative and quantitative, involving generally a discrepancy between resources (time, worker's training and skill, machinery, organizational structure, etc.) and job demands. (3) *Shift work*: fixed afternoon and rotating shifts, which affect time oriented body functions and lead to difficulty in role behaviour (e.g. role of spouse or parent), if the role activities are normally performed during the time of day when the worker is on the shift. (4) *Supervision*: job demands which are unclear or conflicting (role ambiguity and role conflict); close supervision and no autonomy; lack of feedback from supervisor; reports of problems with supervisor. (5) *The organization*: working on the boundary of the organization. (6) *Wages and promotion*: inadequate income; perception of promotional opportunities as unfair or too slow. In the above studies, the obtained relationships are generally stronger for indices of life satisfaction, self-esteem, tension, and the like, and generally weaker for mental health indicators based on psychiatric symptom checklists.

This type of evidence has led Locke (1976) to characterize desirable conditions at work as follows: (1) work represents mental challenge (with which the worker can cope successfully) and leads to involvement and personal interest; (2) work is not physically too tiring; (3) rewards for performance are just, informative, and in line with aspirations; (4) working conditions are compatible with physical needs and they facilitate work goals; (5) work leads to high self-esteem; and (6) agents in the work place help with the attainment of job values.

The convergence of evidence from this extensive literature again should not blind us to the fact that we are talking about moderate effects and modest correlations. For example, Quinn *et al.* (1971) found that the worker's reports of presence of problems in 18 areas of Labour Standards concern (certainly, one good general measure of the work environment) correlated in the low 0·30s with two indices of job satisfaction and even less with several mental health indices. And data from the later national survey (Quinn and Shepard, 1974) revealed that six measures of job related stress (role ambiguity, under-utilization, overload, resource inadequacy, employment insecurity, and non-participation in decisions) had an average (absolute) correlation of 0·20 with three job satisfaction measures (job satisfaction, motivation to work, intention to leave job), and an average correlation of 0·16 with three mental health measures (depressed mood, self-esteem, life satisfaction) (Margolis et al., 1974). And still another national sample study (Kohn and Schooler, 1973) reported the following multiple–partial correlations (controlling on education, income, and occupational status) between twelve facets of occupational conditions (involving organizational locus, occupational self-direction, job pressures, and uncertainty) and: occupational commitment, $r = 0·25$; job satisfaction, $r = 0·32$; anxiety, $r = 0·22$; and self-esteem, $r = 0·16$.

Data on the association between job satisfaction and indices of mental health reveal a suggestive gradient which can be characterized roughly as follows: (1) behavioural (self-reported) indicators such as drug use, alcohol consumption, and cigarette smoking, show negligible associations with job satisfaction (e.g. Caplan et al., 1975; Mangione and Quinn, 1975; Quinn and Shepard, 1974; von Wiegand, 1972). (2) Alienation at work does not seem to generalize (i.e. does not correlate) to other areas of life (e.g. Seeman, 1974; Payne, 1974). (3) Indices based on somatic complaints and symptom checklists generally correlate with job satisfaction in the 0·10 to 0·30 range (e.g. Caplan et al., 1975; Kasl and Cobb, 1971; Langner and Michael, 1963; McDonald and Gunderson, 1974; Quinn et al., 1971; Roman and Trice, 1972). (4) Affect-based measures (anxiety-tension, depression, irritation) yield still higher correlations, while indices of personal happiness and life satisfaction tend to yield the strongest associations with job satisfaction—but still averaging only in the low 0·40s (e.g. Bradburn, 1969; Caplan et al., 1975; Gurin et al., 1960; Kasl and Cobb, 1971; Quinn et al., 1971; Quinn and Shepard, 1974). Exceptions to these four general points should not be expected in national or broad-based samples, but certainly may be encountered in a 'sample of convenience'. And, of course, whenever job satisfaction is operationalized not in the usual way but as worries, problems, upsets at work (in fact, as a mental health indicator for the work setting) then the correlations with mental health indices may be stronger (e.g. Langner and Michael, 1963; Roman and Trice, 1972; Siassi et al., 1974).

It is also interesting to note that there appears to be no evidence that lack of satisfaction in one area of life is compensated for by particularly strong enjoyment or satisfaction in another—at least, in the sense that none of the studies have shown a negative association between a pair of satisfaction or mental health indices.

What is the point of this kind of a broad summary of evidence? Aside from indicating the convergence of evidence regarding various aspects of the work environment, it serves to emphasize the relatively small size of the associations. And these modest associations must be viewed as *upper limits* of any causal effects from work environment to mental health, since significant methodological criticisms would only tend to reduce the estimates of 'true' effects. This criticism is primarily of three kinds: (1) correlations among self-report indices are subject to the criticism that shared 'method variance' (Campbell and Fiske, 1959) and differences in generalized tendency to complain or to be defensive have inflated the 'true' association. (2) Subjective reports of the work environment are so poorly associated with 'objective' data that uni-directional causal interpretations of associations with self-report outcome measures are difficult to make, and the extent to which the 'objective' work environment is involved is unclear. (3) Even if one uses 'objective' data on the work environment (such as job status), associations based on cross-sectional data do not allow convincing causal interpretation or an adequate control for confounding or self-selection variables. (These are obvious and well known criticisms, familiar to all investigators. However, I also believe that they have become part of the 'forest' which we no longer see as we concentrate on one 'tree' at a time.)

One objection to the above summary of evidence is that in drawing primarily on studies using large, representative samples, I have offered generalizations which hide a good deal of variability, depending upon what work setting one is talking about. Accordingly, I will consider briefly three issues which currently draw a good deal of interest and which are more situation-specific: (1) mental health of unskilled and semi-skilled blue collar workers and some associated issues (job enlargement, alienation); (2) studies of role stress, role conflict, and overload, which primarily involve white collar and/or managerial samples; (3) studies of P–E (person–work environment) fit.

As a group, blue collar workers are not appreciably different from the remainder of the US employed population (Quinn *et al.*, 1971; Quinn and Shepard, 1974) on somatic complaints, self-evaluated physical health, depression, self-esteem, zest, and life satisfaction; the biggest difference for these scales was obtained with life satisfaction, on which they were 0·29 standard deviations below the overall sample mean (but only in the earlier of the two surveys). On job satisfaction, blue collar workers were less than two-tenths of a standard deviation below the overall mean (if one averages the findings for two measures of job satisfaction and for the two surveys). Overall then, the blue collar 'blues' are not primarily a function of blue collar jobs but of certain characteristics of workers (e.g. blacks under 30, college educated persons under 30) and of their descriptions (perceptions) of their jobs (Seashore and Barnowe, 1972; Sheppard and Herrick, 1972).

However, the major interest in blue collar workers has been in those who perform routine work, generally machine paced, requiring little skill. Tasks which call for vigilance, no matter how simple they are, are associated with some elevation of noradrenaline; this is especially true of machine paced tasks which require skilled judgements at short intervals (Frankenhauser and Gardell, 1976).

Several studies have indicated that blue collar workers doing machine paced repetitive work have poorer mental health. For example, Kornhauser (1965) found that 13% of machine paced workers, in contrast to 29% of other repetitive semi-skilled workers, were found to have 'good' mental health (i.e. above an arbitrary cut-off). However, the author is reluctant to attribute this difference directly to the nature of the work environment: (1) it appeared to be part of an overall association between job status and mental health (gamma = 0·37); (2) speed and intensity of work were not found to be related to mental health; (3) certain perceptions of the job (chance to use one's abilities, perception of job as interesting, work as important activity) were strongly related to mental health but weakly related to the work environment. A Swedish study of workers doing machine controlled repetitive work (Gardell, 1971) found them to be of poorer mental health (on life satisfaction, feelings of competence and self-esteem, and psychosomatic symptoms) and with lower job satisfaction (particularly perception of work as interesting and perceived personal control over work); comparison groups were a group of craftsmen and those operating complicated mechanical systems. However, a New York study (Roman and Trice, 1972) failed to find any mental health differences between assembly line workers, workers in blue collar manufacturing jobs, and those in a large engineering R & D company.

The study of 23 occupations (Caplan et al., 1975) permits a detailed comparison of data on assemblers in machine paced and non-machine paced jobs, and workers in a variety of other blue collar jobs. I shall present some of the means for selected variables on the two groups of assemblers and a combined group of forklift drivers, machine tenders, continuous flow monitors, and tool and die makers. From data presented in the report, I have computed the means in standard scores (mean = 0, S.S. = 1) derived from a random sample of all of their study occupations, including white collar and professional groups; see Table 1.1. (The data on the four blue collar jobs are a simple mean of the four job means.)

It is evident that assemblers on machine paced jobs describe their work as boring, simple, and demanding little attention. However, their level of job satisfaction is not very different from the other two groups. On three of the mental health measures (somatic complaints, anxiety, depression), they reveal deficits, compared to the other two groups. On the social support measures, the machine paced assemblers are not strikingly different from the other two groups.

Studies of alienation among workers on machine paced or mechanized jobs (e.g. Blauner, 1964; Fried et al., 1972; Kirsch and Langermann, 1972; Shepard, 1971) amply document their high levels of alienation and related outcomes, such as absenteeism. However, in these studies the measures of 'powerlessness', 'meaninglessness', and 'self-estrangement' turn out to be nothing more than workers' accurate descriptions of their jobs: lack of control

Table 1.1

	Assemblers, machine paced	Assemblers, non-machine paced	Other collar wor\
Job complexity	−1·19	−0·91	−0·53
Demands for attention & concentration	−1·14	−0·71	−0·32
Boredom	1·34	0·75	0·49
Work load dissatisfaction	0·76	0·25	0·22
Job dissatisfaction (content free)*	0·66	0·49	0·59
Somatic complaints	0·81	0·35	0·09
Anxiety	0·36	−0·19	0·04
Depression	0·49	0·15	−0·01
Irritation	0·05	0·05	0·03
Social support (other people at work)	−0·44	−0·29	−0·21
Social support (wife, friends, relatives)	−0·30	−0·50	−0·15

*From Quinn and Shepard, 1974.

over pace and over work techniques, the simplicity and repetitiveness of the tasks, and the lack of intrinsic meaning in the work. In my opinion, there is a bit of conceptual legerdemain in this literature since perceptions of job are conceptualized ('alienation', 'self-estrangement') in powerful, value laden terms which suggest mental health outcomes. This also misses one of the crucial points, which is that while workers are able to call their jobs simple and boring, they do not necessarily call themselves more dissatisfied (e.g. the Caplan et al. (1975) data above). Moreover, this appears to be a widespread phenomenon; in a study of car workers in both industrialized and developing countries (Form, 1973) only between 5% to 10% cited monotony as a reason for job dissatisfaction in any country.

Studies of job enlargement–job enrichment (Alderfer, 1969; Evans, 1973; Ford, 1969; Hackman and Lawler, 1971; Hulin and Blood, 1968; Janson, 1975; Vroom, 1969) are in general agreement and suggest that job enlargement leads to increased job satisfaction, particularly in the following areas: use of skills and abilities, opportunity to learn new things, perception of work as meaningful, and amount of responsibility and autonomy. Absenteeism, turnover, and work performance may also be affected. There is also some evidence that these findings may be more applicable to small town workers (versus urban ones) and to workers with stronger needs for growth, challenge, and variety (Hackman and Lawler, 1971; Hulin and Blood, 1968; Turner and Lawrence, 1968). These individual differences might explain why expected benefits of job redesign are sometimes not obtained (e.g. Lawler et al., 1973).

One must be careful to distinguish *job enlargement* (which allows the worker to set his own pace, to inspect his own work, to set up and repair his own machinery, and so on) from mere *job extension*, which only adds similar elements to the job without altering job content (Hulin and Blood, 1968); there is no evidence that job extension has any effects on job satisfaction.

And to the extent that automation brings about job enlargement, the above listed consequences of job enlargement should also hold for automation. However, sometimes automation, even when accompanied by sizeable job enlargement, may have undesirable consequences: need for closer supervision and the resultant lower satisfaction with supervision; reduced opportunity for social interaction because of need for constant and close monitoring; greater work pressures because of higher performance standards more rigidly enforced; and reduced (perceived) job security and increased perception of management as impersonal and disinterested (Faunce, 1958; Mann and Williams, 1962).

In summary, the data on the blue collar workers in routine machine paced jobs present the following picture. Men on dull and monotonous jobs do not seem to misperceive their work: they call their jobs dull and monotonous. Their levels of job satisfaction, however, do not correspond to this description, since they are not much different from other blue collar workers. Yet, when their jobs are changed (enlarged), they do respond with higher job satisfaction, though this is probably not true for all subgroups. The most plausible interpretation of these results is offered by Strauss (1974b) who suggests that workers 'can adjust to non-challenging work, usually by lowering their expectations, changing their need structure, making most of social opportunities on and off the job' (p. 78). Kornhauser (1965) offers a similar interpretation, but with a more pessimistic emphasis: 'The unsatisfactory mental health of working people consists in no small measure of their dwarfed desires and deadened initiative, reduction of their goals and restriction of their efforts to a point where life is relatively empty and only half meaningful' (p. 270). Kornhauser goes on to discuss the two dead-end options for the car worker: maintain high expectations from work, which leads to constant frustration, or limit one's expectations, which leads to a drab existence.

Clearly, what is needed now are studies which directly examine this *process of adaptation* to unfulfilling and unchallenging jobs. This in turn suggests *longitudinal studies*, especially those designed around significant transitions and stages of life cycle. Many questions are begging for answers: (1) Do we understand the role of financial compensation; can money 'substitute' for unfulfilling jobs; is an attitude of instrumentality towards work (job as a means towards other life goals) part of the process of adaptation? These issues are part of an ongoing debate (e.g. Fein, 1973; Herrick, 1972; Opsahl and Dunnette, 1966). (2) Do routine, structured jobs have their own sources of satisfaction to which the workers can turn and come to value—as some have suggested (e.g. Sexton, 1968)? (3) Can social interaction on the job substitute as a source of job satisfaction when the work is intrinsically dull and boring—as some have suggested (e.g. Form, 1973; Strauss, 1974b)? (4) What is the dynamic role of absenteeism and turnover in the overall process of adaptation to an unsatisfactory job? There is a tiresome repetitiousness in the many studies that have looked at the intercorrelations among job satisfaction, performance, turnover, and absenteeism (reviewed in Kahn, 1972;

Lawler, 1970; Porter and Steers, 1973; Robinson *et al.*, 1969; Vroom, 1964 and 1969), but no interest in the important issue of the mental health consequences of the dynamic interplay between absenteeism/turnover and job dissatisfaction. (5) What are the mental health 'costs' of reducing one's aspirations and expectations? Are they only in the area of 'positive mental health' (Jahoda, 1958), such as inadequate self-actualization, or are they also detectable in other areas, such as symptoms and affects? (6) Is there a process of making the work role less salient in the maintenance of the self-concept or self-identity and in self-evaluation and is this part of the adaptation to an unsatisfactory job? For example, Quinn and Shepard (1974) found that, in response to the question 'How much do you think you can tell about a person just from knowing what he or she does for a living?' some 48% of the national sample chose 'nothing' or 'a little' as their answers. And Shepard (1971) found that blue collar workers in mechanized production were the lowest on 'self evaluative involvement', i.e. the degree to which work (versus non-work) activity was most important for self-evaluation. (7) What is the process of maintaining (or enhancing) satisfaction in other life roles when the work role has shrivelled in importance?

Perhaps the most fundamental question underlying these problems is a metatheoretical one, one which cannot be tested directly. Are we postulating a human nature with certain inherent needs (*à la* Maslow) or do we view the work environment (and other social settings) as a significant source of some of these needs; if the latter, then one would view dull and boring jobs not as frustrating certain needs, but as never giving birth to them in the first place.

I wish to turn now to studies of role stress, role conflict, and overload. The model study which gave rise to much of the current work was done almost 15 years ago (Kahn *et al.*, 1964). A good deal of this current work is repetitious and trivial (Hammer and Tosi, 1974; House and Rizzo, 1972; Johnson and Stinson, 1975; Keller, 1975; Lyons, 1971), involving cross-sectional correlations of self-reports of perceived job environments and reactions to these— in general, two sets of constructs with varying amounts of conceptual overlap. These studies reveal the expected negative correlations between role conflict and ambiguity and components of job satisfaction, generally in the -0.20 to -0.50 range (depending on overlap); correlations with mental health measures, such as anxiety and somatic symptoms, are weak or marginal (e.g. House and Rizzo, 1972; Miles and Perreault, 1976).

Very few studies collect repeated information. One such effort (Miles, 1975) was an attempt to test for causal inferences using the method of cross-lagged correlations (for a discussion of this method, see Cook and Campbell (1976); the results provided very little support for the causal interpretation that role conflict and role ambiguity may be viewed as antecedent variables, while job satisfaction and job tension measures may be viewed as outcomes. An opportunistic field study of male users of a university computer just before a 3 week shutdown, and a repeat data collection 5 months later (Caplan and Jones, 1975), revealed that changes in role ambiguity and in subjective quantitative work load were associated with changes in anxiety-tension; these associations were particularly strong among men high on a brief measure of Behaviour Type A.

The most broadly-based data on role stress and work load come from the study of 23 occupations (Caplan *et al.*, 1975). Some of the relevant findings can be summarized as follows: (1) occupations which deviated by about one-third of a standard deviation from the overall mean were: (a) above the mean on *role conflict*: forklift driver, assembler (relief), assembler (non-machine paced), and train dispatcher; (b) below the mean on role conflict: air traffic controller (small airports), scientist, professor, and physician; (c) above the mean on *role ambiguity*: forklift driver, programmer, engineer, and scientist; (d) below the mean on role ambiguity: continuous flow monitor, delivery service courier, train dispatcher, air traffic controller, and physician; (e) above the mean on *workload* (quantitative): train dispatcher, professor in administration, and physician; (f) below the mean on work load (quantitative): assembler (relief), assembler (non-machine paced) continuous flow monitor, tool and die maker, and programmer. In general, these three measures show a surprising lack of association with the blue collar versus white collar distinction, except that those low on work load are mostly blue collar jobs. Moreover, it is not clear what the jobs which are high or low on a particular variable have in common and thus the conditions in the (objective) work setting responsible for these differences are difficult to isolate. (2) Ecological correlations (using means for the 23 occupations) between the three measures of role stress and work load and four mental health measures (somatic complaints, anxiety, depression, and irritation) yielded four of the resultant twelve correlations above $\pm$ 0·40: role ambiguity with anxiety ($r = 0·40$) and with depression ($r = 0·64$), and role conflict with depression ($r = 0·43$) and irritation ($r = 0·46$). (3) At the individual level of analysis (using a random stratified sample of the study subjects), the same twelve intercorrelations yielded five values above $\pm$ 0·20: quantitative work load with irritation ($r = 0·21$), and role conflict with somatic complaints ($r = 0·25$), anxiety ($r = 26$), depression ($r = 0·22$), and irritation ($r = 0·33$).

More detailed analyses of correlates of role stress (Kahn, 1974b: Kahn *et al.*, 1964; French and Caplan, 1972) reveal that conflict, ambiguity, and overload are richly embedded in a network of associations including organizational variables (such as requirements for crossing organizational boundaries, for producing innovative solutions to non-routine problems, and for being responsible for work of others), many diverse (probable) outcome variables (such as various aspects of job satisfaction, job related tension, relations with co-workers and subordinates, and aspects of mental health), and conditioning effects of personality variables (such as anxiety-proneness, flexibility–rigidity).

Despite this richness of suggestive evidence, troublesome areas remain. One concerns the need for more precise operationalization of variables. For example, role ambiguity measures tend to include both unclarity of job demands and also lack of feedback regarding others' evaluation of one's job performance; role conflict measures include both demands which are truly conflicting as well as those which basically lead to overload. Second, links to objective work conditions remain extremely tenuous and this hampers our understanding of the dynamics involved. Third, there has been a good deal of imitation of the Kahn *et al.* (1964) formulation at the cost of neglect of other areas; for example, Klein (1971) opens up a promising area in his study of blue collar workers and the sequence of work pressure change → competitive behaviour and intra-group conflict → low work group cohesiveness. And, fourth, we need more field studies (preferably longitudinal ones) in which the investigator has oppor-tunistically selected a setting because something is going on which is more likely to yield meaningful data on cause–effect relationships: stronger pressures from the work environment, unusually vulnerable subjects, or a situation where most confounding variables are naturally held constant. The Hall and Mansfield (1971) study of three R & D organizations going through a marked decrease in available financial resources, or the Warheit (1974) study of Cape Kennedy personnel under pressure to launch a space vehicle for moon landing (but facing possible job loss if successful) are examples of such studies, of such 'natural experiments'. They can provide much more useful data than the typical cross-sectional study of a steady-state work environment in which significant adaptations have long since taken place.

The last topic which I wish to consider briefly in this review concerns the P–E (person–environment) fit formulation. In this approach (French, 1974; French *et al.*, 1974; Harrison, 1976), two kinds of fit between the individual and his environment are of concern: (1) the match of a person's skills and abilities to the demands and requirements of the job; and (2) the extent to which the needs of the person are supplied in the job environment. Since the empirical work bearing on this formulation is in its infancy, the operationalization of concepts lags far behind the theoretical formulations, and most measures of P–E fit, in fact, consist of asking the subject to characterize the job along a set of dimensions (such as job complexity, work load) and then to indicate his preferences or aspirations—how he would like his job to be. Since the typical job satisfaction measures are generally interpreted to reflect the extent to which the job satisfies a worker's expectations or aspirations, the P–E fit measures may be viewed as more sensitive and more probing job satisfaction indicators: they measure the two components separately and they distinguish two kinds of misfit (too much versus not enough of some job characteristic). Such measures would be especially suitable in longitudinal studies in which one studied adaptation to a work environment: changes in perceptions of the job and in aspirations (expectations) could be assessed separately.

The early work in which there was a separate measurement of personality variables (needs or valued dimensions of self-image) and of the work environ-ment (satisfaction of needs or congruence with self-image) revealed that the discrepancy between the two was not associated with job status (e.g. Argyris, 1960; Wilensky, 1964), which is in contrast to the usual positive association between job satisfaction and status. The independent evidence that men at different occupational levels have different needs and expectations (Armstrong, 1971; Kilpatrick *et al.*, 1964; Taylor, 1968) presumably accounts for these findings. The usefulness of the P–E fit approach is also illustrated by the panel study of time pressure and performance of NASA scientists (Andrews and Farris, 1972): when experienced time pressure was optimal (neither too little nor too much, as reflected by indicated preferences for time pressure), innovation and productivity during a later time period were at their greatest; judged usefulness of the scientists' work, however, was as high when pressure was optimal as when there was too much pressure (actual more than preferred).

In a mailed questionnaire study of male workers in a Canadian city (Coburn, 1975), an objective index of P–E fit was derived from (1) the worker's level of education and (2) US Department of Labour listing of General Educational Development required for the job which the worker held. Men on the extremes of this discrepancy measure (education too low or too high) tended to dislike their jobs more and to have a slightly poorer assessment of their physical health status; reports of 'pressure or stress' went up more or less linearly as education requirements exceeded educational attainment (gamma = 0·10). Other measures, such as general happiness, an index of mental health based on the Langner scale (Langner and Michael, 1963), and a self-report role incapacity index (hospitalizations, illness absences) were not related in a meaningful or significant way. A subjective measure of overload–underload (a single item going from 'job too much' or 'extremely mentally tiring' to 'job dull, monotonous, not challenging') correlated weakly (gamma = 0·12) with the objective discrepancy measures. And as would be expected, this subjective measure showed stronger association with the several 'outcome' measures: personal happiness, self-assessed physical health, and mental health based on the Langner scale were optimal in the middle range of this subjective scale, while dislike of one's job was more or less linearly associated with underload.

The study of 23 occupations (Caplan *et al.*, 1975) developed four measures of P–E fit, involving parallel descriptions of the work environment (E) and personal preferences (P) along four dimensions: quantitative work load, job complexity, responsibility for persons, and role ambiguity. Analysis of associations with various measures of strain (job satisfaction, mental health) revealed that 'optimal' scoring of the P–E fit measures called for taking the absolute difference between P and E on all but quantitative work load (i.e. that difference in either direction is misfit for the three measures, whereas for the fourth good fit = underload and poor fit = overload).

The most general way to evaluate the usefulness of the P–E fit measures in this study is to see what difference it makes if one uses them instead of just the environmental description (E) measures (Harrison, 1976). The results are only mildly encouraging. (1) The P–E fit measure of quantitative work load correlates 0·81 with the E measure, using ecological analysis of 23 occupations, and 0·71, using individual level of analysis; moreover, its correlations with several outcome measures (job dissatisfaction, somatic complaints, depression, anxiety, irritation) do not demonstrate its superiority, except perhaps in the case of depression ($r = 0.27$ for P–E fit, $r = 0.05$ for the E measure). (2) The P–E fit on job complexity reveals that jobs with poor fit are low on complexity ($r = -0.90$); at the individual level, the correlation is -0.41. Its correlations with the five outcome measures suggests that it is more useful than the E measure alone: average correlation of 0.24 involving P–E fit versus 0.10 involving E alone. (3) The P–E fit on responsibility for person reveals that jobs with poor fit tend to involve less responsibility ($r = -0.69$); the correlation for individuals is -0.43. Its correlations with the five outcome measures provide no evidence for its greater usefulness. (4) The P–E fit on role ambiguity is more or less independent of the E measure (ecological $r = 0.23$, individual $r = 0.27$). Its correlations with outcome measures suggest that it is less useful than the E measure. It is very possible that P–E fit on role ambiguity is an ambiguous measure.

Overall, the formulation of job stress as person–environment misfit offers only limited evidence regarding its usefulness. The one area worth pursuing further is job complexity (variety of tasks, working with different groups of people, working on several tasks at different stages of completion). It is perhaps not a coincidence that the earlier section of the review dealing with mental health of blue collar workers on routine jobs, and with job enlargement, revealed the need for greater understanding of the process of adaptation to such jobs. Perhaps the P–E fit approach will be of help here.

Concluding remarks

Inasmuch as this review has already provided many critical comments regarding current evidence and current methodology, and offered many suggestions for further studies, there is little point in collecting these criticisms all in one place and hitting the reader over the head with them again. Instead, I want to give selective emphasis to three points which I feel are worth emphasizing.

First, we need to concentrate on longitudinal studies of the work setting, preferably those designed around 'natural experiments', that is, significant events and transitions, which may better reveal the way the work environment affects health and well-being, and the way individuals adapt to this environment and to changes therein. McGrath (1970b) has rightly pointed out that temporal factors in stress research are nearly always neglected: stress as anticipation, perceived and actual duration, cyclical response capabilities, and so on. Moreover, too much of our evidence is based on studies of short term effects of stress and we are forced to extrapolate that prolonged stress would show prolonged effects. For example, do the biochemical consequences of 75 hours of work and wakefulness among military officers, or of several days of accelerated output among female invoicing clerks (Levi, 1974), predict the effects one would obtain under chronic conditions, or under some cyclical variation of such stress? There is, in fact, some evidence that it is improper to make such extrapolations. In a longitudinal study of plant closing and job loss (Kasl *et al.*, 1977), short term stress effects of the transition from anticipation of plant closing to unemployment (versus prompt re-employment) were not observed as chronic effects under conditions of prolonged unemployment: many of the mental health and physiological variables returned to 'normal' even though unemployment persisted. Finally, such longitudinal studies will get us away from the plethora of hopeless cross-sectional studies which attack extremely complex issues with the weakest of research designs; they are bound to yield uninterpretable findings (e.g. Ferguson, 1973; Shirom *et al.*, 1973; Siassi *et al.*, 1974), in spite of the extensive effort that may go into collecting the data.

Second, we need a frontal attack on the whole issue of defining and measuring environmental stress subjectively and relating it to subjective measures of distress. Earlier in the review I referred to this as 'a self-serving methodological trap ... trivializing a good deal of research'. Frankly, if our conceptualization dictates trivial methodology, let us change the conceptualization; such 'correct' operationalization of concepts is not worth it. It is a good indication of how far we have gone in ignoring the objective work environment when such an excellent and rich report as *Job Demands and Worker Health* (Caplan *et al.*, 1975) provides us with no information about the work settings other than the briefest of occupational titles.

In principle, it should be possible to move away somewhat from the excessive operational circularity of stress and distress measures without doing violence to the subjectivist conceptualization of stress. For example, there is no point in using some 'objective' measure of job demands (such as a fourth level supervisor disclosing to the investigator that company policy demands that a certain piece-rate be achieved on the assembly line) when there is no evidence that such demands have been communicated and accepted. On the other hand, there is no need to use a measure of 'perceived' job demands into which the reactions of the respondent are built: it is a difference between measuring perceived demands by items like 'I am expected to produce 50 pieces an hour' versus items like 'The piece rate demands on this job are too much for me'. In terms of Lewinian theory (Cartwright, 1959), we are only obliged to make sure that the work environment variables we are studying are part of the 'life space' of the person, but we are not obliged to use perceptions which are confounded with the outcome variables we wish to study. It would also be my suspicion that when the objective and perceived work environments have been measured in appropriately commensurate fashion, then a lack of any correlation between the two probably means that the very outcome variables which we are trying to predict (indicators of distress, strain) are influencing the perceptions, rather than the more comforting conclusion that this shows one must use subjective perceptions in order to understand what is going on.

My third point can be stated quite briefly. It is likely that our understanding of the effects of stress at work on health and well-being will be greatly enhanced as we carry out studies which go beyond the immediate confines of the work environment—not just studying associated activities such as driving to work

(Bellet *et al.*, 1969), but viewing issues such as occupational mobility from a broader perspective, that of the family (Olive *et al.*, 1976; Weissman and Paykel, 1972). The growing emphasis on social support coming from family and friends in the study of effects of work environment (Cobb, 1976; Pinneau, 1976) is a move in this direction. In general, we need many more studies which are specifically concerned with interrelationships among life roles, or which study effects of events and changes which cross several life roles. It still remains true that research on work and on the family is quite segregated and that it is quite rare to find a study which focuses on more than one role (Rapoport and Rapoport, 1965).

References

Aitken, R. C. B. (1969) Prevalence of worry in normal aircrew, *Brit. J. Med. Psychol.*, **42**, 283–286.
Alderfer, C. P. (1969) Job enlargement and the organizational context, *Personnel Psychol.*, **22**, 418–426.
Alvarez, W. C., and Stanley, L. L. (1930) Blood pressure in six thousand prisoners and four hundred prison guards, *Arch. Int. Med.*, **46**, 17–39.
Andrews, F. M., and Farris, G. F. (1972) Time pressure and performance of scientists and engineers: a five-year panel study, *Org. Behav. & Hum. Perform.*, **8**, 185–200.
Antonovsky, A. (1968) Social class and the major cardiovascular diseases, *J. chron. Dis.*, **21**, 65–106.
Appley, M. H., and Trumbull, R. (1967) On the concept of psychological stress. In Appley, M. H., and Trumbull, R. (eds), *Psychological Stress*. New York. Appleton-Century-Crofts, pp. 1–13.
Argyris, C. (1960) Individual actualization in complex organizations, *Mental Hygiene*, **44**, 226–237.
Argyris, C. (1964) *Integrating the Individual and the Organization*. New York. Wiley.
Armstrong, T. B. (1971) Job content and context factors related to satisfaction for different occupational levels, *J. Appl. Psychol.*, **55**, 57–65.
Bahnson, C. B. (ed.) (1974) Behavioural factors associated with the etiology of physical disease, *Amer. J. Pub. Hlth*, **64**, 1033–1055.
Barfield, R., and Morgan, J. N. (1969) *Early Retirement: the Decision and the Experience*. Ann Arbor: Institute for Social Research, The University of Michigan.
Barnard, R. J., and Duncan, H. W. (1975) Heart rate and ECG responses of fire fighters, *J. Occup. Med.*, **17**, 247–250.
Barrow, J. G., Quinlan, C. B., Edmands, R. E., and Rodilosso, P. T. (1961) Prevalence of atherosclerotic complications in Trappist and Benedictine monks, *Circulation*, **24**, 881–882 (abstract).
Bellet, S., Roman, L., and Kostis, J. (1969) The effect of automobile driving on catecholamine and adrenocortical excretion, *Amer. J. Cardiol.*, **24**, 365–368.
Berger, A. J (1969) *The Relationship of Self-Perception and Job-Component Perception to Overall Job Satisfaction: a 'Self-Appropriateness' Model of Job Satisfaction*. New York: Unpublished doctoral dissertation, New York University.
Bernacki, E. J. (1975) Uses of the epidemiologic method in occupational medicine, *Conn. Med.*, **39**, 117–118.
Blauner, R. (1960) Work satisfaction and industrial trends in modern society. In Gelenson, W., and Lipset, S. (eds), *Labor and Trend Unionism*. New York: Wiley.
Blauner, R. (1964) *Alienation and Freedom: the Factory Worker and His Industry*. University of Chicago Press.

38

Bonner, K. (1967) Industrial implications of stress. In Levi, L. (ed.), *Emotional Stress*. New York: American Elsevier Publishing Co., 225–232.

Bourne, P. G., Rose, R. M., and Mason, J. W. (1968) 17-OHCS levels in combat, *Arch. Gen. Psychiat.*, **19**, 135–140.

Bradburn, N. (1969) *The Structure of Psychological Well-Being*. Chicago. Aldine.

Brand, R. J., Rosenman, R. H., Sholtz, R. I., and Friedman, M. (1976) Multivariate prediction of coronary heart disease in the Western Collaborative Group Study compared to the findings of the Framingham Study, *Circulation*, **53**, 348–355.

Brenner, M. H. (1973) *Mental Illness and the Economy*. Cambridge, Mass. Harvard University Press.

Brooks, G. W., and Mueller, E. (1966) Serum urate concentrations among university professors, *J.A.M.A.*, **195**, 415–418.

Brouha, L. (1967) *Physiology in Industry*. Oxford. Pergamon Press, 2nd ed.

Bruhn, J. G., Wolf, S., Lynn, T. N., Bird, H. B., and Chandler, B. (1968) Social aspects of coronary heart disease in a Pennsylvania German community. *Soc. Sci. & Med.*, **2**, 201–212.

Buell, P., and Breslow, L. (1960) Mortality from coronary heart disease in California men who work long hours, *J. chron. Dis.*, **11**, 615–626.

Caffrey, B. (1969) Behaviour patterns and personality characteristics related to prevalence rates of coronary heart disease in American monks, *J. chron. Dis.*, **22**, 93–103.

Campbell, A., Converse, P. E., and Rodgers, W. L. (1976) *The Quality of American Life*. New York: Russell Sage Foundation.

Campbell, D. T., and Fiske, D. W. (1959) Convergent and discriminant validation by the multitrait-multimethod matrix, *Psychol. Bull.*, **56**, 81–105.

Cantril, A. H., and Roll, C. W., Jr. (1971) *Hopes and Fears of the American People*. New York: Universe Books.

Caplan, R. D. (1971) *Organizational Stress and Individual Strain: a Social–Psychological Study of Risk Factors in Coronary Heart Disease among Administrators, Engineers, and Scientists*. Ann Arbor: Unpublished doctoral dissertation, The University of Michigan.

Caplan, R. D., Cobb, S., and French, J. R. P., Jr. (1975) Relationship of cessation of smoking with the stress, personality, and social support, *J. Appl. Psychol.*, **60**, 211–219.

Caplan, R. D., Cobb, S., French, J. R. P., Jr., Harrison, R. V., and Pinneau, S. R., Jr. (1975) *Job Demands and Worker Health*. Washington, D. C. HEW Publication No. (NIOSH) 75–160.

Caplan, R. D., and Jones, K. W. (1975) Effects of work load, role ambiguity and Type A personality on anxiety, depression, and heart rate, *J. Appl. Psychol.*, **60**, 713–719.

Cartwright, D. (1959) Lewinian theory as a systematic framework. In Koch, S. (ed.), *Psychology: a Study of a Science*, Vol. 2. New York. McGraw-Hill, pp. 7–91.

Cassel, J. C. (1963) The use of medical records: opportunity for epidemiological studies, *J. Occup. Med.*, **5**, 185–190.

Cassel, J. C. (1971) Summary of major findings of the Evans Country cardiovascular studies, *Arch. Intern. Med.*, **128**, 890–895.

Cassel, J. C. (1974) An epidemiological perspective of psychosocial factors in disease etiology, *Amer. J. Pub. Hlth*, **64**, 1040–1043.

Chapman, J. M., Reeder, L. G., Massey, F. J., Jr., Borun, E. R., Picken, B., Browning, G. G., Coulson, A. A., and Zimmerman, D. H. (1966) Relationships of stress, tranquilizers, and serum cholesterol levels in a sample population under study for coronary heart disease, *Amer. J. Epidemiol.*, **83**, 537–547.

Chinoy, E. (1955) *Automobile Workers and the American Dream*. Garden City, N.Y. Doubleday.

Christenson, W. N., and Hinkle, L. E., Jr. (1961) Differences in illness and prognostic signs in two groups of young men, *J.A.M.A.*, **177**, 247–253.

Cobb, S. (1974) Role responsibility: the differentiation of a concept. In McLean, A. (ed.), *Occupational Stress*. Springfield, Ill. C. C. Thomas, pp. 62–69.

Cobb, S. (1976) Social support as a moderator of life stress, *Psychosom. Med.*, **38**, 300–314.

Cobb, S., and Rose, R. M. (1973) Hypertension, peptic ulcer, and diabetes in air traffic controllers, *J.A.M.A.*, **224**, 489–492.

Coburn, D. (1975) Job-worker incongruence: consequences for health, *J. Hlth & Soc. Behav.*, **16**, 198–212.

Comstock, G. W. (1971) Fatal arteriosclerotic heart disease, water hardness at home, and socioeconomic characteristics, *Amer. J. Epidemiol.*, **94**, 1–10.

Cook, T. D., and Campbell, D. T. (1976) The design and conduct of quasi-experiments and true experiments in field settings. In Dunnette, M. D. (ed.), *Handbook of Industrial and Organizational Psychology*. Chicago. Rand McNally, pp. 223–326

Creech, J. L., and Johnson, M. N. (1974) Angiosarcoma of liver in the manufacture of polyvinyl chloride, *J. Occup. Med.*, **16**, 150–151.

Daubs, J. (1973) The mental health crisis in opthalmology, *Amer. J. Optom. & Arch. Am. Acad. Optom.*, **50**, 816–822.

Davis, L. E., and Cherns, A. B. (eds) (1975) *The Quality of Working Life*. New York. The Free Press.

Dawis, R. V., England, G. W., and Lofquist, L. H. (1964) *Minnesota Studies in Vocational Rehabilitation. XV. A Theory of Work Adjustment*. Minneapolis. Industrial Relations Center, University of Minnesota.

Dohrenwend, B. S., and Dohrenwend, B. P. (eds) (1974) *Stressful Life Events*. New York. Wiley.

Dubin, R. (1956) Industrial workers' worlds: a study of the 'central life interests' of industrial workers, *Soc. Problems*, **3**, 131–142.

Editorial (1975), *J. Hum. Stress*, **1**, 3.

Ellard, J. (1974) The disease of being a doctor, *Med. J. Aust.*, **2**, 318–323.

Engel, G. L. (1962) *Psychological Development in Health and Disease*. Philadelphia. Saunders.

Enterline, P. E. (1976) Pitfalls in epidemiological research, *J. Occup. Med.*, **18**, 150–156.

Erikson, E. H. (1956) The problem of ego identity, *J. Amer. Psychoanal. Assn*, **4**, 56–121.

Evans, M. G. (1973) Notes on the impact of Flextime in a large insurance company, *Occup. Psychol.*, **47**, 237–240.

Faunce, W. A. (1958) Automation in the automobile industry: some consequences for in-plant social structure, *Amer. Sociol. Rev.*, **23**, 401–407.

Fein, M. (1973) The real needs and goals of blue collar workers, *The Conference Board RECORD*, February 1973, 26–33.

Feinstein, A. R. (1968) Clinical epidemiology, *Ann. Intern. Med.*, **69**, 807–820, 1037–1061, 1287–1312.

Ferguson, D. (1973) A study of neurosis and occupation, *Brit. J. Industr. Med.*, **30**, 187–198.

Ford, R. N. (1969) *Motivation Through Work Itself*. New York: American Management Association.

Form, W. H. (1973) Auto workers and their machines: a study of work, factory and job dissatisfaction in four countries, *Social Forces*, **52**, 1–15.

Frankenhauser, M., and Gardell, B. (1976) Underload and overload in working life: outline of a multidisciplinary approach, *J. Hum. Stress*, **2**, 35–46.

Frankenhauser, M., Nordheden, B., Myrsten, A. L., and Post, B. (1971) Psycho-physiological reactions to understimulation and overstimulation, *Acta Psychol.*, **35**, 298–308.

French, J. R. P., Jr. (1974) Person role fit. In McLean, A. (ed.), *Occupational Stress*. Springfield, Ill. C. C. Thomas, pp. 70–79.

French, J. R. P., Jr., and Caplan, R. D. (1970) Psychosocial factors in coronary heart disease, *Industr. Med. & Surg.*, **39**, 383–397.

French, J. R. P., Jr., and Caplan, R. D. (1972) Organizational stress and individual strain.

In Marrow, A. J. (ed.), *The Failure of Success*. New York. AMACOM, pp. 30–66.

French, J. R. P., Jr., Rodgers, W., and Cobb, S. (1974) Adjustment as person–environment fit. In Coelho, G. V., Hamburg, D. A., and Adams, J. E. (eds), *Coping and Adaptation*. New York. Basic Books, pp. 316–333.

Fried, J., Weitman, M., and Davis, M. K. (1972) Man-machine interaction and absenteeism, *J. Appl. Psychol.*, **56**, 428–429.

Friedman, E. H., and Hellerstein, H. K. (1968) Occupational stress, law school hierarchy and coronary artery disease in Cleveland attorneys, *Psychosom. Med.*, **30**, 72–86.

Friedman, E. W., and Havinghurst, R. J. (1954) *The Meaning of Work and Retirement*. University of Chicago Press.

Friedman, M. D. (1969) *Pathogenesis of Coronary Artery Disease*. New York. McGraw-Hill.

Friedman, M. D., and Rosenman, R. H. (1959) Association of specific overt behaviour pattern with blood and cardiovascular findings, *J.A.M.A.*, **169**, 1286–1296.

Friedman, M. D., and Rosenman, R. H. (1974) *Type A Behaviour and Your Heart*. New York. Knopf.

Friedman, M. D., Rosenman, R. D., and Carroll, V. (1958) Changes in serum cholesterol and blood clotting time in men subjected to cyclic variation of occupational stress, *Circulation*, **17**, 852–861.

Gaffney, W. R. (1973) Epidemiological studies in industry, *J. Occup. Med.*, **15**, 782–785.

Gardell, B. (1971) Alienation and mental health in the modern industrial environment. In Levi, L. (ed.), *Society, Stress and Disease*, vol. I. London. Oxford University Press, pp. 148–180.

Gardner, W., and Taylor, P. (1975) *Health and Work*. New York. Wiley.

Gechman, A. S. (1974) Without work, life goes . . ., *J. Occup. Med.*, **16**, 749–751.

Groen, J. J. (1971) Social change and psychosomatic disease. In Levi, L. (ed.), *Society, Stress and Disease*, vol. I. London. Oxford University Press, pp. 91–109.

Groen, J. J., and Bastiaans, J. (1975) Psychosocial stress, interhuman communication, and psychosomatic disease. In Spielberger, C. D., and Sarason, I. G. (eds), *Stress and Anxiety*, vol. I. Washington, DC. Hemisphere Publishing Corp., pp. 27–49.

Groen, J. J., and Drory, S. (1967) Influence of psychosocial factors on coronary heart disease, *Path. Microbiol.*, **30**, 779–788.

Groen, J. J., Tijong, K. B., Koster, M., Willebrands, A. F., Verdonck, G., and Pierloot, M. (1962) The influence of nutrition and ways of life on blood cholesterol and the prevalence of hypertension and coronary heart disease among Trappist and Benedictine monks, *Amer. J. Clin. Nutr.*, **10**, 456–470.

Gross, E. (1970) Work, organization, and stress. In Levine, S., and Scotch, N. A. (eds), *Social Stress*. Chicago. Aldine, pp. 54–110.

Guralnick, L. (1963) *Mortality by Occupation and Cause of Death* (No. 3), *Mortality by Industry and Cause of Death* (No. 4), *Mortality by Occupational Level and Cause of Death* (No. 5), *Among Men 20 to 64 Years of Age, U.S. 1950*. USDHEW PHS. Vital Statistics–Special Reports, vol. 53.

Gurin, G., Veroff, J., and Feld, S. (1960) *American View Their Mental Health*. New York. Basic Books.

Hackman, J. R., and Lawler, E. E., III (1971) Employee reactions to job characteristics, *J. Appl. Psychol.*, **55**, 259–286.

Hall, D. T., and Mansfield, R. (1971) Organizational and individual response to external stress, *Admin. Sci. Quart.*, **16**, 533–547.

Hamilton, A., and Hardy, H. L. (1974) *Industrial Toxicology*. Action, Mass. Publishing Sciences Group, 3rd ed.

Hammer, W. C., and Tosi, H. L. (1974) Relationship of role conflict and role ambiguity to job involvement measures, *J. Appl. Psychol.*, **59**, 497–499.

Harris, L. (1965) 'Pleasant' retirement expected, *Washington Post*, 28 November.

Harrison, R. V. (1976) Job stress as person–environment misfit. Presented at a symposium on Job Demands and Worker Health, held at the 84th Annual Convention of the American Psychological Association, Washington, DC, September 1976.

Herrick, N. Q. (1972) Who's unhappy at work and why?, *Manpower*, US Department of Labour, January 1972.

Hinkle, L. E., Jr. (1973) The concept of 'stress' in the biological and social sciences, *Sci., Med. & Man*, 1, 31–48.

Hinkle, L. E., Jr., Benjamin, B., Christenson, W. N., and Ullmann, D. S. (1966) Coronary heart disease, *Arch. Environ. Hlth*, 13, 312–321.

Hinkle, L. E., Jr., Dohrenwend, B. P., Elinson, J., Kasl, S. V., McDowell, A., Mechanic, D., and Syme, L. S. (1976) Social determinants of human health. In *Preventive Medicine, USA*. New York. Prodist, pp. 89–146.

Hinkle, L. E., Jr., Whitney, L. H., Lehman, E. W., Dunn, J., Benjamin, B., King, R., Plakun, A., and Fehinger, B. (1968) Occupation, education, and coronary heart disease, *Science*, 161, 238–246.

Horan, P. M., and Gray, B. H. (1974) Status inconsistency, mobility, and coronary heart disease, *J. Hlth & Soc. Behav.*, 15, 300–310.

House, J. S. (1972) *The Relationship of Intrinsic and Extrinsic Work Motivations to Occupational Stress and Coronary Heart Disease Risk*. Ann Arbor. Unpublished doctoral dissertation, The University of Michigan.

House, J. S. (1974a) The effects of occupational stress on physical health. In O'Toole, J. (ed.), *Work and the Quality of Life*. Cambridge, Mass. The MIT Press, pp. 145–170.

House, J. S. (1974b) Occupational stress and coronary heart disease: a review and theoretical integration, *J. Hlth & Soc. Behav.*, 15, 12–27.

House, R. J., and Rizzo, J. R. (1972) Role conflict and ambiguity as critical variables in a model of organizational behaviour, *Organiz. Behav. & Hum. Perform.*, 7, 467–505.

Hulin, C. L., and Blood, M. R. (1968) Job enlargement, individual differences and worker responses, *Psychol. Bull.*, 69, 41–55.

Indik, B. P. (1963) Some effects of organization size on member attitudes and behaviour, *Human Relat.*, 16, 369–384.

Jahoda, M. (1958) *Current Concepts of Positive Mental Health*. New York. Basic Books.

Janson, R. (1975) A job enrichment trial in data processing in an insurance organization. In Davis, L. E., and Cherns, A. B. (eds), *The Quality of Working Life*, vol. 2. New York. The Free Press, pp. 300–314.

Jenkins, C. D. (1971) Psychologic and social precursors of coronary disease, *New Engl. J. Med.*, 284, 244–255 and 307–317.

Jenkins, C. D., Rosenman, R. H., and Friedman, M. (1966) Components of the coronary-prone behaviour pattern: their relation to silent myocardial infarction and blood lipids, *J. Chron. Dis.*, 19, 599–609.

Jenkins, C. D., Rosenman, R. H., and Zyzanski, S. J. (1974) Prediction of clinical coronary heart disease by a test for the coronary-prone behaviour pattern, *New Engl. J. Med.*, 290, 1271–1275.

Jenkins, C. D., Zyzanski, S. J., and Rosenman, R. H. (1971) Progress toward validation of a computer-scored test for Type A Coronary-Prone Behaviour Pattern, *Psychosom. Med.*, 33, 193–202.

Jenkins, C. D., Zyzanski, S. J., and Rosenman, R. H. (1976) Risk of new myocardial infarction in middle-aged men with manifest coronary heart disease, *Circulation*, 53, 342–347.

Johnson, T. W., and Stinson, J. E. (1975) Role ambiguity, role conflict, and satisfaction: moderating effects of individual differences, *J. Appl. Psychol.*, 60, 329–333.

Kagan, A. (1971) Epidemiology and society, stress and disease. In Levi, L. (ed.), *Society, Stress, and Disease*, vol. I. London. Oxford University Press, pp. 36–48.

Kahn, R. L. (1972) The meaning of work: interpretation and proposals for measurement.

In Campbell, A., and Converse, P. E. (eds), *The Human Meaning of Social Change*. New York. Russell Sage Foundation, pp. 159–203.

Kahn, R. L. (1974a) On the meaning of work, *J. Occup. Med.*, **16**, 716–719.

Kahn, R. L. (1974b) Conflict, ambiguity, and overload: three elements in job stress. In McLean, A. (ed.), *Occupational Stress*. Springfield, Ill. C. C. Thomas, pp. 47–61.

Kahn, R. L., and Quinn, R. P. (1970) Role stress: a framework for analysis. In McLean, A. (ed.), *Mental Health and Work Organizations*. Chicago. Rand McNally, pp. 50–115.

Kahn, R. L., Wolfe, D. M., Quinn, R. P., Snoek, J. D., and Rosenthal, R. A. (1964) *Organizational Stress: Studies in Role Conflict and Ambiguity*. New York. Wiley.

Kaplan, B. H., Cassel, J. C., Tyroler, H. A., Cornoni, J. C., Kleinbaum, D. G., and Hames, C. G. (1971) Occupational mobility and coronary heart disease, *Arch. Int. Med.*, **128**, 938–942.

Kasl, S. V. (1973) Mental health and the work environment: an examination of the evidence, *J. Occup. Med.*, **15**, 509–518.

Kasl, S. V. (1974) Work and mental health. In O'Toole, J. (ed.), *Work and the Quality of Life*. Cambridge, Mass. The MIT Press, pp. 171–196.

Kasl, S. V., and Cobb, S. (1966) Health behaviour, illness behaviour, and sick role behaviour, *Arch. Environ. Hlth*, **12**, 246–266 and 531–541.

Kasl, S. V., and Cobb, S. (1971) Physical and mental health correlates of status incongruence, *Social Psychiat.*, **6**, 1–10.

Kasl, S. V., Cobb, S., and Thompson, W. D. (1977) Duration of stressful life situation and reactivity of psychological and physiological variables: can one extrapolate chronic changes from reaction to acute stress? Presented at the Annual Meeting of the American Psychosomatic Society, Atlanta, March 1977.

Kasl, S. V., and French, J. R. P., Jr. (1962) The effects of occupational status on physical and mental health, *J. Soc. Issues*, **18**, 3, 67–89.

Keller, R. T. (1975) Role conflict and ambiguity: correlates with job satisfaction and values, *Personnel Psychol.*, **28**, 57–64.

Kilpatrick, F., Cummings, M., and Jennings, M. (1964) *The Image of the Federal Service*. Washington, DC. The Brookings Institution.

King, H. (1970) Health in the medical and other learned professions, *J. chron. Dis.*, **23**, 257–281.

Kirsch, B. A., and Langermann, J. L. (1972) An empirical test of Robert Blauner's ideas on alienation in work as applied to different type jobs in a white collar setting, *Sociol. & Soc. Res.*, **56**, 180–194.

Kitagawa, E. M., and Hauser, P. M. (1973) *Differential Mortality in the United States; a Study in Socioeconomic Epidemiology*. Cambridge, Mass. Harvard University Press.

Klein, S. M. (1971) *Workers Under Stress*. Lexington: University Press of Kentucky.

Kohn, M. L., and Schooler, C. (1973) Occupational experience and psychological functioning: an assessment of reciprocal effects, *Amer. Soc. Rev.*, **38**, 97–118.

Kornhauser, A. (1965) *Mental Health of the Industrial Worker*. New York. Wiley.

Kroes, W. H., Margolis, B. L., and Hurrell, J. J. (1974) Job stress in policemen, *J. Police Sci. & Admin.*, **2**, 145–155.

Kryter, K. D. (1972) Non-auditory effects of environmental noise, *Amer. J. Pub. Hlth*, **62**, 389–398.

Landy, F. J., and Trumbo, D. A. (1976) *Psychology of Work Behaviour*. Homewood, Ill. Dorsey Press.

Langner, T. S., and Michael, S. T. (1963) *Life Stress and Mental Health*. New York. The Free Press.

Lawler, E. E., III (1970) Job attitudes and employee motivation: theory, research, and practice, *Personnel Psychol.*, **23**, 223–237.

Lawler, E. E., III, Hackman, J. R., and Kaufman, S. (1973) Effects of job redesign: a field experiment, *J. Appl. Soc. Psychol.*, **3**, 49–62.

Lazarus, R. S. (1966) *Psychological Stress and the Coping Process*. New York. McGraw-Hill.

Lazarus, R. S. (1971) The concepts of stress and disease. In Levi, L. (ed.), *Society, Stress and Disease*, vol. I. London. Oxford University Press, pp. 53–58.

Lebovits, B. Z., Shekelle, R. B., Ostfeld, A. M., and Paul, O. (1967) Prospective and retrospective psychological studies of coronary heart disease, *Psychosom. Med.*, **29**, 265–272.

Lee, R. E., and Schneider, R. F. (1958) Hypertension and arteriosclerosis in executive and nonexecutive personnel, *J.A.M.A.*, **167**, 1447–1450.

Lehman, E. W. (1967) Social class and coronary heart disease: a sociological assessment of the medical literature, *J. chron. Dis.*, **20**, 381–391.

Lehman, E. W., Schulman, J., and Hinkle, L. E., Jr. (1967) Coronary deaths and organizational mobility, *Arch. Environ. Hlth*, **15**, 455–461.

Lehr, I., Messinger, H. B., and Rosenman, R. H. (1973) A sociobiological approach to the study of coronary heart disease, *J. chron. Dis.*, **26**, 13–30.

Levi, L. (1974) Stress, distress, and psychosocial stimuli. In McLean, A. A. (ed.), *Occupational Stress*. Springfield, Ill. C. C. Thomas, pp. 31–46.

Lipowski, Z. J. (1975) Physical illness, the patient, and his environment: psychosocial foundations in medicine. In Reiser, M. F. (ed.), *Organic Disorders and Psychosomatic Medicine*. Vol. 4, *American Handbook of Psychiatry*. New York. Basic Books, pp. 3–42.

Locke, E. A. (1976) The nature and causes of job satisfaction. In Dunnette, M. D. (ed.), *Handbook of Industrial and Organizational Psychology*. Chicago. Rand McNally, pp. 1297–1349.

Loether, H. J. (1965) The meaning of work and adjustment to retirement. In Shostak, A. B., and Gomberg, W. (eds), *Blue Collar World*. Englewood Cliffs, NJ Prentice-Hall, pp. 525–533.

Lofquist, L. H., and Dawis, R. V. (1969) *Adjustment to Work*. New York. Appleton-Century-Crofts.

Lyons, T. F. (1971) Role clarity, need for clarity, satisfaction, tension, and withdrawal, *Org. Behav. & Hum. Perform.*, **6**, 99–110.

McCord, C. P. (1948) Life and death by the minute, *Industr. Med.*, **17**, 377–382.

McDonald, B. W., and Gunderson, E. K. E. (1974) Correlates of job satisfaction in naval environments, *J. Appl. Psychol.*, **59**, 371–373.

McGrath, J. E. (1970a) A conceptual formulation for research on stress. In McGrath, J. E. (ed.), *Social and Psychological Factors in Stress*. New York. Holt, Rinehart, Winston, pp. 10–21.

McGrath, J. E. (1970b) Major substantive issues: time setting, and the coping process. In McGrath, J. E. (ed.), *Social and Psychological Factors in Stress*. New York. Holt, Rinehart, Winston, pp. 22–40.

McGrath, J. E. (1976) Stress and behaviour in organizations. In Dunnette, M. D. (ed.), *Handbook of Industrial and Organizational Psychology*. Chicago. Rand McNally, pp. 1351–1395.

McLean, A. (1974) Occupational 'stress'—a misnomer. In McLean, A. (ed.), *Occupational Stress*. Springfield, Ill. C. C. Thomas, pp. 98–105.

MacMahon, B., and Pugh, T. F. (1970) *Epidemiology: Principles and Methods*. Boston: Little, Brown.

McMichael, A. J. (1976) Standardized mortality ratios and the 'healthy worker effect': scratching beneath the surface, *J. Occup. Med.*, **18**, 165–168.

Maddison, D. (1974) Stress on the doctor and his family, *Med. J. Aust.*, **2**, 315–318.

Mangione, T. W., and Quinn, R. P. (1975) Job satisfaction, counter productive behaviour, and drug use at work, *J. Appl. Psychol.*, **60**, 114–116.

Mann, F. C., and Williams, L. K. (1962) Some effects of the changing work environment in the office, *J. soc. Issues*, **18**, 3, 90–101.

44

Margolis, B. L. (1973) Stress is a work hazard, too, *Industr. Med. & Surg.*, **42**, 20–23.

Margolis, B. L., Kroes, W. H., and Quinn, R. P. (1974) Job stress: an unlisted occupational hazard, *J. Occup. Med.*, **16**, 659–661.

Marks, R. U. (1967) Social stress and cardiovascular disease: a review of empirical findings, *Milbank Mem. Fund. Quart.*, **45**, 2, part 2, 51–108.

Matsumoto, Y. S. (1970) Social stress and coronary heart disease in Japan: a hypothesis, *Milkbank Mem. Fund Quart.*, **48**, 1, 9–36.

Mausner, J. S., and Bahn, A. K. (1974) *Epidemiology: an Introductory Text*. Philadelphia, Pa. W. B. Saunders.

Mausner, J. S., and Steppacher, R. C. (1973) Suicide in professionals: a study of male and female psychologists, *Amer. J. Epidemiol.*, **98**, 436–445.

Mayers, M. R. (1969) *Occupational Health*. Baltimore, Md. Williams & Wilkins Co.

Medalie, J. H., Snyder, M., Groen, J. J., Neufeld, H. N., Goldbourt, U., and Riss, E. (1973) Angina pectoris among 10,000 men, *Amer. J. Med.*, **55**, 583–594.

Miles, R. H. (1975) An empirical test of causal inference between role perceptions of conflict and ambiguity and various personal outcomes, *J. Appl. Psychol.*, **60**, 334–339.

Miles, R. H., and Perreault, W. D., Jr. (1976) Organizational role conflict: its antecedents and consequences, *Organiz. Behav. & Hum. Perform.*, **17**, 19–44.

Miller, D. R. (1963) The study of social relationships: situation, identity, and social interaction. In Koch, S. (ed.), *Psychology: a Study of a Science*, vol. 5, New York. McGraw-Hill, pp. 639–737.

Morris, J. N., Heady, J. A., and Barley, R. G. (1952) Coronary heart disease in medical practitioners, *Brit. J. Med.*, **1**, 503–520.

Morris, J. N., Heady, J. A., and Raffle, A. B. (1956) Physique of London busmen, *Lancet*, **2**, 569–578.

Morris, J. N., Heady, J. A., Raffle, P. A. B., Roberts, C. G., and Parks, J. W. (1953) coronary heart disease and physical activity of work, *Lancet*, **2**, 1111–1113.

Morse, N. E., and Weiss, R. S. (1955) The function and meaning of work and the job, *Amer. Sociol. Rev.*, **20**, 191–198.

Mott, P. E., Mann, F. C., McLaughlin, Q., and Warwick, D. P. (1965) *Shift Work*. Ann Arbor. University of Michigan Press.

Mueller, E. F. (1965) *Psychological and Physiological Correlates of Work Overload Among University Professors*. Ann Arbor. Unpublished doctoral dissertation. The University of Michigan.

National Center for Health Statistics (1965) *Coronary Heart Disease in Adults, U.S. 1960–1962*. Washington, DC. Vital and Health Statistics, PHS Publication no. 1000, series 11, no. 10.

National Center for Health Statistics (1966) *Hypertension and Hypertensive Heart Disease in Adults, U.S., 1960–1962*. Washington, DC. Vital and Health Statistics, PHS Publication no. 1000, series 11, no. 13.

National Center for Health Statistics (1967) *Serum Cholesterol Levels of Adults, U.S., 1960–1962*. Washington, DC. Vital and Health Statistics, PHS Publication no. 1000, series 11, no. 22.

Neel, R. (1955) Nervous stress in the industrial situation, *Personnel Psychol.*, **8**, 405–416.

Olive, L. E., Kelsey, J. E., Visser, M. J., and Daly, R. T. (1976) Moving as perceived by executives and their families, *J. Occup. Med.*, **18**, 546–550.

Opsahl, R. L., and Dunnette, M. D. (1966) The role of financial compensation in industrial motivation, *Psychol. Bulll.*, **66**, 94–118.

Orth-Gomer, K. (1974) Ischemic heart disease as result of psychosocial processes, *Soc. Sci. & Med.*, **8**, 39–45.

Orzack, L. H. (1959) Work as a 'central life interest' of professionals, *Soc. Problems*, **7**, 125–132.

Ostfeld, A. M., Lebovitz, B. Z., Shekelle, R. B., and Paul, O. (1964) A prospective study of the relationship between personality and coronary heart disease, *J. chron. Dis.*, **17**, 265–276.

O'Toole, J. (ed.) (1974a) *Work and the Quality of Life*. Cambridge, Mass. The MIT Press.

O'Toole, J. (1974b) Work in America and the great job satisfaction controversy, *J. Occup. Med.*, **16**, 710–715.

Paffenbarger, R. S., Jr., Wolf, P. A., Notkin, J., and Thorne, M. C. (1966) Chronic disease in former college students. I. Early precursors of fatal coronary heart disease, *Amer. J. Epidem.*, **83**, 314–328.

Palmore, E. B. (1969) Physical, mental and social factors in predicting longevity, *Gerontologist*, **9**, 2, part I, 103–108.

Paykel, E. S., Myers, J. K., Dienelt, M. N., Klerman, G. L., Lindenthal, J. L., and Pepper, M. P. (1969) Life events and depression, *Arch. Gen. Psychiat.*, **21**, 753–760.

Payne, D. E. (1974) Alienation: an organizational–societal comparison, *Social Forces*, **53**, 274–282.

Payne, R., and Pugh, D. S. (1976) Organizational structure and climate. In Dunnette, M. D. (ed.), *Handbook of Industrial and Organizational Psychology*. Chicago. Rand McNally, pp. 1125–1173.

Pell, S., and d'Alonzo, C. A. (1963) Acute myocardial infarction in a large industrial population, *J.A.M.A.*, **185**, 831–838.

Pepitone, A. (1967) Self, social environment, and stress. In Appley, M. H., and Trumbull, R. (eds), *Psychological Stress*. New York. Appleton-Century-Crofts, pp. 182–199.

Pflanz, M. (1971) Epidemiological and sociocultural factors in the etiology of duodenal ulcer. In Weiner, H. (ed.), *Duodenal Ulcer*. vol. 6, *Advances in Psychosomatic Medicine*. Basel. S. Karger, pp. 121–151.

Pinneau, S. R. (1976) Effects of social support on occupational stresses and strains. Presented at a symposium on Job Demands and Worker Health, held at the 84th Annual Convention of the American Psychological Association, Washington, DC, September 1976.

Porter, L. W. (1962) Job attitudes in management. I. Perceived deficiencies in need fulfilment as a function of job level, *J. Appl. Psychol.*, **46**, 375–384.

Porter, L. W., and Lawler, E. E. (1965) Properties of organization structure in relation to job attitudes and job behaviour, *Psychol. Bull.*, **64**, 23–51.

Porter, L. W., and Steers, R. M. (1973) Organizational, work, and personal factors in employee turnover and absenteeism, *Psychol. Bull.*, **80**, 151–176.

Proceedings of the Conference on Epidemiologic Research in Occupational Health (1962), *J. Occup. Med.*, **4**, 567–650 (special supplement, October 1962).

Quinn, R. P., Seashore, S., Kahn, R., Mangione, T., Campbell, D., Staines, G., and McCullough, M. (1971) *Survey of Working Conditions*. Washington, DC. US Government Printing Office, document no. 2916–0001.

Quinn, R. P., and Shepard, L. J. (1974) *The 1972–73 Quality of Employment Survey*. Ann Arbor. Institute for Social Research, The University of Michigan.

Rabkin, J. G., and Struening, E. L. (1976) Life events, stress, and illness, *Science*, **194**, 1013–1020.

Rapoport, R., and Rapoport, R. (1965) Work and family in contemporary society, *Amer. Sociol. Rev.*, **30**, 381–394.

Reeder, L. G., Schrama, P. G. M., and Dirken, J. M. (1973) Stress and cardiovascular health: an international cooperative study—I, *Soc. Sci. & Med.*, **7**, 573–584.

Reim, B., Glass, D. C., and Singer, J. E. (1971) Behavioural consequences of exposure to uncontrollable and unpredictable noise, *J. Appl. Soc. Psychol.*, **1**, 44–56.

Reynolds, R. C. (1974) Community and occupational influences in stress at Cape Kennedy: relationships to heart disease. In Eliot, R. S. (ed.), *Stress and the Heart*. Mount Kisco, NY. Futura Publishing, pp. 33–49.

Robinson, J. P., Athanasiou, R., and Head, K. B. (eds) (1969) *Measures of Occupational*

46

Attitudes and Occupational Characteristics. Ann Arbor. Institute for Social Research, The University of Michigan.

Robinson, J. P., and Converse, P. E. (1972) Social change reflected in the use of time. In Campbell, A., and Converse, P. E. (eds), *The Human Meaning of Social Change*. New York. Russell Sage Foundation, pp. 17–86.

Roman, P. H., and Trice, H. M. (1972) Psychiatric impairment among 'Middle Americans'. Surveys of work organizations, *Social Psychiat.*, 7, 157–166.

Rosenman, R. H., Brand, R. J., Jenkins, C. D., Friedman, M., Straus, R., and Wurm, M. (1975) Coronary heart disease in the Western Collaborative Group Study: final follow-up experience of 8½ years, *J.A.M.A.*, 233, 872–877.

Rosenman, R. H., and Friedman, M. (1958) The possible relationship of occupational stress to clinical coronary heart disease, *Calif. Med.*, 89, 169–174.

Rosenman, R. H., and Friedman, M. (1961) Association of specific behaviour pattern in women with blood and cardiovascular findings, *Circulation*, 24, 1173–1184.

Rosenman, R. H., Friedman, M., Straus, R., Wurm, M., Kositchek, R., Hahn, W., and Werthessen, N. T. (1964) A predictive study of coronary heart disease: the Western Collaborative Group Study, *J.A.M.A.*, 189, 15–22.

Rubin, R. T. (1974) Biochemical and endocrine responses to severe psychological stress. In Gunderson, E. K. E., and Rahe, R. H. (eds), *Life Stress and Illness*. Springfield, Ill. C. C. Thomas, pp. 227–241.

Ruff, G. E., and Korchin, S. J. (1967) Adaptive stress behaviour. In Appley, M. H., and Trumbull, R. (eds), *Psychological Stress*. New York. Appleton-Century-Crofts, pp. 297–306.

Russek, H. I. (1962) Emotional stress and coronary heart disease in American physicians, dentists, and lawyers, *Amer. J. Med. Sci.*, 243, 716–725.

Russek, H. I. (1965) Stress, tobacco, and coronary disease in North American professional groups, *J.A.M.A.*, 192, 189–194.

Russek, H. I., and Zohman, B. L. (1958) Relative significance of heredity, diet, and occupational stress in coronary heart disease of young adults, *Amer. J. Med. Sci.*, 235, 266–275.

Sales, S. M. (1969) Organizational role as a risk factor in coronary disease, *Ad. Sci. Quart.*, 14, 325–336.

Sales, S. M., and House, J. (1971) Job dissatisfaction as a possible risk factor in coronary heart disease, *J. chron. Dis.*, 23, 861–873.

Sayles, L., and Strauss, G. (1966) *Human Behaviour in Organizations*. Englewood Cliffs, NJ. Prentice-Hall.

Schär, M., Reeder, L. G., and Dirken, J. M. (1973) Stress and cardiovascular health: an international cooperative study-II. The male population of a factory in Zurich, *Soc. Sci. & Med.*, 7, 585–603.

Schuckit, M. A., and Gunderson, E. K. E. (1973) Job stress and psychiatric illness in the U.S. Navy, *J. Occup. Med.*, 15, 884–887.

Scott, R., and Howard, A. (1970) Models of stress. In Levine, S., and Scotch, N. A. (eds), *Social Stress*. Chicago. Aldine, pp. 259–278.

Seashore, S. E., and Barnowe, J. T. (1972) Collar color doesn't count, *Psychol. Today*, 6, 3, 53–54, 80–82.

Seeman, M. (1974) Alienation and engagement. In Campbell, A., and Converse, P. E. (eds), *The Human Meaning of Social Change*. New York. Russell Sage Foundation, pp. 467–527.

Sells, S. B. (1970) On the nature of stress. In McGrath, J. E. (ed.), *Social and Psychological Factors in Stress*. New York. Holt, Rinehart, Winston, pp. 134–139.

Sexton, W. P. (1968) Industrial work: who calls it psychologically devastating?, *Manag. Personnel Quart.*, 6, 2–8.

Shekelle, R. B. (1976) Status inconsistency, mobility and CHD: a reply to Horan and Gray, *J. Hlth & Soc. Behav.*, 17, 83–87.

Shekelle, R. B., Ostfeld, A. M., and Paul, O. (1969) Social status and incidence of coronary heart disease, *J. chron. Dis.*, **22**, 381–394.

Shepard, J. M. (1971) *Automation and Alienation*. Cambridge. The MIT Press.

Shepard, R. J. (1974) *Men at Work : Applications of Ergonomics to Performance and Design*. Springfield, Ill. C. C. Thomas.

Sheppard, H. L., and Herrick, N. Q. (1972) *Where Have All the Robots Gone? Worker Dissatisfaction in '70's*. New York. The Free Press.

Shirom, A., Eden, D., Silberwasser, S., and Kellermann, J. J. (1973) Job stress and risk factors in coronary heart disease among five occupational categories in kibbutzim, *Soc. Sci. & Med.*, **7**, 875–892.

Siassi, I., Crocetti, G., Spiro, H. R. (1974) Loneliness and dissatisfaction in a blue collar population, *Arch. Gen. Psychiat.*, **30**, 261–265.

Singer, R., and Rutenfranz, J. (1971) Attitudes of air traffic controllers at Frankfurt airport towards work and the working environment, *Ergonomics*, **14**, 633–639.

Sleight, R. B., and Cook, K. G. (1974) *Problems in Occupational Safety and Health : a Critical Review of Select Worker Physical and Psychological Factors*. Cincinnati. HEW Publication no. (NIOSH) 75–124.

Smith, R. C. (1973) Comparison of job attitudes of personnel in three air traffic control specialities, *Aerospace Med.*, **44**, 919–927.

Smith, T. (1967) Sociocultural incongruity and change: a review of empirical findings, *Milbank Mem. Fund Quart.*, **45**, 2, part 2, 109–116.

Stellman, J. M., and Daum, S. M. (1973) *Work is Dangerous to Your Health*. New York. Pantheon Books.

Sterling, T. D., and Weinkman, J. J. (1976) Smoking characteristics by type of employment, *J. Occup. Med.*, **18**, 743–754.

Strauss, G. (1974a) Is there a blue-collar revolt against work? In O'Toole, J. (ed.), *Work and the Quality of Life*. Cambridge Mass. The MIT Press, pp. 40–69.

Strauss, G. (1974b) Workers: attitudes and adjustments. In the American Assembly, Columbia University, *The Worker and the Job: Coping with Change*. Englewood Cliffs, NJ. Prentice-Hall, pp. 73–98.

Struening, E. L., and Guttentag, M. (eds) (1975) *Handbook of Evaluation Research*, vol. I. Beverly Hills. Sage Publications.

Susser, M. (1967) Causes of peptic ulcer: a selective epidemiologic review, *J. chron. Dis.*, **20**, 435–456.

Susser, M. (1973) *Causal Thinking in the Health Sciences. Concepts and Strategies of Epidemiology*. New York. Oxford University Press.

Syme, L. S., Borhani, N. O., and Buechley, R. W. (1965) Cultural mobility and coronary heart disease in an urban area, *Amer. J. Epidem.*, **82**, 334–346.

Syme, S. L., Hyman, M. M., and Enterline, P. E. (1964) Some social and cultural factors associated with the occurrence of coronary heart disease, *J. chron. Dis.*, **17**, 277–289.

Tausky, C., and Piedmont, E. B. (1967/1968) The meaning of work and unemployment: implications for mental health, *Int. J. Soc. Psychiat.*, **14**, 44–49.

Taylor, L. (1968) *Occupational Sociology*. New York: Oxford University Press.

Theorell, T., and Rahe, R. (1972) Behaviour and life satisfactions characteristics of Swedish subjects with myocardial infarction, *J. chron. Dis.*, **25**, 139–147.

Thomas, C. B., and Greenstreet, R. L. (1973) Psychological characteristics in youth as predictors of five disease states: suicide, mental illness, hypertension, coronary heart disease, and tumor, *Johns Hopkins Med. J.*, **132**, 16–43.

Turner, A. N., and Lawrence, P. R. (1968) *Industrial Jobs and the Worker*. Cambridge, Mass. Harvard University Graduate School of Business Administration.

Tyroler, H. A., and Cassel, J. (1964) Health consequences of culture change. II The effect of urbanization on coronary heart mortality in rural residents, *J. chron. Dis.*, **17**, 167–177.

48

Veroff, J., and Feld, S. (1970) *Marriage and Work in America: a Study of Motives and Roles.* New York. Van Nostrand Reinhold.

Vroom, V. H. (1964) *Work and Motivation.* New York. Wiley.

Vroom, V. H. (1969) Industrial social psychology. In Lindzey, G., and Aronson, E. (eds), *Handbook of Social Psychology,* vol. 5. Reading, Mass. Addison-Wesley, pp. 196–268.

Wan, T. (1971) Status stress and morbidity: a sociological investigation of selected categories of work-limiting chronic condition, *J. chron. Dis.,* **24**, 453–468.

Wardwell, W. I., and Bahnson, C. B. (1973) Behavioural variables and myocardial infarction in the southeastern Connecticut Heart Study, *J. chron. Dis.,* **26**, 447–461.

Wardwell, W. I., Hyman, M., and Bahnson, C. B. (1968) Socio-environmental antecedents to coronary heart disease in 87 white males, *Soc. Sci. & Med.,* **2**, 165–183.

Warheit, G. J. (1974) Occupation: a key factor in stress at the manned space center. In Eliot, R. S. (ed.), *Stress and the Heart.* Mount Kisco, N. Y. Futura Publishing, pp. 51–65.

Weissman, M. M., and Paykel, E. S. (1972) Moving and depression in women, *Society,* **9**, 24–28.

Weitz, J. (1970) Psychological research needs on the problems of human stress. In McGrath, J. E. (ed.), *Social and Psychological Factors in Stress.* New York. Holt, Rinehart, Winston, pp. 124–133.

Wessman, A. E. (1956) *A Psychological Inquiry into Satisfaction and Happiness.* Princeton, NJ. Unpublished doctoral dissertation, Princeton University.

White, K. L., and Henderson, M. M. (1976) *Epidemiology as a Fundamental Science.* New York. Oxford University Press.

Wiegand, R. A. von (1972) Alcoholism in industry (U.S.A.), *Brit. J. Addict.,* **67**, 181–187.

Wilensky, H. L. (1964) Varieties of work experience. In Borow, H. (ed.), *Man in a World at Work.* Boston, Mass. Houghton-Mifflin, pp. 125–154.

Wilson, W. (1967) Correlates of avowed happiness, *Psychol. Bull.,* **67**, 294–306.

Wolf, S. (1971) Psychosocial forces in myocardial infarction and sudden death. In Levi, L. (ed.), *Society, Stress, and Disease,* vol. I. London. Oxford University Press, pp. 324–330.

Work in America (1973) Report of a Special Task Force to the Secretary of Health, Education and Welfare, Cambridge, Mass. The MIT Press.

Zander, A., and Quinn, R. P. (1962) The social environment and mental health: a review of past research at the Institute for Social Research, *J. soc. Issues,* **18**, 3, 48–66.

Zohman, B. L. (1973) Emotional factors in coronary disease, *Geriatrics,* **28**, 110–119.

Zyzanski, S. J., and Jenkins, C. D. (1970) Basic dimensions within the coronary-prone behaviour pattern, *J. chron. Dis.,* **22**, 781–795.

PART II

Factors in the Person's Environment

Chapter 2

Blue Collar Stressors

E. Christopher Poulton

University of Cambridge

Summary

There are both objective and subjective measures of stress, but the subjective measures are likely to be biased. Insufficient light and glare both reduce working efficiency. A few people cannot tolerate flickering displays. Noise produces industrial deafness. It prevents people from hearing what they want to listen to. Intermittent noise is distracting. But noise may arouse people and make them work more efficiently. Vibration blurs vision and interferes with delicate movements. But vertical vibration at 5 Hz helps to keep people alert. Slow rotary accelerations produce motion sickness. Heat usually reduces working efficiency, but may increase efficiency for a brief period. Cold hands and feet are clumsy. Gusty winds blow people around and interfere with skilled movements. Industrial processes produce dusts, mists, fumes, vapours, and gases which can harm the human body when they are breathed or get on the skin. Ionizing radiation, and electromagnetic radiation of very short wavelength, can also harm the human body. Breathing air under pressure produces nitrogen narcosis, and can produce acute oxygen poisoning. The reduced oxygen in the air high above the ground reduces the efficiency of the brain, and eventually produces unconsciousness. Rapid compression can be painful when a person has a common cold. Decompression can injure a person if it is too rapid. Heavy physical work reduces the efficiency of the brain and produces muscular fatigue, especially in people who are not physically fit. The arousal produced by intense fear also causes inefficiency. Having too much to do all at once, and having too little to do, both reduce working efficiency. People work less efficiently than usual when they are short of sleep. They also work less efficiently between 1 and 4 o'clock in the early morning, unless they are used to working then. In the absence of any valid evidence, it is safest to assume that the combined effect of a number of stressors is the sum of the individual effects.

Introduction. Subjective and objective measures of stress

In dealing with stressors at work, the manager has available both subjective judgement of stress, and objective measures. Both kinds of information can be valuable to him, but he need not necessarily give them equal weight. There are a number of examples where the subjective judgements of stress conflict with the objective measures:

(1) In passing a road vehicle going in the opposite direction at night on a two-lane road, undipped headlamps produce more discomfort glare than dipped headlamps. Yet they make it easier to see unlighted obstacles in the road.
(2) People may complain about the noise at work. Yet noise can increase the rate of work, and can help to maintain vigilance in prolonged boring tasks. Music while you work is an example.
(3) Vertical vibration at 5 Hz can help to maintain alertness, although people may complain of it.
(4) A raised body temperature can increase the rate of work for a brief period without affecting accuracy appreciably, although people may believe that their performance is worse.
(5) Protective clothing may be discarded as uncomfortable. Yet it may be essential for health, or even for survival in hostile environments.

In coming to a decision in these cases, a manager clearly needs to give most weight to the objective measures. But he needs to be aware of the subjective judgements of stress, because they are likely to influence people's behaviour in other ways. A stress may increase efficiency at work, but may encourage discontent, absenteeism, and dropping out from the job. The optimal decision may be some form of compromise.

A difficulty with subjective judgements of stress is that they may be based upon a rule which most people know and agree on, but which does not happen to apply in the particular circumstances under investigation. In the examples just given, the well known rules are that glare, noise, vibration, heat, and discomfort reduce efficiency. Usually this is the case, but not always. In assessing the validity of the subjective judgements, the manager needs to be aware of possible sources of bias.

The central tendency of judgement is another bias in subjective judgements of stress. People have been asked to rate noises for acceptability on a scale ranging from quiet, through acceptable and noisy, to excessively noisy. Noise intensities near the middle of the range of noise intensities tend to be judged just acceptable, whatever their actual values.

The central tendency of judgement makes it virtually impossible to obtain an unbiased estimate of the just acceptable noise level. If each person is asked to judge only a single noise, his judgement will be biased by the range of noise intensities which he is used to hearing. He will tend to accept a noise which is less intense than the average he is used to, and reject a noise which is more intense. The central tendency of judgement biases all subjective judgements of acceptability, whether of noise, glare, vibration, temperature, or anything else (Poulton, 1977b).

Poor visibility

Too little light

Table 2.1 shows the amount of light which is required for various kinds of work. The tasks at the top of the table involve seeing minute details and small differences in brightness contrast. If there is insufficient light, people have to devise and learn special strategies to overcome the inadequate visual cues. It makes the tasks more time consuming and more frustrating.

Table 2.1 Recommended minimal levels of illumination

Minimum luminance in nits*	Kind of visual task	Examples
1000—600	Exceptionally severe tasks with minute detail	Inspecting very small instruments; watch making
600—400	Very severe prolonged tasks with very small detail	Gauging very small parts; hosiery mending
300	Severe prolonged tasks with small detail	Fine assembly and machining; weaving thin fibres
200	Fairly severe tasks with small detail	Drawing offices; cutting and sewing clothes
100	Ordinary tasks with medium detail	General offices; general assembly
60	Rough tasks with large detail	Stores; heavy machinery assembly
30	Casual seeing	Passages; cloakrooms

(After Hopkinson and Collins, 1970, Table 9.2)

*Candela per square metre, cd/m^2.

Glare

Figure 2.1 shows how glare reduces the visibility of objects. Both the display being looked at and the glare source form images on the retina at the back of the eye. The bright glare source also produces a cone of scattered light within the eye, which is represented by the dotted lines. The glare reduces the visibility of the display when the image of the display falls within the cone of scattered light.

Glare is a greater handicap when looking at a dark display than when looking at a bright display. This is because the amount of scattered light from the source of the glare is relatively large compared with the light entering the eye from a dark display. Whereas the scattered light is only a small proportion of the light entering the eye from a bright display.

The disability produced by glare depends also upon the square of the angle

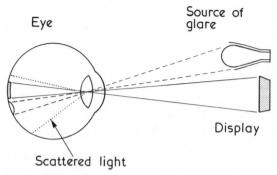

Figure 2.1 The light scattered within the eye by a
source of glare located close to the display being
looked at

between the display and the source of the glare. Doubling the angle reduces
the disability by a factor of 4. The reduction in glare with the increase in visual
angle is seen in driving at night. The headlamps of an approaching car which
is more or less directly ahead produce the greatest disability. When the distance
of the approaching car is reduced to half, four times as much light is received
from its headlamps. But the headlamps move over to the side as the
car approaches. So the disability becomes a lot less, in spite of the increase
in light received from the headlamps.

In Figure 2.1 the lamp which produces the glare shines directly into the
eye. But glare is often caused by reflected light. If a display is covered by glass,
the glass may reflect light into the person's eyes from a source of light behind
the person's head. Instruments mounted in panels used to have shiny metal
edges. They are a source of glare if they reflect light into the person's eyes while
he is reading the instruments.

People may complain of glare which is too small to have any measurable
effect upon their work. The British Illuminating Engineering Society has a
code of maximum recommended levels of glare, which is based upon subjective
measures of discomfort (Hopkinson and Collins, 1970). Unfortunately recommendations based upon discomfort do not necessarily provide the optimum
visibility. Contrary to popular belief, a car driver can see better if both he and the
approaching driver use their full headlights, instead of dipped headlights.
A pedestrian or other object at the side of the road without its own source of
light can be seen about twice as far ahead when the drivers pass each other
with undipped headlights. This is an extreme example of comfort not being
compatible with optimum visibility. But it is a point which needs to
be remembered when considering glare which is simply uncomfortable.

Flicker

The light given out by an ordinary filament electric lamp depends upon the
voltage of the mains supply. If the voltage of the mains fluctuates as a result

of sudden transient increases in demand, the light will fluctuate. Fluorescent strip lights discharge at twice the mains frequency, 50 Hz in Great Britain. So when they are not functioning properly the light may flicker at 100 Hz. Fluorescent tubes flicker close to each end when the phosphor is wearing out.

The displays of television tubes are usually painted at half the mains frequency. With the 50 Hz British mains supply, alternate lines are painted 25 times per second. The remaining lines are painted the other 25 times per second. With an electronic display system the face of the tube may not be painted more than perhaps twelve times per second. If the phosphor which coats the face of the tube stays bright for $\frac{1}{12}$ second, flicker will not be visible. But phosphor which persists as long as this leaves ghosts each time the display changes. In selecting the persistence of the phosphor to coat the face of the display, the manufacturer has a choice between flicker and ghosts. He is likely to prefer the flicker.

One person in every 5000 or 10 000 people can have an epileptic attack when exposed to flickering light at frequencies between 3 and 100 Hz. The worst frequencies are between 15 and 20 Hz. Sitting close to a flickering television screen is the commonest cause. Other people are likely to complain of flicker, so it should be avoided if possible. But if it cannot easily be avoided, at least it should not affect the efficiency of most people. To produce reliable changes in performance in ordinary people, the light has to be turned right off and on again at a frequency below 10 Hz. The few people who cannot tolerate the flicker should be removed to other jobs. It may be the job, rather than the flicker, which they really object to.

Noise

Table 2.2 gives the approximate noise levels of some common sources of sound. In factories the noise is greater when a number of noisy machines like metal punches or perforators are placed close together. Impulsive noises are produced by mechanical hammers, by blasting, and by supersonic aircraft.

Table 2.2

Effect	Sound pressure level in dB (A)	Example
Pain	140	
	120	Near a jet aircraft at take-off
Bad work	100	Near a pneumatic drill
Deafness	80	In a busy street
Raised voice	60	In a busy office
	40	In a public library
Threshold	0	

Note: 0 dB represents 20 micronewtons per square metre (20μ N/m^2, $0\cdot00002$ N/M^2 or $0\cdot0002$ dynes/em^2).

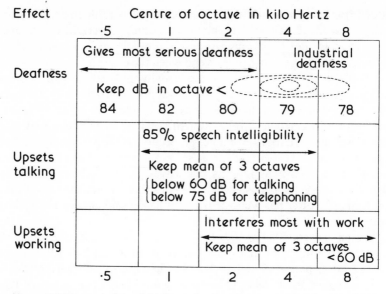

Figure 2.2 The main harmful effects of noise upon man (after Poulton, 1970)

Industrial deafness

Noise in one octave produces most deafness in the octave one higher. The middle section of Figure 2.2 shows that it is the three octaves centred on 1, 2, and 4 kHz which are responsible for most of the intelligibility of speech. So the most serious hearing losses are produced by noise in the three octaves one octave lower, centred on 0·5, 1, and 2 kHz, as indicated in the top section of the figure. To prevent deafness here in normal people, the average sound pressure level at work has to be kept below 84 to 80 dB in each of the three octaves, as shown in the figure (Burns, 1973).

Masking of speech

The middle section of Figure 2.2 shows that noise is most effective in masking speech in the three octaves centred on 1, 2, and 4 kHz. About 85% of the intelligibility of speech comes from these three octaves. If speech in these three octaves is masked by loud noise, people cannot hear the consonants which enable them to distinguish one word from another.

The average intensity of the noise in these three octaves is called the speech interference level. Figure 2.3 shows the maximum distance at which it is possible to talk to someone at various speech interference levels. When the speech interference level is too great, a talker has to raise his voice or shout in order to be heard. For comfortable conversation, the speech interference level should be kept below 60 dB. This corresponds to an overall noise level of about 70 dB (A).

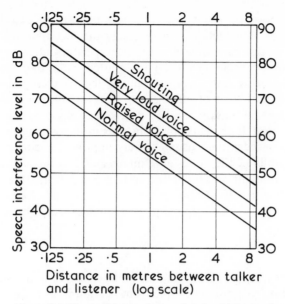

Figure 2.3 The speech interference levels which permit talkers at various distances to speak to each other with only slight difficulty (after Poulton, 1970)

Interference with work

Continuous noise isolates a person from his normal auditory environment. We have just seen that in noise a listener cannot hear what people are saying. Noise also masks the inner speech which a person uses in thinking, and in keeping track of what he is doing. A person cannot hear himself think in intense noise.

Noise also masks the auditory feedback cues coming from the equipment which a person is using. In quiet these bangs, taps, clicks, squeaks, and scrapes are used as cues. They tell a person when he has successfully completed a particular operation. He can use them to time the start of his next operation. In noise a person may not be able to hear these cues. So he has to use his eyes and his other senses more. When his eyes and his other senses are fully occupied already, he is likely to miss the help which the auditory cues can give him. As a result, the amount of spoilt work is likely to increase. So is the number of accidents at work, because warning signals are less easy to hear (Poulton, 1976).

Noise has a second kind of detrimental effect upon a person's work. It distracts him from what he is doing. He attends to the noise for a moment, instead of attending to the work. This tends to produce spoilt work and accidents. Continuous noise is most likely to distract a person when it first starts. As it continues, he gradually gets used to it. He is distracted less and less.

Intermittent noise does not lose its power to distract, especially when it occurs irregularly. Distraction is most likely the first time the intermittent noise comes on. But each time it occurs, the person's attention may switch to the noise for an instant. Irregular intermittent noise does not have to be very intense in order to distract people, and so degrade their performance.

Noise has a third kind of effect upon work, which tends to oppose the detrimental effects of masking and of distraction. Noise increases a person's behavioural arousal. It prevents him from relaxing and going to sleep. It makes him feel more on edge than usual. It may improve his concentration. This explains the results of the quite large number of experiments in which continuous or intermittent noise is found to improve performance. Music while you work for about half an hour mid-morning and mid-afternoon often has a similar effect. It helps to keep people at their jobs when the work is boring and routine.

Annoyance

When questioned, people often complain of the effects of noise. Noise interferes with conversation. It prevents people from hearing what is said on television or radio. Unexpected noises are distracting. The arousing effects of noise are not welcome when people want to relax at home, or go to sleep.

However, little attention is usually paid to the beneficial effects of noise. In obtaining subjective judgements of the effects of noise, the rating scales usually contrast acceptable with noisy, inoffensive with annoying, or unobjectionable with objectionable. Ratings such as bracing or stimulating are not provided. People are not given the opportunity of indicating that noise can be beneficial, if they happen to notice that it is.

Vibration and motion

Figure 2.4 shows the sources of vibration which are most likely to affect people, and the maximum levels of vibration which they produce. In describing the effects upon the human body of various levels of vibration, the intensity of the vibration is usually given in terms of the acceleration at various frequencies. This is because the greatest vibration which people will tolerate depends primarily upon the size of the acceleration, rather than simply upon the amplitude of the vibration. However, the amount of blurring of vision and of shaking of the hands depends primarily upon the amplitude of the vibration, rather than simply upon the acceleration. In Figure 2.4 the amplitude is represented by the sloping lines. The figure shows that vehicles like farm tractors, cars, and heavy goods vehicles vibrate mostly between 1 and 10 Hz. Light aircraft and helicopters vibrate mostly between 5 and 100 Hz. Hand tools vibrate mostly at frequencies above 100 Hz.

Resonance of the human body

The amplitude of vibration of the human body depends partly upon the ampli-

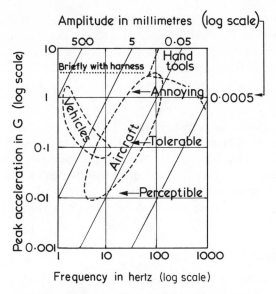

Figure 2.4 The maximum levels of vibration produced by some common sources (after Poulton, 1975)

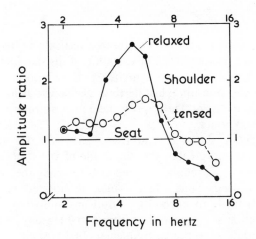

Figure 2.5 The effect of tensed and relaxed trunk muscles upon the amplitude of vertical vibration of the shoulders of a seated man. The seat vibrates vertically at the amplitude called 1 on the ordinate (after Guignard, 1965)

tude of the vibration to which it is exposed. In addition, the human body has its own natural frequencies of vibration, which depend upon its mass and its structure. The amplitude of the vibration at certain frequencies is reduced by the human body. The amplitude at other frequencies is greatly increased, a phenomenon called resonance.

The resonant frequency of the human body to vertical vibration is at about 5 Hz. The unbroken function in Figure 2.5 shows that the amplitude of the vertical vibration of the shoulder at 5 Hz is about 2·5 times the amplitude of vibration of the seat when a person is relaxed.

Blurred vision

The head rotates when the body is vibrated vertically, because the join between the head and neck is behind the centre of gravity of the head. The rotation of the head blurs vision a good deal more than simple vertical vibration does. This explains why reading is a lot more difficult if the head is vibrated vertically than if the print is vibrated vertically by the same amount. The additional rotary vibration of the head which occurs when it is vibrated increases the amount of blurring of the print.

Shaky hands and feet

Vibration shakes the hands. It makes small fine movements in the direction of the vibration difficult to perform accurately. You notice this if you try to write in a train, car or bus. It is difficult to compensate for the vibration.

Muscle tension and alertness

Figure 2.5 shows that when the man is vibrated vertically at frequencies around 5 Hz, he can reduce the amplitude of vibration of his shoulders by tensing his trunk muscles. Whenever he starts to relax, the vibration of his shoulders increases and shakes him up. This alerting mechanism helps him to remain vigilant in dull routine tasks. The improvement in performance has been shown to last for at least 3 hours.

However the figure shows that at frequencies of 3 Hz and less, and at frequencies of 7 Hz and greater, the amplitude of vibration of the shoulders is smaller when the trunk muscles are relaxed. Relaxing the muscles is a good way of going to sleep. Thus when a man is vibrated vertically at these frequencies, he is likely to do badly at dull unstimulating tasks. It follows that vertical vibration at frequencies of from 4 to 6 Hz may help to keep a man alert. Whereas vertical vibration at frequencies of 3 Hz and below, and at 7 Hz and above, is likely to reduce alertness (Poulton, 1977a).

A modern heavy goods vehicle may have a well designed cab with little vibration and little noise. It may be comfortably warm. In driving in the dark at night on a motorway there may be practically no other traffic. Ideal conditions like these may make the driver feel that he is sailing in the air, especially if he is sleepy. This could be dangerous. A driver who feels like this would be well advised to open his window, to let in some noise and a cool, buffeting wind. This will help to prevent him from dropping off to sleep. Vertical vibration at frequencies around 5 Hz can have a similar beneficial effect.

Vibration and comfort

Figure 2.4 gives a rough indication of the accelerations at frequencies up to 30 Hz which people judge to be perceptible, tolerable, annoying, and intolerable except for brief periods with a harness. Different experimenters have obtained very different results, depending upon the range of levels of vibration which they have presented to their groups of observers. Peak accelerations judged on average to be perceptible vary from 0·003 to 0·3 g, a ratio of 1 to 100. Peak accelerations judged intolerable or alarming vary from 0·3 to 3 g, a ratio of 1 to 10.

Long term effects of vibration

People who work with vibrating hand tools year after year can gradually receive injuries to their hands. In Raynaud's disease the hands become more sensitive to cold than usual. They go white as soon as the person's body or his hands become cold. Raynaud's disease is produced by frequencies of 50 to 100 Hz. Pneumatic drills can do this.

In Dart's disease the hands become blue, swollen, and painful. It is produced by frequencies above 200 Hz.

Motion sickness

Motion sickness is produced by rotary accelerations with frequencies below 1 Hz. The worst frequency is about 0·15 Hz, which is produced by a swing 12 m high. Other examples are a ship heaving and rotating in all directions around its centre of gravity in heavy seas, an aircraft heaving and rotating around its centre of gravity in turbulent air, and a car rapidly turning a corner.

Rotating the head when travelling in a rotating vehicle increases the probability of motion sickness. This is due to the three semi-circular canals of the inner ear, which are sensitive to rotary accelerations of the head in the three dimensions. When the head is facing the direction of motion of a car turning a corner it is rotated as the car turns. This stimulates the semi-circular canals which are sensitive to rotary acceleration in the horizontal plane. If the passenger suddenly tilts his head sideways or forward, the rotation of the car suddenly stimulates the semi-circular canals which are sensitive to sideways or forward rotation of the head. The sudden stimulation produces a quick but large rotary acceleration. The effect upon the corresponding semi-circular canals is greater when the car is cornering more rapidly, and when the head is turned more quickly. The rotary accelerations which result from the combination of the vehicle rotation and the head rotation help to produce motion sickness.

Heat, cold, and wind

Cooling the human body

The human body is a machine which produces heat like any other machine.

The heat has to be got rid of, or the person eventually dies from heat collapse or heat stroke. Heavy work and exercise increase the amount of heat produced by the human body. In summer, radiation from the sun heats the body. Heating by radiation occurs also in repairing the lining of a hot furnace, and in fighting a fierce fire if the fireman is unable to remain close to the ground away from the radiant heat.

In a cool environment the human body loses by radiation more heat than it receives from the environment. The body also loses heat by warming the air and objects which touch it (conduction), provided they are cooler than the skin. These methods of losing heat are not possible when the surrounding air and objects are too warm, as in a factory during a heatwave in summer.

In a hot environment heat can be lost only by the evaporation of sweat, which cools the skin. If the air is saturated with water vapour, as in badly ventilated mines and in compartments of ships which are not ventilated, the human body cannot lose heat by the evaporation of sweat. If it is hot, the body has no way of losing heat, and so gradually heats up.

Air movement cools the human body by changing the air touching the skin (convection). The air which the skin has warmed by conduction, and moistened by the evaporation of sweat, is replaced by cool dry air. The air movement helps the processes of cooling to continue effectively. Thus the cooling of the body depends upon the temperature of the surroundings, the humidity of the air close to the skin, and upon the movement of the air close to the skin.

Figure 2.6 shows the new Effective Temperature (ET*) or Subjective

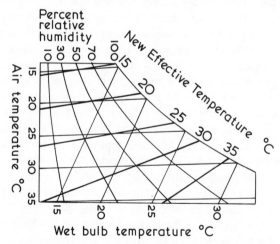

Figure 2.6 The new Effective Temperature (ET*) or Subjective Temperature. It is defined as the air temperature when the relative humidity is 50% and the air movement is about 0·1 m/s (drawn by permission of the American Society of Heating, Refrigerating and Air-conditioning Engineers Inc. (ASHRAE), from *Handbook of Fundamentals*. New York, 1972)

Temperature for any room or factory with a small amount of air movement, about 0·1 metre per second. New ET* is the air temperature when the relative humidity is 50%. All the points on any one of the thick lines of new ET* give the same feeling of warmth to people who simply sit around.

Heat, behavioural arousal, and performance

Figure 2.7 illustrates the effect of the time spent in heat upon a person's level of behavioural arousal. As a general rule people work more efficiently when they are more aroused and alert, especially in dull routine tasks and tasks which require speed. But for difficult tasks which require a lot of thought, people may work less efficiently if they are too highly aroused.

The figure shows that on first entering a hot space a person's level of behavioural arousal is likely to increase. The heat stimulates the face and any other exposed areas of skin. The stimulation temporarily increases behavioural arousal. Thus on first entering a hot space a person may work more efficiently than usual.

When the initial effect of entering the heat wears off, the person's level of behavioural arousal depends upon whether or not the heat increases the deep body temperature. In spaces with new ETs* ranging from about 35 to 45 °C, the temperature of the body should not rise unless the person is wearing too many clothes. So the level of behavioural arousal is likely to fall, as indicated by the lower unbroken function in Figure 2.7. The person gradually works less and less efficiently. This is what most people expect to happen when they feel too hot.

At and above a new ET* of about 45 °C the temperature of the body gradually rises. Here the person's level of behavioural arousal is likely to remain raised, as indicated by the broken function in the figure. The person may continue to work at least as efficiently as he does in the cool, although difficult tasks which require a lot of thought are likely to be performed less effectively than usual.

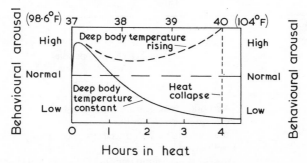

Figure 2.7 Level of behavioural arousal after various times
in heat (after Poulton, 1977b)

64

In one experiment trainee pilots had their body temperatures raised to 38·5°C (101·3°F) while keeping their skin comfortably cool. In this condition the group of pilots worked reliably faster and more efficiently. Yet when questioned at the end, ten of the 16 men who worked faster when hot reported that they worked more slowly. Here the subjective judgements contradict the measures of performance. The problems of using subjective judgements are discussed in the Introduction.

Figure 2.7 shows that behavioural arousal remains high until the deep body temperature reaches about 40°C (104°F). At this point the person is likely to collapse, and so cannot continue to work. Just before a person collapses he may become highly aroused and excited, and refuse to complete the job he has been given to do in the heat. This is probably a built-in safety mechanism, because if the person does not escape before he collapses, he never will unless someone is available to carry him out.

Comfortable temperatures for light and heavy work

Table 2.3 shows how the new ET* or Subjective Temperature relates to the efficiency of work and to comfort. There are considerable differences between people. At the most comfortable temperature of a group of people, about 5% of them will be either too hot or too cold. About 20% of the group will be comfortable at a temperature 6°C below the optimum. Another 20% will be comfortable at a temperature 6°C above the optimum.

Figure 2.8 shows how the most comfortable new ET* is affected by the insulation of the clothes worn, and by the heaviness of the work performed. Look up the insulation of the clothes worn in clo in Table 2.4. Look up the heaviness of the work in watts per square metre of surface area in Table 2.5, and read off the most comfortable new ET* in Figure 2.8. For example, Table 2.3 shows that the British maximum comfortable new ET* for sedentary work is about 20°C. For office work producing 80 W/m² of heat (Table 2.5), Figure 2.8 shows that this means wearing clothes with an insulation of 1 clo unit.

Table 2.3

New ET* or Subjective Temperature in °C	Effect upon people
45	Deep body temperature rises at rest
35	Performance deteriorates
30	Tasks which are dull or require speed may improve for brief periods
25	American maximum comfort for sedentary work
20	British maximum comfort for sedentary work
15	Upper limit of comfort for heavy work

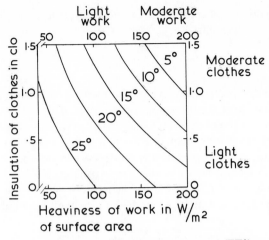

Figure 2.8 The new Effective Temperature (ET*) at which people are comfortable when performing work of various heavinesses wearing clothes with various amounts of insulation. The heaviness of the work can be determined from Table 2.5. The insulation of the clothes can be determined from Table 2.4 (after McIntyre, 1973)

Table 2.4

Insulation in clo	Clothes worn
0	No clothes
0·2	Light sleeveless dress, cotton underwear
0·5	Light trousers, short sleeve shirt
0·7	{ Warm long sleeve dress, full length slip { Light trousers, vest, long sleeve shirt
1·0	Jacket, light trousers, vest, long sleeve shirt
1·5	Heavy three-piece suit, long underwear

(After McIntyre, 1973, Table 2.)

Table 2.5

Heat production in W/m² of surface area	Heaviness of work
45	Lying half asleep
60	Sitting at rest
75	Office work
90	Light work standing
170	Walking at 5 kph (3 mph)
250	Heavy manual work
320	Digging

(After McIntyre, 1973, Table 1.)

Table 2.4 shows that this corresponds to wearing a jacket with light trousers, a vest, and a long sleeve shirt.

Performance in the cold

As the body cools, the temperature of the hands and feet falls more rapidly than the temperature of the remainder of the body. This is a protective mechanism which prevents the body from losing heat too rapidly. The hands and feet become numb. Precise movements of the hands take longer to make, and are made less accurately. The person has to depend more upon his eyes to tell him exactly what his fingers are doing. Unfortunately thick warm gloves may make the hands just as clumsy as they are when cold without gloves. If a person walks over rough ground with cold feet, he is more likely to stumble.

Performance in wind

Wind is met in outdoor jobs like working on the open deck of a fishing trawler, farming in the fields, and in delivering milk or newspapers to people's homes. It is a problem in working on high buildings, and in maintaining plant out of doors like the distillation columns of oil refineries, electricity pylons, and overhead telephone wires. Tower blocks of offices or flats in cities catch the wind which blows 30 to 50 metres above the ground, and bring it down to ground level.

A characteristic of wind is that it comes in gusts, not at a steady rate. A person may enter the wind unexpectedly as he leaves a doorway, or walks past the corner of a building. A sudden unexpected gust of wind is difficult to compensate for. People who suddenly walk into a wind are liable to be blown off course. They sometimes lose their balance. This can happen with windspeeds of only about 8 metres per second, or force 4 to 5 on the Beaufort wind scale.

Skilled activities take longer in the wind. Accurate aiming movements are more difficult. In reaching for an object, it may be possible with practice to compensate for a steady wind by aiming a little up-wind. But an unpredictable gusty wind cannot be compensated for (Poulton, Hunt, Mumford, and Poulton, 1975).

Harmful atmospheric pollution

Many industrial processes produce harmful substances which pollute the environment at work. The harmful substances in the air enter the human body through the mouth, nose, and lungs, or through the skin. In mining and quarrying, and in working with abrasives, the dust in the air may contain quartz. When breathed year after year, quartz dust produces a fibrosis of the lungs called silicosis. In working with asbestos, the dust contains asbestos fibres. Asbestos dust produces fibrosis of the lungs and can cause cancer. Organic dusts are produced in machining hardwood and leather, and in preparing natural fibres in the textile industry. They also can cause cancer.

Metal fumes and vapours are produced by heating and cleaning metals. Poisonous fumes are produced in burning and partly burning fuels. Small quantities of industrial chemicals and solvents escape and pollute the air. In spraying crops, the droplets contain the pesticide. The pesticide may be harmful to the human body as well as to the pests. Different substances damage different kinds of human tissue. The effects may occur almost at once, or may develop only slowly after years of exposure. Some substances can cause cancer many years later (Gardner and Taylor, 1975).

Ionizing radiation

Radioactive materials are used to produce electric power in nuclear power stations. They are used also to destroy cancer cells in the human body, and to produce tracer chemicals for studying living tissues. Radioactive materials give off ionizing radiations of several kinds. The energy in the radiation damages living tissue by ionizing it. Radiation can also cause cancer.

The small alpha particles or helium nuclei are used in industry to monitor the thickness of thin films of paper and polythene. They can penetrate human tissues to a depth of only 0·1 mm. The penetrating gamma (γ) rays or deep X-rays are used to detect faults in welded metal, and for other detection devices used in industry. They are used also to sterilize medical equipment and food. X-rays are used in medical diagnosis. Both gamma rays and X-rays are used to destroy cancer cells in the human body.

Harmful electromagnetic radiation

Figure 2.9 shows the range of electromagnetic radiation. We have already dealt with the gamma (γ) rays and X-rays at the bottom of the figure. Ultraviolet radiation is emitted during welding. It is used in a number of chemical processes, and in inspecting materials for faults which glow in ultraviolet light. Ultra-violet radiation harms living tissues only on the surface of the human body, because it does not penetrate very far. It causes conjunctivitis, sun burn, and cancer of the skin.

Electromagnetic radiation of longer wavelength damages the human body only by overheating it. Laser beams of light are used in cutting and welding, and in photography. A laser beam will burn the retina at the back of the eye if it accidentally shines into the eye. It can cause severe blindness if the eye turns and looks at it.

Infra-red radiation occurs for long periods while hot objects are cooling down. This happens after blowing glass, after shaping metal objects by heating them, and while kilns and furnaces are cooling down. Like light, infra-red radiation does not penetrate far into the human body. It heats mainly the skin.

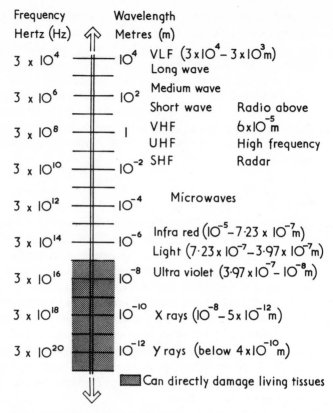

Figure 2.9 Kinds of electromagnetic radiation (after Poulton, 1970)

In contrast, microwaves and radar both penetrate deeply into the body. They heat the deep tissues almost as much as they heat the skin. Microwave ovens are used in cooking because they heat the inside of the joint without burning the surface. The eyes are particularly easily damaged by infra-red and microwave radiation. The longer wavelengths used for radio do not carry enough energy to overheat and damage the body (Gardner and Taylor, 1975).

Increased and reduced pressure

Increased atmospheric pressure

The pressure of water upon a skin diver increases rapidly as he dives, because water is 770 times as dense as air. This is illustrated by the calibrations on the two sides of the lower half of Figure 2.10. In tunnelling under water and in sinking a caisson in water, the pressure of the air in the tunnel or caisson has to correspond to the pressure of the depth of water outside. This is to prevent water from flooding the tunnel or caisson. When air is compressed, it contains

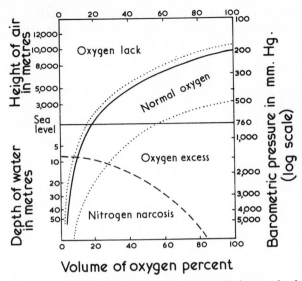

Figure 2.10 Safe proportions of oxygen and nitrogen in the
air breathed at various heights above sea level, and at various
depths or pressures (after Poulton, 1975)

a greater concentration of oxygen, nitrogen, and any harmful gases which
happen to be in it.

Air normally contains about 21% of oxygen. This means that the partial
pressure of the oxygen is 0·21 atmospheres. When the pressure of the oxygen
in the air breathed reaches 1 atmosphere, performance has been found to
deteriorate on a sensitive task. When the pressure reaches 2 atmospheres,
there is a risk of a fit or convulsion. This is caused by the irritant effect on the
brain of the excessive amount of oxygen. The risk of a fit starts when breathing
air at a pressure of about 10 atmospheres, or a depth of 90 metres of water.
It is probably wisest to keep the partial pressure of the oxygen breathed below
0·6 atmospheres or three times the normal, in order to avoid possible but
less obvious effects of oxygen poisoning. This also reduces the risk of fire,
which increases as the partial pressure of the oxygen increases. It means
keeping above the lower dotted curve in Figure 2.10 sloping down towards
the left.

Practically all the remaining 79% of the air is normally nitrogen. Nitrogen
behaves like an anaesthetic when it is breathed under pressure. Nitrogen
narcosis has been found to degrade the performance of a sensitive task at
a pressure of 2 atmospheres absolute. This is the pressure at a depth of water
of 10 metres. The pressures at which nitrogen narcosis can be a danger are
indicated by the broken function at the bottom of Figure 2.10 sloping down
to the right. At a pressure of 10 atmospheres absolute, or a depth of 90 metres,
the nitrogen narcosis is so severe that divers are incapable of being responsible
for their own safety. In working at pressures greater than 2 atmospheres

absolute, divers should therefore breathe a mixture of oxygen and helium, instead of air. This is because helium is less narcotic than nitrogen.

Reduced oxygen pressure at height

Figure 2.10 shows that the air pressure falls the farther up a mountain one climbs and the higher one flies an aircraft. Thus at height the air contains a lower pressure of oxygen. The performance of a task which requires a certain amount of physical work is a sensitive test for lack of oxygen. On a test of this kind, performance at sea level deteriorates when the proportion of oxygen is reduced from the normal 21% to 17%. Seventeen per cent of oxygen at sea level is equivalent to the amount of oxygen at 1500 metres above sea level. In order to avoid a fall in efficiency produced by lack of oxygen, it is therefore necessary to keep below the higher dotted function sloping up to the right in Figure 2.10.

Harmful effects of changes in pressure

When a person is compressed, air has to be able to enter the air spaces of the middle ear and of the sinuses connected to the nose. It may be possible to force air into the air spaces by holding the nose and blowing hard. If air cannot enter, it is exceedingly painful. Blood is sucked into the air spaces. The ear drums may burst. To prevent this, people with colds or blocked noses or ears should not be compressed.

When a person is decompressed, air has to leave the air spaces of the middle ear and sinuses. Fortunately this usually gives less trouble. During decompression the main problem is decompression sickness.

In compressed air the body gradually takes up the extra oxygen, and nitrogen or helium, which is breathed in through the lungs. When a person is decompressed, the gas gradually leaves the body. Much of the extra oxygen is used by the body. It is the nitrogen, or helium if it is breathed instead of nitrogen, which can be dangerous if a person is decompressed too rapidly. The nitrogen or helium appears as bubbles of gas in the tissues of the body. The commonest complaint is pain in and around the joints, usually the knees, caused by minute bubbles of gas. It is described as 'the bends'. It indicates that the person has been decompressed too rapidly, before the excess nitrogen or helium has had a chance to escape from the body through the lungs.

If the bubbles appear in the bloodstream, it is far more serious. They are carried by the blood, and get stuck in the small blood vessels. Here they block the supply of oxygen to the tissues. The tissues may die. If the tissues are essential to life, like the heart or parts of the brain, the person dies soon after the tissues die. If the bone dies close to a joint, the bone may collapse after a year or two under the strain of normal use. This aseptic necrosis of the bone causes severe pain and disability in the joint. The risk of decompression sickness can be greatly reduced by gradual decompression.

Heavy work and physical fitness

Table 2.5 gives examples of light and heavy work. Rescue operations during an emergency may involve particularly heavy work: forcing a passage into the emergency area, and carrying out the injured people.

The brain functions most efficiently in jobs which require a certain amount of physical work. A person who sits still without moving, tends to drop off to sleep. Having to perform a certain amount of physical work helps to keep the person alert and awake.

But the efficiency of the brain is reduced during and immediately after heavy work. The lungs and heart can supply the body with only a limited amount of oxygen. If the muscles make excessive demands upon the oxygen which is available, the brain has to go short.

Becoming physically fit increases the capacity of the mechanism which keeps the body supplied with oxygen. Thus a physically fit person is able to perform heavy work without as great a loss of brain efficiency as a less fit person. Remaining at rest in bed for a week or two reduces the capacity of the mechanism which supplies the oxygen. It reduces the efficiency of the brain during exercise.

Prolonged physical work causes fatigue in the muscles which do the work, especially if the person is not used to excercising the muscles so much. The person may feel too tired to work any longer without a rest. Precise movements of fatigued muscles are made less accurately. But a task performed by muscles which are not fatigued should be carried out as efficiently as ever, unless the brain is short of oxygen.

Perceived danger

People who work on tall buildings and structures run the risk of falling to the ground and being killed. Rescue operations in blazing buildings, and after mining disasters underground, are also dangerous. Warfare between armed gangs in the streets is a danger to people whose work involves using the streets. Emergencies while flying may lead to disaster. So may parachuting.

Dangerous emergencies are often occasions when it is important that people should work with maximum efficiency. Yet when people are afraid, they tend to perform less efficiently than usual. This has been shown by a simulated emergency in an aircraft. A group of recruits who had recently joined the US Army performed less efficiently during a simulated emergency than a group which performed the same tasks when there was no emergency.

However, people differ in their reactions to danger. In another simulation, one recruit at a time was left in an isolated outpost. He heard a series of explosions coming nearer, and was told over the radio that artillery shells were landing outside their designated area. He must repair his radio transmitter so that he could be located. Ten of the 24 recruits left the outpost before they had completed the job. But the 14 who remained worked almost as efficiently as a control group which was not stressed. So it may be possible to select people who will work efficiently during dangerous rescue operations.

Training and experience can both reduce the effect of perceived danger upon performance. In one investigation parachute jumpers were tested just before they ascended to make their jumps. A group of novices who had not been very thoroughly trained, performed very much worse before their first jump than they had done the previous day. Whereas a group of men who had jumped before, and a group of well trained novices, both performed only a little worse than they had done the previous day.

Curiously enough, training and experience have relatively little effect upon the body's reactions to the stress. Most experienced parachute jumpers still have heart rates of 150 or more beats per minute just before they pull the rip cord which opens the parachute, compared with a heart rate at rest which is about 72 beats per minute. So the stress is still present, even after practice (Reid, Doerr, Doshier and Ellertson, 1971).

Work overload and underload

Transient work overload

Work overload and underload often result from the irregular flow of work. Short bursts of speed are required when a person receives work from a number of sources which function independently. Several people may put finished articles onto the same moving belt as it passes them. By chance there will sometimes be a bunch of articles close together, and sometimes a gap without any articles. The inspector who examines the articles will sometimes have a lot of articles to inspect all at once, and sometimes none to inspect. The work load can be evened out by arranging for the articles to collect in a store. The inspector can then take the articles from the store and examine them in his own time.

In suburban railways there are predictable periods of peak load while everyone is travelling to work in the morning, and travelling back home in the evening. At these times there are queues at ticket offices and at the barriers where tickets are collected. Air traffic controllers have periods of peak load soon after breakfast, and again at teatime. The peak loads correspond to the most popular times for starting and completing flights. Telephone girls answering enquiries, and putting through calls, have their peak period in the middle of the morning. This is the time by which executives have been through their morning's mail, and are busy answering it, or organizing their day's activities.

Occasional panics

A number of organizations have a central co-ordinator who is in touch by special telephone or radio with people scattered over a wide area. Examples are the police, the fire service, and the ambulance service. Another example is the specialized services of an airline at an airport, which have to get each aircraft back in the air as quickly as possible with its new load of fuel, refreshments, passengers, and freight.

Occasional panics occur when there is a major calamity. The co-ordinator at the centre of the communications network suddenly receives more messages than he can handle. While he is answering calls, he has to assess the situation and decide upon the best overall course of action. He has then to give instructions as quickly as he can to the people on his communications network. The co-ordinator is the unavoidable bottleneck in the system. While he is under this stress, he has to decide the best emergency measures to take.

Some organizations have a central control room where visual displays show the state of a network of outstations. Examples are the grid control centres of the electricity generating boards, and the control-rooms of an automatic oil refinery or chemical plant. The difficulty here is that a fault in one part of the system may rapidly produce faults in other parts of the system, because the parts of the system are linked together and depend upon each other. For safety and to avoid costly repairs, each part of the system is designed to close down automatically as soon as it ceases to function properly. Unless the controller can take the appropriate action almost at once to compensate for the original fault, he may see the parts of the system rapidly closing down in front of his eyes, without being able to prevent it. With electricity networks, this causes a blackout over a considerable area of the country, which may last for several hours. With an oil refinery or chemical plant, it may take 2 or 3 days to start the plant up again after a shut down. As soon as a fault occurs, the controller has therefore to assess its nature, and decide what, if anything, can be done to prevent the whole system from closing down. He may have only a few seconds in which to make the correct decision.

Having to do several things at once

A driver in an unfamiliar part of the country has to watch the road signs which tell him his route. He does this while he is driving his vehicle, and watching out for traffic on the road ahead, and in his rear mirror. A driver who is not aware of the risk he is taking, may drive while he is talking earnestly to a passenger, talking over a radio telephone, or dictating letters.

An aircraft pilot has to fly his aircraft, or monitor the autopilot if his aircraft is on automatic control. He has also to keep in touch with ground control over his radio. If he does not carry a navigator, he may have to work out and check his route as he goes. If he is flying visually, he has to look out for other aircraft and perhaps mountain peaks. He has also to monitor his aircraft instruments, to check that nothing is amiss.

On a busy day a foreman may have a telephone call from a manager asking for information. While he is hunting up the information, someone else rings, also wanting to know something. So the foreman scribbles a note about it, and returns to the first query. Then the telephone rings again with another query. Finally perhaps the boss comes in before the first query has been fully dealt with. He takes the foreman off for an hour's consultation, and leaves him with a list of urgent jobs which have to be done right away, before returning to the day's work.

The risk of having to do several things at once is that some essential task gets omitted, or gets forgotten until it is too late. A driver may be so preoccupied with reading the road signs, or watching in his rear mirror the heavy goods vehicle directly behind him, that he fails to notice a vehicle coming at him in the opposite direction, right in the middle of his own lane. The aircraft pilot may get lost, and not notice that his fuel gauge is reading empty. The foreman may lose track of some of the queries he receives by telephone. The way to avoid omitting routine checks is to have a check list, either written down or carried in the head. Go through it from time to time, to ensure that nothing has been forgotten. Pilots have printed check lists which they work through before take off. The way to ensure that a message is not forgotten, is to write it down somewhere, where it will be seen before it is too late.

Work underload

Work underload occurs in the same jobs as work overload, during the periods when there is little or nothing to do. An air traffic controller, a telephone girl waiting to answer queries or put through calls, a controller in the grid control room of an electricity generating board, and a processman in an automatic oil refinery or chemical plant, all have periods of work underload. So does the airline pilot flying by autopilot over the mid-Atlantic, and the helmsman on the bridge of a supertanker on automatic control in the mid-Atlantic. The periods of work underload are more frequent and last longer at night, because there is less happening then.

The difficulty at night is that there may not be enough stimulation to keep the person alert. The jobs can be described as 'waiting for nothing to happen'. The person becomes bored and inefficient. He is likely to have brief lapses of attention even if he sits looking conscientiously at his instruments all the time. The person may even fall asleep for a period of time. At night sleepiness is especially likely if the person is not used to working at night, or if he cannot get adequate sleep at home in the day owing to interruptions by a noisy young family.

Night shifts and loss of sleep

A number of industrial processes cannot be stopped overnight or at weekends. Furnaces stay hot for hours or days, and take hours or days to heat up. Chemical and petrochemical plants may take 2 or 3 days to start up. So may nuclear power stations. Once they are working smoothly, it would be folly to shut them down. Plant which is new and extremely expensive has to be operated continuously over the 24 hours, 7 days per week, otherwise it may not pay for itself before it becomes obsolete. Road, rail, and air transport all operate throughout the 24 hours. So do community services like hospitals, and the police and fire services.

Standing shifts

People do not work very efficiently between 1 and 4 o'clock in the morning if they are usually asleep at this time. The most efficient system of shifts has day people who work always during the day, and night people who work always at night. The night people get used to working at night and sleeping during the day. It makes several weeks to get really used to the inverted rhythm of sleeping and waking. Once this has been done, people working at night should be as efficient as people working during the day, although some of the body's 24-hour physiological rhythms may take several months to adapt fully to the inversion.

The difficulty is that few people are willing to become efficient night-time workers. For most people their off-duty activities are more important to them than the efficiency of their work. They want to spend their free time doing things with their family and friends, at the times when their family and friends do them. On their days or weekends off, they stay awake in the day and go to bed at night. They never let themselves adapt properly to working at night. So night work remains stressful and inefficient, because it always occurs at the time when the people want to be asleep. As a result, it may not be possible to get enough people to work always at night, even when special incentives are offered.

Rotating shifts

When working at night cannot be avoided, rotating shifts may be more popular than standing shifts. In the shift system of Figure 2.11 a person works during

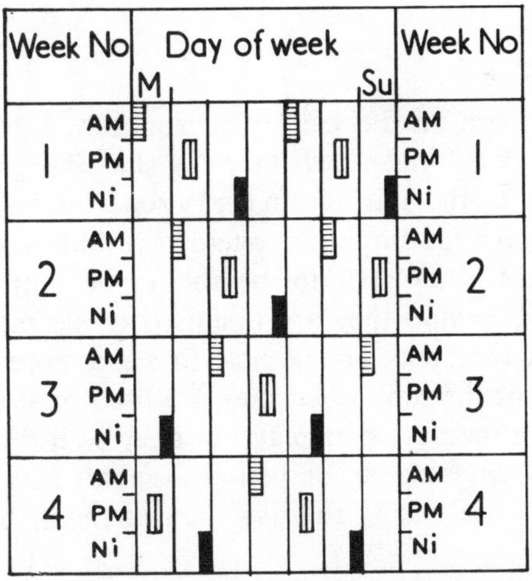

Figure 2.11 A simple 8-hour rotating shift system. The 4 weeks are manned consecutively by four separate teams, who return to week 1 after week 4

the day the first 24 hours, during the evening the second 24 hours, and during the night the third 24 hours. He then has 24 hours off duty before he works again during the day. The 168 hours in the week are divided between four teams of people. Each team works a different one of the four weekly schedules, and then continues with the schedule of the week below. After week 4 the schedule restarts with week 1. Each person works an average of $5\frac{1}{4}$ shifts of 8 hours per week, making a total of 42 hours.

The difficulty with the rotating system of Figure 2.11 is that people never get more than 24 hours off duty at a stretch. This is because each shift is separated from the next shift by 24 hours, instead of the usual 16 hours which separates periods of work always at the same time of day. People who work the conventional 5 days per week at the same time each day, get 64 hours off every weekend; whereas with the rotating shift system the extra 8 hours between each shift, and having $5\frac{1}{4}$ shifts per week instead of the usual 5 working days, cuts the break at the weekend to 24 hours like the break between any other shift and the next.

More popular rotating shift systems providing 42 hours work per week lack one or more of the three advantages of the shift system of Figure 2.11 which promote efficiency. Shifts are lengthened beyond 8 hours; less than 24 hours off duty is given to prepare and recover from night shifts; or less than 16 hours off duty is given between day shifts. These modifications allow occasional longer breaks of 3 or more days consecutively off duty. Again this reflects the greater value which people set on their off-duty activities than on their efficiency at work. They are willing to accept stressful periods of relatively inefficient work for the sake of the longer breaks afterwards (Tejmar, 1976).

Loss of sleep

People who work only in the day can suffer from loss of sleep. They may not go to bed early enough before an early morning shift. They may be kept awake by children crying, or by the noises from heavy road vehicles or aircraft.

People who work on a rotating shift system have additional problems before and after a night shift. They may not be able to sleep much during the day before a night shift, because they are not used to sleeping during the day. After the night shift they may not be able to sleep more than a few hours, because again it is not the time when they are used to sleeping. Also if they sleep too long during the day, they may not sleep well the next night before work the day after. There may be competing social attractions during the day. There is also more noise during the day than at night, both from children and from traffic.

Rotating shift systems do not usually deprive people of all sleep for a period as long as 24 hours. But the effects of sleep debts cumulate over successive 24-hour periods. Sleep debts of 2 hours on each of 3 consecutive days are not as detrimental as a single sleep debt of 6 hours, but they may be sufficient to reduce a person's efficiency when he performs a routine task.

A person is likely to work less efficiently than usual when he has lost 3 hours or more sleep during the previous 24 hours. He may become drowsy. He may have lapses of attention lasting a second or two, during which he is out of touch with his surroundings. He may even drop off to sleep. This is most likely to happen at times when the person would normally be asleep, like between 1 and 4 o'clock in the early morning.

The effects of loss of sleep are particularly likely to appear in jobs where the person is not actively doing anything. In watching a number of instruments which stay within their accepted limits, a man in a control room may have no actions to take. In inspecting finished products for faults as they move past on a conveyor belt, the inspector has nothing to do unless he happens to detect a fault. Unfortunately it is these kinds of job which are often run 24 hours a day on a rotating shift system, and so are likely to be performed by people who are short of sleep.

In an emergency a person can probably work as efficiently as ever, provided he has not been totally deprived of sleep over the last 24 hours. But he has to be sufficiently alert to recognize the emergency, in order to react to it as an emergency. Most of the time he is likely to be less efficient than usual when he feels sleepy (Poulton et al., 1978).

Combined environmental stresses

A person may be subjected to a number of stresses at the same time. People who work on powerful machines are exposed to the noise, vibration, and heat of the machines all at once. Rescue operations may involve heavy physical work, danger, and heat if there is a fire. People who live and work in a noisy environment may not sleep well at night owing to the noise. The next day they work in the noise when they are short of sleep. This raises the question of how stresses combine. Can a person tolerate as much noise when he is also vibrated and hot?

A simple assumption is that the effects of a number of stresses sum. If noise, vibration, and heat each reduce the efficiency of work by 10%, the effect of all three stresses combined will reduce the efficiency by about 30%.

This additive assumption does not hold if a person has only a limited ability to compensate for stress. When he is subjected to a single stress, his efficiency is perhaps reduced by only 10% because he is able to try harder and so to compensate for much of the adverse effects. He then has no spare effort available to compensate for additional stresses. If so, when he is subjected to all three stresses at once, his efficiency will be reduced by considerably more than 30%.

The effect of a combination of stresses could be less than the sum of the separate effects. Both noise, and loss of sleep the previous night, could reduce the efficiency of work by 10%. One of the effects of noise is to increase behavioural arousal and help a person stay awake and alert. The arousing effect of the noise could counteract the sleepiness produced by not sleeping well the previous night. If so, the effect of the two stresses could be less than

78

the sum of the two separate effects. Efficiency might be reduced by only 15%, instead of by the full 20%.

At present it is not possible to decide between these three alternatives. It is therefore safest to accept the middle alternative, because it is the least likely to be far from the truth. This is the alternative which assumes that the effect of a combination of stresses is about the sum of the separate effects.

Transfer between conditions

There are a number of difficulties in evaluating the results of investigations of combinations of stresses. The principal difficulty is that the same people are given a number of stresses and combinations of stresses in turn, in different random or balanced orders. The effect upon a person of one stress or combination of stresses depends upon the stress conditions which he has met previously in the investigation.

When a person performs badly in a particularly unfavourable condition, he may perform better than he would do otherwise on his next condition. The increased effort which he exerts to perform well in the unfavourable condition carries over to his next condition, which would not otherwise encourage so great on effort. Transfer between conditions makes the results of an investigation impossible to interpret unambiguously (Poulton and Edwards, 1974).

References

American Society of Heating, Refrigerating and Air-conditioning Engineers Inc. (ASHRAE) (1972) *Handbook of Fundamentals.* New York.
Burns, W. (1973) *Noise and Man.* London. Murray, 2nd ed.
Gardner, W., and Taylor, P. (1975) *Health at Work.* London. Associated Business Programmes.
Guignard, J. C. (1965) Vibration. In Gillies J. A. (ed.), *A Textbook of Aviation Physiology.* Oxford. Pergamon Press, chapter 29, pp. 813–894.
Hopkinson, R. G., and Collins, J. B. (1970) *The Ergonomics of Lighting.* London. Macdonald.
McIntyre, D. (1973) A guide to thermal comfort, *Appl. Ergonomics,* 4, 66–72.
Poulton, E. C. (1970) *Environment and Human Efficiency.* Ill, Thomas, Springfield.
Poulton, E. C. (1975) Stresses and hazards. In Elliott E. (ed.), *Human Factors for Designers of Naval Equipment.* London. Medical Research Council, chapter 5.
Poulton, E. C. (1976) Continuous noise interferes with work by masking auditory feedback and inner speech, *Appl. Ergonomics,* 7, 79–84.
Poulton, E. C. (1977a) A built-in alerting mechanism for sleepy drivers, *Appl. Ergonomics,* 8, in preparation.
Poulton, E. C. (1977b) Subjective assessments are almost always biased, sometimes completely misleading, *Brit. J. Psychol.,* 68, in press.
Poulton, E. C., and Edwards, R. S. (1974) Interactions, range effects, and comparisons between tasks in experiments measuring performance with pairs of stresses: mild heat and 1 mg of 1-hyoscine hydrobromide, *Aerospace Med.,* 45, 735–741.
Poulton, E. C., Hunt, G. M., Carpenter, A., and Edwards, R. S. (1978) The performance of junior hospital doctors following reduced sleep and long hours of work, *Ergonomics,* 21, in preparation.

Poulton, E. C., Hunt, J. C. R., Mumford, J. C., and Poulton, J. (1975) The mechanical disturbance produced by steady and gusty winds of moderate strength: skilled performance and semantic assessments, *Ergonomics*, **18**, 651–673.

Reid, D. H., Doerr, J. E., Doshier, H. D. and Ellertson, D. G. (1971) Heart rate and respiratory rate response to parachuting: physiological studies of military parachutists via FM/FM telemetry-II, *Aerospace Med.*, **42**, 1200–1207.

Tejmar, J. (1976) Shift work round the clock in supervision and control, *Appl. Ergonomics*, **7**, 66–74.

Chapter 3

Sources of Managerial and White Collar Stress

Cary L. Cooper
Judi Marshall

University of Manchester
Institute of Science and Technology

Life in complex industrial organizations can be a great source of stress for managers. Increasingly, as Brummet, Pyle, and Flamholtz (1968) suggest, managers are suffering extreme physiological symptoms from stress at work, such as disabling ulcers or coronary heart disease (CHD), which force them to retire prematurely from active organizational life before they have had an opportunity to fully actualize their potential. These and other stress related effects (e.g. tension, poor adjustment, etc.) also feed into the family, becoming potential sources of disturbance and thus pervading the whole quality of life of the individual. The mental and physical health effects of job stress are not only disruptive influences on the individual manager, but also a 'real' cost to the organization, on whom many individuals depend: a cost which is rarely, if ever, seriously considered either in human or financial terms by organizations, but one which they incur in their day-to-day operations. In order to do something positive about managerial stressors at work, it is important to be able to identify them. The success of any effort to minimize stress and maximize job satisfaction will depend on accurate diagnosis, for different stressors will require different action. Any approach to stress reduction in an organization which relied on one particular approach (e.g. transcendental meditation or job enrichment), without taking into account the differences within work groups or divisions, would be doomed to failure. A recognition of the possible sources of management stress, therefore, may help us to arrive at suggestions of ways of minimizing its negative consequences. It was with this in mind that we decided to bring together the research literature in the field of management and organizational stress in a framework that would help us to more clearly identify sources of stress on managers.

One of the main problems currently facing research workers in the field of stress is that there is no integrated framework or conceptual map of the area. Much of the early stress research came from two sources: (1) from work carried out in 'crisis' situations such as stress in battle the stress effects of major illness or bereavement, etc., which focused heavily on the assessment of physical and mental symptoms exhibited in these unique circumstances; (2) from the 'company doctor' literature, which was geared essentially to the needs of industry and based on intuition rather than substantiated fact. These studies were usually descriptive reports by individual industrial medical officers on, for example, the relationship of poor physical conditions at work and worker apathy or stress, or of work overload and nervous complaints by workers and managers, etc. In the last 10–15 years, however, there has been a determined effort by social scientists to consider more systematically the sources of management and organizational stress (Cooper and Marshall, 1976). The framework offered in this chapter is basically an attempt to integrate the findings of this new wave of research. Much of this work will be in the field of managerial stress. However, from an examination of the 'shop floor' studies it would appear that most of the factors to be discussed here are applicable to the labour force as a whole.

A study of the literature reveals a formidable list of over 40 interacting factors which might be sources of managerial stress—those to be dealt with here were drawn mainly from a wider body of theory and research in a variety of fields; medicine, psychology, management sciences, etc.[1] Additional material has been drawn from exploratory studies carried out at UMIST. Seven major categories of stress can be identified. Figure 3.1 is an attempt to represent these diagrammatically; below they will be dealt with in a natural progression from individual-centred to total environment-centred.

Factors intrinsic to the job

Factors *intrinsic to the job* were a first and vital focus of study for early researchers in the field, and in 'shop floor' (as opposed to management) studies are still the main preoccupation. Stress can be caused by too much or too little work, time pressures and deadlines, having too many decisions (Sofer, 1970), fatigue from the physical strains of the work environment (e.g. assembly line), excessive travel, long hours, having to cope with changes at work and the expenses (monetary and career) of making mistakes (Kearns, 1973). It can be seen that every job description includes factors which for some individuals at some point in time will be a source of pressure. Two factors have received the major part of research effort in this area (the others being more speculative than proven sources of stress): working conditions and work overload.

Working conditions

A great deal of work has been done linking the working conditions of a particular job to physical and mental health. Kornhauser (1965) found, for example, that poor mental health was directly related to unpleasant work conditions, the necessity to work fast and to expend a lot of physical effort, and to excessive

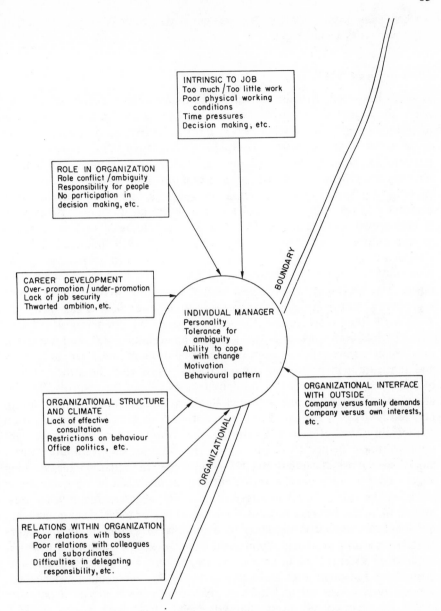

Figure 3.1 Sources of managerial stress

and inconvenient hours. There is increasing evidence (Marcson, 1970; Shepard, 1971) that physical health, as well, is adversely affected by repetitive and dehumanizing environments (e.g. paced assembly lines). Kritsikis *et al.* (1968), for example, in a study of 150 men with angina pectoris in a population of over 4000 industrial workers in Berlin, reported that a larger number of these workers came from work environments employing conveyor line systems than any other work technology.

Work overload

A more important stressor for managers than working conditions is work overload. Research into work overload has been given substantial empirical attention. French and Caplan (1973) have differentiated overload in terms of *quantitative* and *qualitative* overload. Quantitative refers to having 'too much to do', while qualitative means work that is 'too difficult'. (The complementary phenomena of quantitative and qualitative underload are also hypothesized as potential sources of stress but with little or no supportive research evidence.) Miller (1960) has theorized that 'overload' in most systems leads to breakdown, whether we are dealing with single biological cells or managers in organizations. In an early study, French and Caplan (1970) found that objective quantitative overload was strongly linked to cigarette smoking (an important risk factor or symptom of CHD). Persons with more phone calls, office visits, and meetings per given unit of work time were found to smoke significantly more cigarettes than persons with fewer such engagements. In a study of 100 young coronary patients, Russek and Zohman (1958) found that 25% had been working at two jobs and an additional 45% had worked at jobs which required (due to work overload) 60 or more hours per week. They add that although prolonged emotional strain preceded the attack in 91% of the cases, similar stress was only observed in 20% of the controls. Breslow and Buell (1960) have also reported findings which support a relationship between hours of work and death from coronary disease. In an investigation of mortality rates of men in California, they observed that workers in light industry under the age of 45, who are on the job more than 48 hours a week, have twice the risk of death from CHD compared with similar workers working 40 or under hours a week. Another substantial investigation on quantitative work load was carried out by Margolis *et al.* (1974) on a representative national sample of 1496 employed persons, 16 years of age or older. They found that overload was significantly related to a number of symptoms or indicators of stress: escapist drinking, absenteeism from work, low motivation to work, lowered self-esteem, and an absence of suggestions to employers. The results from these and other studies (Quinn *et al.*, 1971; Porter and Lawler, 1965) are relatively consistent and indicate that this factor is indeed a potential source of occupational stress that adversely affects both health and job satisfaction.

There is also some evidence that (for some occupations) 'qualitative' overload is a source of stress, and this is particularly relevant to managers. French *et al.* (1965) looked at qualitative and quantitative work overload in a large university. They used questionnaires, interviews, and medical examinations to obtain data on risk factors associated with CHD for 122 university administrators and professors. They found that one symptom of stress, low self-esteem, was related to work overload but that this was different for the two occupational groupings. Qualitative overload was not significantly linked to low self-esteem among the administrators but was significantly correlated for the professors. The greater the 'quality' of work expected of the professor the lower the self-esteem. They also found that qualitative and quantitative overload were correlated to achievement orientation. And more interestingly, in a follow-up study, that achievement orientation correlated very strongly with serum uric acid (Brooks and Mueller, 1966). Several other studies have reported an association of qualitative work overload with cholesterol level; a tax deadline for accountants (Friedman et al., 1958), and medical students performing a medical examination under observation (Dreyfuss and Czackes, 1959). French and Caplan (1973) summarize this research by suggesting that both qualitative and quantitative overload produce at least nine different symptoms of psychological and physical strain: job dissatisfaction, job tension, lower self-esteem, threat, embarrassment, high cholesterol levels, increased heart rate, skin resistance, and more smoking. In analysing this data, however, one cannot ignore the vital interactive relationship of the job and manager or employee; objective work overload, for example, should not be viewed in isolation but relative to the individual's capacities and personality.

Such caution is sanctioned by much of the American and some English literature which shows that overload is not always externally imposed. Many managers (perhaps certain personality types more than others) react to overload by working longer hours (Uris, 1972). For example, in reports on an American study it was found that 45% of the executives investigated worked all day, in the evenings, and at weekends, and that a further 37% kept weekends free but worked extra hours in the evenings. In many companies this type of behaviour has become a norm to which everyone feels they must adhere.

Role in the organization

Another major source of managerial stress is associated with a person's role at work. A great deal of research in this area has concentrated on role ambiguity and role conflict, since the seminal investigations of the Survey Research Center of The University of Michigan which were reported in the classic book *Organizational Stress: Studies in Role Conflict and Ambiguity* (Kahn et al., 1964).

Role ambiguity

Role ambiguity exists when an individual has inadequate information about his work role, that is, where there is 'lack of clarity about the work objectives associated with the role, about work colleagues' expectation of the work role and about the scope and responsibilities of the job'. Kahn et al. (1964) found in their study that men who suffered from role ambiguity experienced lower job satisfaction, high job related tension, greater futility, and lower self-confidence. French and Caplan (1970) found, at one of NASA's bases (Goddard Space Flight Center), in a sample of 205 volunteer engineers, scientists, and administrators, that role ambiguity was significantly related to low job satisfaction and to feelings of job related threat to one's mental and physical well-being. This also related to indicators of physiological strain such as increased blood pressure and pulse rate. Margolis *et al.* (1974) also found a number of significant relationships between symptoms or indicators of physical and mental ill health with role ambiguity in their representative national sample ($n = 1496$). The stress indicators related to role ambiguity were depressed mood, lowered self-esteem, life dissatisfaction, job dissatisfaction, low motivation to work, and intention to leave job. These were not very strong relationships but, nevertheless, statistically significant, and they do indicate that 'lack of role clarity' may be one among many potential stressors at work.

Kahn (1973) feels that it is now time to separate out distinctive elements of role ambiguity for individual treatment (just as he and his research team have done for 'overload' and 'responsibility'). He suggests that two components are involved—those of 'present ambiguity' and 'future prospects of ambiguity' (much of the material he assigns to the latter is here classified as career development stress)—but he has not yet empirically substantiated this differentiation.

Role conflict

Role conflict exists when an 'individual in a particular work role is torn by conflicting job demands or doing things he/she really does not want to do or does not think are part of the job specification'. The most frequent manifestation of this is when a person is caught between two groups of people who demand different kinds of behaviour or expect that the job should entail different functions. Kahn *et al.* (1964) found that men who suffered more role conflict had lower job satisfaction and higher job related tension. It is interesting to note that they also found that the greater the power or authority of the people 'sending' the conflicting role messages, the more role conflict produced job dissatisfaction. This was related to physiological strain as well, as the Goddard study (French and Caplan, 1970) illustrates. They telemetered and recorded the heart rate of 22 men for a 2-hour period while they were at work in their offices. They found that the mean heart rate for an individual was strongly related to his report of role conflict. A larger and medically more sophisticated study by Shirom *et al.* (1973) found similar results. Their research is of particular interest as it tries to look simultaneously at a wide variety of potential stressors. They collected data on 762 male kibbutz members aged 30 and above, drawn from 13 kibbutzim throughout Israel. They examined the relationships between CHD (myocardial infarction, angina pectoris, and coronary insufficiency), abnormal electrocardiographic readings, CHD risk factors (systolic blood pressure, pulse rate, serum cholesterol levels, etc.), and potential sources of occupational stress (work overload, role ambiguity, role conflict, lack of physical activity). Their data was broken down by occupational groups: agricultural workers, factory groups, craftsmen, and white collar workers. It was found that there was a significant relationship between role conflict and CHD (specifically, abnormal electrocardiographic readings), but for the white collar workers only. In fact, as we moved down the ladder from occupations requiring great physical exertions (e.g. agriculture) to those requiring least (e.g. white collar), the greater was the relationship between role ambiguity/conflict and abnormal electrocardiographic findings. Role conflict was also significantly related to an index of ponderosity (excessive weight for age and height). It was also found that as we go from occupations involving excessive physical activities to those with less such activity, CHD (myocardial infarction; angina pectoris, and coronary insufficiency increased significantly. Drawing together this data, it might be hypothesized that managerial and professional occupations are more likely to suffer occupational stress from role related stress and other interpersonal dynamics and less from the physical conditions of work.

A more quantified measure of role conflict itself is found in research reported by Mettlin and Woelfel (1974). They measured three aspects of interpersonal influence—discrepancy between influences, level of influence, and number of influences—in a study of the educational and occupational aspirations of high school students. Using the Langner Stress Symptom questionnaire as their index of stress, they found that the more extensive and diverse an individual's interpersonal communications network the more stress symptoms he showed. The organizational role which is at a boundary—i.e. between departments or between the company and the outside world—is, by definition, one of extensive communication nets and of high role conflict. Kahn et al. (1964) suggest that such a position is potentially highly stressful. Other researchers have provided empirical support for this suggestion; Margolis and Kroes (1974), for example, found that foremen (high role conflict-prone job) are seven times as likely to develop ulcers as shopfloor workers.

Responsibility

Another important potential stressor associated with one's organizational role is 'responsibility for people'. One can differentiate here between 'responsibility for people' and 'responsibility for things' (equipment, budgets, etc.). Wardwell et al. (1964) found that responsibility for people was significantly more likely to lead to CHD than responsibility for things. Increased responsibility for people frequently means that one has to spend more time interacting with others, attending meetings, working alone and, in consequence, as in the Goddard study (French and Caplan, 1970), more time in trying to meet deadline pressures and schedules. Pincherle (1972) also found this in their UK study of 2000 executives attending a medical centre for a medical check-up. Of the 1200 managers sent by their companies for their annual examination, there was evidence of physical stress being linked to age and level of responsibility; the older and more responsible the executive, the greater the probability of the presence of CHD risk factors or symptoms. Other research (Terhuxe, 1963) has also established this link. The relationship between age and stress related illness could be explained, however, by the fact that as the executive gets older he may be troubled by stressors other than increased responsibility, for example, as Eaton (1969) suggests, by (1) a recognition that further advancement is unlikely, (2) increasing isolation and narrowing of interests, and (3) an awareness of approaching retirement. Nevertheless, the finding by French and Caplan in the Goddard study does indicate that responsibility for people must play some part in the process of stress, particularly for clerical, managerial, and professional workers. They found that responsibility for people was significantly related to heavy smoking, diastolic blood pressure, and serum cholesterol levels—the more the individual had responsibility for 'things' as opposed to 'people' the lower were each of these CHD risk factors.

Other role stressors

Having too little responsibility (Brook, 1973), lack of participation in decision making, lack of managerial support, having to keep up with increasing standards of performance and coping with rapid technological change are other potential role stressors mentioned repeatedly in the literature but with little supportive research evidence. Variations between organizational structures will determine the differential distribution of these factors across differing occupational groups. Kay (1974) does suggest, however, that (independent of employing organization) some pressures are to be found more at middle than at other management levels. He depicts today's middle manager as being particularly hard pressed:

(1) by pay compression, as the salaries of new recruits increase;
(2) by job insecurity—they are particularly vulnerable to redundancy or forced, premature retirement;
(3) by having little real authority at their high levels of responsibility;
(4) by feeling 'boxed in'.

When interviewed it is those pressures intrinsic to the job and due to role organization which managers consider to be the most legitimate sources of stress *vis-à-vis* their jobs. Typically they are referred to as 'what I'm paid for', 'why I'm here', and even when they cause severe disruption, the implication is that they cannot be legitimately avoided. In many companies, in fact, there are institutional ways in which these problems can be handled—for example, deadlines are set unrealistically early to allow a margin of error, decisions are made by groups so that no one individual has to take full responsibility, the employee is allowed to neglect certain tasks (e.g. filing) if he is busy, work can be reallocated within a department if one member is seen to be doing more than his fair share. The manager, however, may not always perceive himself as free to use these fail-safe mechanisms.

Relationships at work

A third major source of stress at work has to do with the nature of relationships with one's boss, subordinates, and colleagues. A number of behavioural scientists (Argyris, 1964; Cooper, 1973) have suggested that good relationships between members of a work group are a central factor in individual and organizational health. Nevertheless very little research work has been done in this area to either support or disprove this hypothesis. French and Caplan (1973) define poor relations as 'those which include low trust, low supportiveness, and low interest in listening to and trying to deal with problems that confront the organizational member'. The most notable studies in this area are by Kahn *et al.* (1964), French and Caplan (1970), and Buck (1972). Both the Kahn *et al.* and French and Caplan studies came to roughly the same conclusion, that mistrust of persons one worked with was positively related to high role ambiguity, which led to inadequate communications between people and to 'psychological strain in the form of low job satisfaction and to feelings of job-related threat to one's well being'. It was interesting to note, however, in the Kahn *et al.* study, that poor relations with one's subordinates was significantly related to feelings of threat with colleagues and superiors but not in relationship to threat with subordinates.

Relationships with superior

Buck (1972) focused on the attitude and relationship of workers and managers to their immediate boss using Fleishman's leadership questionnaire on consideration and initiating structure. The consideration factor was associated with behaviour indicative of friendship, mutual trust, respect, and a certain warmth between boss and subordinate. He found that those workers who felt that their boss was low on 'consideration' reported feeling more job pressure. Workers who were under pressure reported that their boss did not give them criticism in a helpful way, played favourites with subordinates, ' "pulled rank" and took advantage of them whenever they got a chance'. Buck concludes that the 'considerate behaviour of supervisors appears to have contributed significantly inversely to feelings of job pressure'.

Relationships with subordinates

Officially, one of the most critical functions of a manager is his supervision of other people's work. It has long been accepted that an 'inability to delegate' might be a problem but now a new potential stressor is being introduced in the manager's interpersonal skills—he must learn to 'manage by participation'. Donaldson and Gowler (1975) point to the factors which may make today's zealous emphasis on participation a cause of resentment, anxiety, and stress for the manager concerned:

(1) mismatch of formal and actual power,

(2) the manager may well resent the erosion of his formal role and authority (and the loss of status and rewards),
(3) he may be subject to irreconcilable pressures—e.g. to be both participative and to achieve high production,
(4) his subordinates may refuse to participate.

Particularly for those with technical and scientific backgrounds (a 'things orientation'), relationship can be a low priority (seen as 'trivial', 'petty', time consuming and an impediment to doing the job well) and one would expect their interactions to be more a source of stress than those of 'people-oriented' managers.

Relationships with colleagues

Besides the obvious factors of office politics and colleagues' rivalry we find another element here: stress can be caused not only by the pressure of relationships but also by its opposite—a lack of adequate social support in difficult situations (Lazarus, 1966). At highly competitive managerial levels it is likely that problem sharing will be inhibited for fear of appearing weak; and much of the (American) literature particularly mentions the isolated life of the top exccecutive as an added source of strain.

Morris (1975) encompasses this whole area of relationships in one model— what he calls the 'cross of relationships' (Figure 3.2). While he acknowledges the differences between relationships on the various continua, he feels that the focal manager must bring all four into 'dynamic balance' in order to be able to deal with the stress of his position. Morris's suggestion seems 'only sensible' when we see how much of his work time the manager spends with other people. In a research programme to find out exactly what managers do (a relative mystery) Minzberg (1973) showed just how much of their time is spent in interaction. In an intensive study of a small sample of chief executives he found that in a large organization a mere 22% of time was spent in desk work sessions, the rest being taken up by telephone calls (6%), scheduled meetings (59%), unscheduled meetings (10%), and other activities (3%). In small organizations basic desk work played a larger part (52%) but nearly 40% was still devoted to face-to-face contacts of one kind or another. Despite

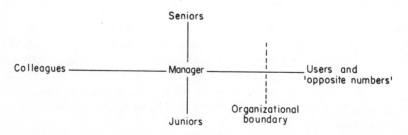

Figure 3.2 The cross of relationships

its obvious importance and the inclusion of 'relationship' measures in many multivariate studies there is little 'in depth' research available in this area.

Career development

Two major clusters of potential stressors can be identified in this area:

(1) lack of job security; fear of redundancy, obsolescence or early retirement, etc.;
(2) status incongruity; under- or over-promotion, frustration at having reached one's career ceiling, etc.

For many managers their career progression is of overriding importance— by promotion they earn not only money but also status and the new job challenges for which they strive. Typically, in the early years at work, this striving and the aptitude to come to terms quickly with a rapidly changing environment is fostered and suitably rewarded by the company. Career progression is, perhaps, a problem by its very nature. For example, Sofer (1970) found that many of his sample believed that 'luck' and 'being in the right place at the right time' play a major role.

At middle age, and usually middle management levels, career becomes more problematic and most executives find their progress slowed, if not actually stopped. Job opportunities become fewer, those jobs that are available take longer to master, past (mistaken?) decisions cannot be revoked, old knowledge and methods become obsolete, energies may be flagging or demanded for family activities, and there is the 'press' of fresh young recruits to face in competition. Both Levinson (1973) and Constandse (1972)—the latter refers to this phase as 'the male menopause'—depict the manager as suffering these fears and disappointments in 'silent isolation' from his family and work colleagues.

The fear of demotion or obsolescence can be strong for those who know they have reached their 'career ceiling'—and most will inevitably suffer some erosion of status before they finally retire. Goffman (1952) extrapolating from a technique employed in the con-game 'cooling the mark out' suggests that the company should bear some of the responsibility for taking the sting out of this (felt) failure experience.

From the company perspective, on the other hand, McMurray (1973) puts the case for not promoting a manager to a higher position if there is doubt that he can fill it. In a syndrome he labels 'the executive neurosis', he describes the over-promoted manager as grossly overworking to keep down a top job and at the same time hiding his insecurity—he points to the consequences of this for his work performance and the company. Age is no longer revered as it was—it is becoming a 'young man's world'. The rapidity with which society is developing (technologically, economically, and socially) is likely to mean that individuals will now need to change career during their working life (as companies and products are having to do). Such trends breed uncertainty and research suggests that older workers look for stability (Sleeper, 1975). Unless managers adapt their expectations to suit new circumstances 'career development' stress, especially in later life, is likely to become an increasingly common experience.

Erikson and Gunderson of the US Navy Neuropsychiatric Unit are developing a comprehensive research programme in the US Navy to assess this problem systematically, which they term 'status congruence' or the matching of one individual's advancement with his experience ability. In an earlier study they found (Arthur and Gunderson, 1965) that promotional lag was significantly related to psychiatric illness. Later they found (Erikson et al., 1972) that Navy personnel experience greater job satisfaction when their rates of advancement exceeded (although not excessively) their expectation; dissatisfaction increased as advancement rates were retarded. Those who were least successful with regard to advancement tended to perceive the greatest amount of stress in their lives. In a more recent study Erikson et al. (1973) found among a sample of over 9000 Navy ratings that (1) status congruency was negatively related to the incidence of psychiatric disorder and (2) that status congruency was positively related to military effectiveness.

The issue of status congruency has also been researched from a sociological perspective, that is, the incongruity between an individual's social status and that of his parents, or social class differences between his parents. Shekelle et al. (1969), for example, in a prospective study of a medically examined industrial population, discovered that men were at a significantly higher risk of CHD when their social class in childhood, or the wife's social class in her childhood, was higher or lower than the class level that they presently shared. Kasl and Cobb (1967) also found that parental status stress appears to be a variable having 'strong, long-term effects on physical and mental health of adult offspring'. Berry (1966) found among a 6131 national sample that a small amount of variance in morbidity rate (incidence of hospitalization) was explained by status inconsistency. Jackson (1962) reached a more differentiated conclusion about status incongruence 'that all forms of status inconsistency are psychologically disturbing, but response to stress varies with relative positions of inconsistent person's achieved and ascribed status ranks'. More and more evidence is growing that social status stress is a problem in Western, highly mobile society. As Wan (1971) summarizes, the rationale for stress induced by status inconsistency is that 'role conflict generated from incompatible expectations of a social position may yield psychological disturbances and frustrations which in turn form part of the stress-disease linkage'.

Organizational structure and climate

A fifth potential source of managerial stress is simply 'being in the organization' and the threat to an individual's freedom, autonomy, and identity this poses. Problem areas such as little or no participation in the decision making process, no sense of belonging, lack of effective consultation, poor communications, restrictions on behaviour, and office politics are some of those with the most impact here. An increasing number of research investigations are being conducted in this area, particularly into the effect of employee participation in the work place. This research development is contemporaneous with a growing movement in North America and in the EEC countries of worker participation programmes, involving autonomous work groups, worker directors, and a greater sharing of the decision making process throughout the organization. The early work on participation was in terms of its' effect on production and attitudes of workers. For example, Coch and French (1948) examined the degrees of participation in a sewing factory. They found the greater the participation the higher was the productivity, the greater the job satisfaction, the lower the turnover and the better the relationship between boss and subordinate. These findings were later supported by a field experiment in a footwear factory in Southern Norway where greater participation led to significantly more favourable attitudes by workers towards management and more involvement in their jobs (French et al., 1960).

The research more relevant to our interests here, however, is the recent work on lack of participation and stress related disease. In the Goddard study (French and Caplan, 1970), for example, they found that people who reported greater opportunities for participation in decision making reported significantly greater job satisfaction, low job related feelings of threat, and higher feelings of self-esteem. Buck (1972) found that both managers and workers who felt 'under pressure' most, reported that their supervisors 'always ruled with an iron hand and rarely tried out new ideas or allowed participation in decision making'. Managers who were under stress also reported that their supervisors never let the persons under them do their work in the way they thought best. Margolis et al. (1974) found that non-participation at work, among a national representative sample of over 1400 workers, was the most consistent and significant predictor or indicator of strain and job related stress. They found that non-participation was significantly related to the following health risk factors: overall poor physical health, escapist drinking, depressed mood, low self-esteem, low life satisfaction, low job satisfaction, low motivation to work, intention to leave job, and absenteeism from work. Kasl (1973) also found that low job satisfaction was related to non-participation in decision making, inability to provide feedback to supervisors, and lack of recognition for good performance; and that poor mental health was linked to close supervision and no autonomy at work (Quinn et al., 1971). Neff (1968) has highlighted the importance of lack of participation and involvement by suggesting that 'mental health at work is to a large extent a function of the degree to which output is under the control of the individual worker'. To summarize, the research above seems to indicate that greater participation leads to lower staff turnover, higher productivity, and that when participation is absent, lower job satisfaction and higher levels of physical and mental health risks may result.

We have seen, however (Donaldson and Gowler, 1975), that it may be difficult to satisfy the needs of all levels of the workforce with the *same* change programme. There is, therefore, reason to approach this topic with caution, particularly as the studies quoted relied on correlational analysis for their conclusions and the inferences to causality that can be drawn are limited.

Extra-organizational sources of stress

The sixth and final 'source' of external job stress is more of a 'catch-all' for all those interfaces between life outside and life inside the organization that might put pressure on the manager: family problems (Pahl and Pahl, 1971), life crises (Dohrenwend and Dohrenwend, 1974), financial difficulties, conflict of personal beliefs with those of the company, and the conflict of company with family demands. Despite repeated calls to researchers to acknowledge that the individual 'functions as a totality' (Wright, 1975a), the practical problems of encompassing the 'whole person' in one research plan, usually leave those who try with either incomprehensibly complex results or platitudinous generalizations. Most studies, then, have only one life area as the focus of study.

The area which has received most research interest is that of the manager's relationship with his wife and family. (It is widely agreed that managers have little time for 'outside activities' apart from their families. Writers who have examined their effects on the local community (Packard, 1975) have pointed to the disruptive effects of the executive's lack of involvement.) The manager has two main problems *vis-à-vis* his family:

(1) the first is that of 'time-management' and 'commitment-management'. Not only does his busy life leave him few resources with which to cope with other people's needs, but in order to do his job well the manager usually also needs support from others to cope with the 'background' details of house management, etc., to relieve stress when possible, and to maintain contact with the outside world;
(2) the second, often a result of the first, is the spill-over of crises or stresses in one system which affect the other.

As these two are inseparable we shall go on to discuss them together.

Marriage patterns

The 'arrangement' the manager comes to with his wife will be of vital importance to both problem areas. Pahl and Pahl (1971) found that the majority of wives in their middle class sample saw their role in relation to their husband's job as a supportive, domestic one; all said that they derived their sense of security from their husbands (only two men said the same of their wives). Barber (1976), interviewing five directors' wives, finds similar attitudes. Gowler and Legge (1975) have dubbed this bond 'the hidden contract', in which the wife agrees to act as a 'support team' so that her husband can fill the demanding job to which he aspires. Handy (1975) supports the idea that this is 'typical' and that it is the path to career success for the manager concerned. Based on individual psychometric data he describes a number of possible marriage-role combinations. In his sample of top British executives (in mid-career) and their wives he found that the most frequent pattern (about half the 22 couples interviewed) was the 'thrusting male–caring female'. This he depicts as highly role segregated with the emphasis on 'separation', 'silence', and complementary activities. Historically both the company and the manager have reaped benefits from maintaining the segregation of work and home implicit in this pattern. The company thus legitimates its demand for a constant work performance from its employee, no matter what his home situation, and the manager is free to pursue his career but keeps a 'safe haven' to which he can return to relax and recuperate. The second and most frequent combination was 'involved–involved'—a dual career pattern, with the emphasis on complete sharing. This, while potentially extremely fulfilling for both parties, requires energy inputs which might well prove so excessive that none of the roles involved is fulfilled successfully.

It is unlikely that the patterns described above will be negotiated explicitly or that they will in the long term be 'in balance'. Major factors in their continuing evolution will be the work and family demands of particular life stages. A recent report by the British Institute of Management, *The Management Threshold* (Beattie *et al.*, 1974), for example, highlights the difficult situation of the young executive who, in order to build up his career, must devote a great deal of time and energy to his job just when his young housebound wife, with small children, is also making pressing demands. The report suggests that the executive fights to maintain the distance between his wife and the organization, so that she will not be in a position to evaluate the choices he has to make; paradoxically he does so at a time when he is most in need of sympathy and understanding. Guest and Williams (1973) examined the complete career cycle in similar terms, pointing out how the demands of the different systems change over time. The addition of role-disposition and personality-disposition variations to their 'equations' would, however, make them even more valuable.

Mobility

Home conflicts become particularly critical in relation to managerial relocation and mobility. Much of the literature on this topic comes from the United States where mobility is much more a part of the national character than in the UK (Pierson, 1972), but there is reason to believe that here, too, it is an increasingly common phenomenon.

At an individual level the effects of mobility on the manager's wife and family have been studied. Researchers agree that whether she is willing to move or not, the wife bears the brunt of relocations, and they conclude that most husbands do not appreciate what this involves. American writers point to signs that wives are suffering and becoming less co-operative. Immundo (1974) hypothesizes that increasing divorce rates are seen as the upwardly aspiring manager races ahead of his socially unskilled, 'stay-at-home' wife. Seidenberg (1973) comments on the rise in the ratio of female to male alcoholics in the United States from 1:5 in 1962 to 1:2 in 1973 and asks the question, 'Do corporate wives have souls?' Descriptive accounts of the frustrations and loneliness of being a 'corporate wife' in the US and UK proliferate. Increasing teenage delinquency and violence is also laid at the door of the mobile manager and the society which he has created.

Constant moving can have profound effects on the life style of the people concerned—particularly on their relationships with others. Staying only 2 years or so in one place, mobile families do not have time to develop close ties with the local community. Immundo (1974) talks of the 'mobility syndrome', a way of behaving geared to developing only temporary relationships. Packard (1975) describes ways in which individuals react to the type of fragmenting society this creates, e.g. treating everything as if it is temporary, being indifferent to local community amenities and organizations, living for the 'present' and becoming adept at 'instant gregariousness'. He goes on to point out the likely consequences for local communities, the nation, and the rootless people involved.

Pahl and Pahl (1971) suggest that the British reaction is, characteristically, more reserved and that many mobiles retreat into their nuclear family. This conclusion is supported, at a theoretical level, by Parsons (1943) who is concerned that this places even greater demands for stability, identity, and emotional support on this, already often precarious, institution. Managers, particularly, do not become involved in local affairs due both to lack of time and to an appreciation that they are only 'short-stay' inhabitants. Their wives find participation easier (especially in a mobile rather than a static area) and a recent survey on Middle Class Housing Estate Study (1975) suggested that, for some, involvement is a necessity to compensate for their husband's ambitions and career involvement which keep him away from home. From the company's point of view, the way in which a wife does adjust to her new environment can affect her husband's work performance. Guest and Williams (1973) illustrate this by an example of a major international company who, on surveying 1800 of their executives in 70 countries, concluded that the two most important influences on overall satisfaction with the overseas assignment were the job itself and, more importantly, the executives' wives adjustment to the foreign environment. Clinical evidence suggesting that one partner's problems may even contribute to the mental ill health of the other comes from work done at Edinburgh University (Kreitman, 1968).

Despite the importance of the work, home interface and the real problem that it poses to most managers and their wives at some time or another, there is a distinct lack of controlled research work to suggest how conflict affects both work performance and marriage or how crises or triumphs in one system 'feed back' to influence the other.

Characteristics of the individual

Sources of pressure at work evoke different reactions from different people. Some people are better able to cope with these stressors than others; they adapt their behaviour in a way that meets the environmental challenge. On the other hand, some people are more characterologically predisposed to stress, that is, they are unable to cope or adapt to the stress provoking situation. Many factors may contribute to these differences—personality, motivation, being able or ill equipped to deal with problems in a particular area of expertise, fluctuations in abilities (particularly with age), insight into one's own motivations and weaknesses, etc. It would be useful to examine, therefore, those characteristics of the individual that research evidence indicates are predisposers to stress. Most of the research in this area has focused on personality differences between high and low stressed individuals. This research has taken two principal directions: one has concentrated on examining the relationship between various psychometric measures (primarily using the MMPI and 16PF) and stress related disease (primarily coronary heart disease (CHD)); and the other on stress- or coronary-prone behaviour patterns and the incidence of disease. Jenkins (1971a, 1971b) provides an extensive and excellent review of these studies which we will summarise here.

Psychometric measures

In the first category, there were six studies which utilized the MMPI. The result of these six studies (Bakker and Levenson, 1967; Ostfeld *et al.*, 1964; Lebovits *et al.*, 1967; Brozek *et al.*, 1966; Bruhn *et al.*, 1969; Mordkoff and Rand, 1968) seems to be that before their illness patients with coronary disease differ from persons who remain healthy on several MMPI scales, particularly those in the 'neurotic' triad of hypochondriasis (Hs), depression (D), and hysteria (Hy). The occurrence of manifest CHD increases the deviation of patients' MMPI scores further and, in addition, there is ego defence breakdown. As Jenkins (1971a) summarizes 'patients with fatal disease tend to show greater neuroticism (particularly depression) in prospective MMPI's than those who incur and survive coronary disease'. There are three major studies utilizing the 16PF (Bakker, 1967; Finn *et al.*, 1969; Lebovits *et al.*, 1967). All three of these report emotional instability (low Scale C), particularly for patients with angina pectoris. Two studies report high conformity and submissiveness (Factor E) and desurgency/seriousness (Factor F), and two report high self-sufficiency (Factor Q2). Bakker's angina patients are similar to Finn's sample with CHD in manifesting shyness (Factor H) and apprehensiveness (Factor O). The results from all three studies portray the patients with CHD or related illness as emotionally unstable and introverted, which is consistent with the six MMPI studies. The limitation of these studies is that they are, on balance, retrospective. That is, that anxiety and neuroticism may well be reactions to CHD and other stress related illnesses rather than precursors of it. Paffenbarger *et al.* (1966) did an interesting prospective study in which they linked university psychometric data on students with death certificates filed years later. They found a number of significant precursors to fatal CHD, one of which was a high anxiety/neuroticism score for the fatal cases.

Kahn *et al.* (1964), adopting a more selective approach to personality measurement, came up with some more practically orientated results than those of the above general explorations. They examined a sample of managers on a series of personality variables: extroversion versus introversion, flexibility versus rigidity, inner versus outer directedness, open versus closed mindedness, achievement status versus security oriented—and related these to job stress. The following gives an indication of some of their results: (1) outer-directed people were more adaptable and more highly reality oriented than inner-directed; (2) 'rigids' and 'flexibles' perceived different types of situations as stressful, the former being more susceptible to rush jobs from above and dependence on other people, while the latter were more open to influence from other people, and thus easily became overloaded; (3) achievement seekers showed significantly more independence and job involvement than did security seekers.

Behaviour patterns

The other research approach to individual stress differences began with the work of Friedman and Rosenman (Friedman, 1969; Rosenman *et al.*, 1964, 1966) in the early 1960s and developed later showing a relationship between behavioural patterns and the prevalence of CHD. They found that individuals manifesting certain behavioural traits were significantly more at risk to CHD. These individuals were later referred to as the 'coronary-prone behaviour pattern Type A' as distinct from Type B (low risk of CHD). Type A was found to be the overt behavioural syndrome or style of living characterized by 'extremes of competitiveness, striving for achievement, aggressiveness, haste, impatience, restlessness, hyperalertness, explosiveness of speech, tenseness of facial musculature and feelings of being under pressure of time and under the challenge of responsibility'. It was suggested that 'people having this particular behavioural pattern were often so deeply involved and committed to their work that other aspects of their lives were relatively neglected' (Jenkins, 1971b). In the early studies, persons were designated as Type A or Type B on the basis of clinical judgements of doctors and psychologists or peer ratings. These studies found higher incidence of CHD among Type A than Type B. Many of the inherent methodological weaknesses of this approach were overcome by the classic Western Collaborative Group Study (Rosenman *et al.*, 1964, 1966). It was a prospective (as opposed to the earlier retrospective studies) national sample of over 3400 men free of CHD. All these men were rated Type A or B by psychiatrists after intensive interviews, without knowledge of any biological data about them and without the individuals being seen by a heart specialist. Diagnosis was made by an electrocardiographer and an independent medical practitioner, who were not informed about the subjects' behavioural patterns. They found the following result: after $2\frac{1}{2}$ years from the start of the study, Type A men between the ages of 39–49 and 50–59, had 6·5 and 1·9 times respectively the incidence of CHD than Type B men. They also had the following risk factors of high serum cholesterol levels, elevated beta-lipoproteins, decreased blood clotting time, and elevated daytime excretion of norepinephrine. After $4\frac{1}{2}$ years of the follow-up observation in the study, the *same* relationship of behavioural pattern and incidence of CHD was found. In terms of the clinical manifestations of CHD, individuals exhibiting Type A behavioural patterns had significantly more incidence of acute myocardial infarction (and of clinically unrecognized myocardial infarction) and angina pectoris. Rosenman *et al.* (1967) also found that the risk of recurrent and fatal myocardial infarction was significantly related to Type A characteristics. Quinlan and his colleagues (Quinlan, *et al.*, 1969) found the same results among Trappist and Benedictine monks. Monks judged to be Type A coronary-prone cases (by a double-blind procedure) had 2·3 times the prevalence of angina and 4·3 times the prevalence of infarction as compared to monks judged Type B. Many other studies (Bortner and Rosenman, 1967; Zyzanski and Jenkins, 1970) have been conducted with roughly the same findings.

Researchers at the Institute of Social Research, The University of Michigan, have focused on A type characteristics, as a central personality measure in many of their studies. Sales (1969) developed a 49-item questionnaire test of Type A; a 9-item rationalization is now also available (Vickers, 1973). Using the Sales version, Caplan *et al.* (1975b) found no significant correlations between personality 'pure' and the 'strains' measured (job dissatisfaction, somatic complaints, anxiety, depression, irritation, physical and behavioural 'stress' correlates). Their expectation to find relationships at interactive levels, instead, is borne out by previous research experience. Caplan and Jones (1975), for example, report on the mediating role of personality. In their study of 13 male users of a university computer system in a 'stressful' time before a 23-day shutdown, they found confirmation of previous findings that role ambiguity was positively associated with anxiety, depression, and resentment, and work load with anxiety, and that these relationships were greatest for Type A personalities. In a further study (Caplan, Cobb, and French, 1975) the team investigated the relationship between smoking and A type personality and shed light on 'A's' ability to modify his coronary-prone behaviour. Caplan *et al.* report that only a fifth of those who try to give up smoking are successful. Following a questionnaire survey of 200 administrators, engineers, and scientists at NASA, they tried to relate 'quitting' to job stress, personality, and social support. They found that 'quitters' had the lowest levels on quantitative work load, responsibility, and social support and that they scored low on Type A characteristics. Care must be taken in interpreting these correlational results (it may well be that As seek out high work loads). One conclusion can, however, be drawn unequivocally: A type personalities are less likely to give up smoking than are B types (as the authors point out, over time this will lead to an increase in the association between smoking and risk of CHD);

thus it would appear that the former's characteristics are so fundamental that they are unable to help themselves (if helped they must be!). Payne (1975) has this in mind when he expresses the need (in somewhat rarefied tones) for a social system of trust and support which would 'manipulate the degree of environmental pressures so as to give a pinprick to the comfortable B-types and respite to the harassed A's'.

Further confirmation of the legitimacy of the behaviour pattern approach comes from the two final studies to be mentioned here. The first started from a more basic level than that above by taking a check list of 25 'habits of nervous tension' (Thomas and Ross, 1967). The 1085 medical student subjects were asked to indicate which of these corresponded to their reactions when 'in situations of undue pressure or stress'. While highly individual patterns of response were found it was possible:

(1) to derive 8 factors (by factor analysis) from the total 25 items—these were 'activity', 'appetite', 'irritation', 'viseral reaction', 'general stress', 'dependency', 'compulsivity', and 'stimulation'; they suggest dimensions on which to base further research;
(2) to relate individual items to serum cholesterol levels—5 items were significantly different for high and low cholesterol groups. Low cholesterol subjects more often reported 'loss of appetite', 'exhaustion', 'nausea', and 'anxiety', and high cholesterol subjects, 'urge to eat'.

The second study is much more assumptive in approach. Gernill and Heister (1972) set out to investigate the relationship between 'Machiavellianism' (a tendency to manipulate and persuade others, to initiate and control in group situations and generally 'be a winner'), job strain, job satisfaction, positional mobility, and perceived opportunities for formal control. High Machiavellian scorers were, overall, much less happy in their jobs—showing more job strain, less dissatisfaction, and lower perceived opportunities for formal control—than low scorers. Explanation of these results is not easy (largely because the researchers failed to reach the underlying elements in a complex situation). These differences could be (1) perceptual, due to a basic Machiavellian cynicism; (2) because of the subjects' ways of operating which are likely to cause frustration, or (3) because they worked for formalized organizations and not in the ambiguous environments in which they flourish.

To summarize, while psychometric measures do show relationships with stress measures, the macro approach of behaviour patterns offers more practically applicable data. The doubtful reliability of psychometric tests also makes their use in causal research less intuitively appealing than that of behavioural measures.

A research technique which stands somewhat alone by explicitly incorporating personal characteristics into job stress measures (and, at the same time, reduces the number of variables in, and therefore the complexity of, multivariate analysis) is discussed by Van Harrison (1975) and French (1973). They assess 'person–environment fit' by asking subjects to indicate 'desired' and 'actual' levels of work load, work complexity, responsibility, ambiguity, etc., in their jobs, and then taking the difference between scores on the various dimensions as their measures. (Some other questionnaires do contain this evaluative element implicitly.) This approach has been relatively successful and P–E fit has proved to be an equally good or more powerful predictor of stress (job dissatisfaction, anxiety, depression, etc.) than either elements separately (although there are still some unsolved problems of analysis).

The management of stress

Cooper and Marshall (1976) have argued that understanding the sources of managerial pressure, as we have tried to do here, is only the first step in stress reduction. Next, we must begin to explore 'when' and 'how' to intervene. There are a number of changes that can be introduced in organizational life to begin to manage stress at work, for example:

(1) To re-create the social, psychological, and organizational environment in the work place to encourage greater autonomy and participation by managers in *their* jobs.
(2) To begin to build the bridges between the work place and the home; providing opportunities for the manager's wife to understand better her husband's job, to express her views about the consequences of his work on family life, and to be involved in the decision making process of work that affects all members of the family unit.
(3) To utilize the well developed catalogue of social and interactive skill training programmes to help clarify role and interpersonal relationship difficulties within organizations.
(4) And more fundamentally, to create an organizational climate to encourage rather than discourage communication, openness, and trust—so that individual managers are able to express their inability to cope, their work related fears, and are able to ask for help if needed.

There are many other methods and approaches of coping and managing stress, depending on the sources activated and the interface between these sources and the individual make-up of the manager concerned—these will, however, be dealt with more systematically and in greater detail in the section of this book which deals with stress reduction methods. Nevertheless, one important point that must always be kept in mind in coping with and managing organizational stress is, as Wright (1975b) so aptly summarizes, that 'the responsibility for maintaining health should be a reflection of the basic relationship between the individual and the organization for which he works; it is in the best interests of both parties that reasonable steps are taken to live and work sensibly and not too demandingly'.

Note

1. Some of the research literature reviewed here was drawn from an article published by the authors in the *Journal of Occupational Psychology*, 1976, **49**, 11–28. We would like to thank the British Psychological Society for permission to use some of this material.

102

References

Argyris, C. (1964) *Integrating the Individual and the Organization.* New York. Wiley.
Arthur, R. J., and Gunderson, E. K. (1965) Promotion and mental illness in the Navy, *Journal of Occupational Medicine*, **7**, 452–456.
Bakker, C. B. (1967) Psychological factors in angina pectoris, *Psychosom.*, **8**, 43–49.
Bakker, C. B., and Levenson, R. M. (1967) Determinants of angina pectoris, *Psychosom. Med.*, **29**, 621–633.
Barber, R. (1976) Who would marry a director?, *Director*, March issue, 60–62.
Beattie, R. T., Darlington, T. G., and Cripps, D. M. (1974) *The Management Threshold.* BIM Paper OPN 11.
Bellotto, S. (1971) Keeping fit on the executive level, *International Administrative Management*, **32**, 62–63.
Berry, K. J. (1966) *Status Integration and Morbidity.* Unpublished Ph.D. thesis, Corvallis. University of Oregon.
Bortner, R. W., and Rosenman, R. H. (1967) The measurement of pattern A behavior, *J. chron. Dis.*, **20**, 525–533.
Breslow, L., and Buell, P. (1960) Mortality from coronary heart disease and physical activity of work in California, *J. chron. Dis.*, **11**, 615–626.
Brook, A. (1973) Mental stress at work, *The Practitioner*, **210**, 500–506.
Brooks, G. W., and Mueller, E. F. (1966) Serum urate concentrations among university professors, *J. Amer. Med. Assoc.*, **195**, 415–418.
Brozek, J., Keys, A., and Blackburn, H. (1966) Personality differences between potential coronary and non-coronary patients, *Annals of New York Academy of Science*, **134**, 1057–1064.
Bruhn, J. G., Chandler, B., and Wolf, S. (1969) A psychological study of survivors and nonsurvivors of myocardial infarction, *Psychosom. Med.*, **31**, 8–19.
Brummet, R. L., Pyle, W. C., and Flamholtz, E. G. (1968) Accounting for human resources, *Michigan Business Review*, **20**, 2, 20–25.
Buck, V. (1972) *Working Under Pressure.* London. Staples Press.
Caplan, R. D., Cobb, S., and French, J. R. P. (1975a) Relationships of cessation of smoking with job stress, personality and social support, *J. of Applied Psychology*, **60**, 2, 211–219.
Caplan, R. D., Cobb, S., French, J. R. P., Harrison, R. Van, and Pinneau, S. R. (1975) *Job Demands and Worker Health: Main Effects and Occupational Differences.* NIOSH Research Report.
Caplan, R. D., and Jones, K. W. (1975) Effects of workload, role ambiguity and type-A personality on anxiety, depression and heart rate, *J. of Applied Psychology*, **60**, 6, 713–719.
Clutterbuck, D. (1973) How I learned to stop worrying and love the job, *International Management*, **28**, 8, 27–29.
Coch, L., and French, J. R. P. (1948) Overcoming resistance to change, *Hum. Relat.*, **11**, 512–532.
Constandse, W. J. (1972) A neglected personnel problem, *Personnel Journal*, **51**, 2, 129–133.
Cooper, C. L. (1973) *Group Training for Individual and Organizational Development.* Basel, Switzerland. S. Karger.
Cooper, C. L., and Marshall, J. (1976) Occupational sources of stress: a review of the literature relating to coronary heart disease and mental ill health, *Journal of Occupational Psychology*, **49**, 11–28.
Dohrenwend, B. S., and Dohrenwend, B. P. (1974) *Stressful Life Events.* New York. Wiley.
Donaldson, J., and Gowler, D. (1975) Prerogatives, participation and managerial stress, In Gowler, D., and Legge, K. (eds), *Managerial Stress.* Epping, Gower Press.
Doyle, C. (1975) Stress isn't such a killer after all, *Observer*, 9 November.
Dreyfuss, F., and Czackes, J. W. (1954) Blood cholesterol and uric acid of healthy medical

students under stress of examination, *Arch. Int. Med.*, **103**, 708.

Eaton, M. T. (1969) The mental health of the older executive, *Geriat.*, **24**, 126–134.

Erikson, J., Edwards, D., and Gunderson, E. K. (1973) Status congruency and mental health, *Psychological Reports*, **33**, 395–401.

Erikson, J., Pugh, W. M., and Gunderson, E. K. (1972) Status congruency as a predictor of job satisfaction and life stress, *Journal of Applied Psychology*, **56**, 523–525.

Finn, F., Hickey, N., and O'Doherty, E. F. (1969) The psychological profiles of male and female patients with CHD, *Irish J. Med. Sci.*, **2**, 339–341.

French, J. R. P. (1973) Person–role fit, *Occupational Mental Health*, **3** (1).

French, J. R. P., and Caplan, R. D. (1970) Psychosocial factors in coronary heart disease, *Indus. Med.*, **39**, 383–397.

French, J. R. P., and Caplan, R. D. (1973) Organizational stress and individual strain. In Marrow, A. J. (ed.), *The Failure of Success*. New York. AMACOM, pp. 30–66.

French, J. R. P., Israel, J., and As, D. (1960) An experiment in participation in a Norwegian factory, *Hum. Relat.*, **13** (1), 3–20.

French, J. R. P., Tupper, C. J., and Mueller, E. I. (1965) *Workload of University Professors.* Unpublished research report, Ann Arbor, Mich. The University of Michigan.

Friedman, M. (1969) *Pathogenesis of Coronary Artery Disease.* New York. McGraw-Hill.

Friedman, M., Rosenman, R. H., and Carroll, V. (1958) Changes in serum cholesterol and blood clotting time in men subjected to cyclic variations of occupational stress, *Circulation*, **17**, 852–861.

Gernill, G. R., and Heister, W. J. (1972) Machiavellianism as a factor in managerial job strain, job satisfaction and upward mobility, *Academy of Management J.*, **15**, 1, 51–62.

Goffman, E. (1952) On cooling the mark out, *Psychiatry*, **15** (4), 451–463.

Gowler, D., and Legge, K. (1975) Stress and external relationships—the 'hidden contract'. In Gowler, D., and Legge, K. (eds), *Managerial Stress*. Epping. Gower Press.

Guest, D., and Williams, R. (1973) How home affects work, *New Society*, 18 January.

Handy, C. (1975) Difficulties of combining family and career, *The Times*, London, Sept. 22nd, p. 16.

Harrison, R. Van (1975) Job stress and worker health: person–environment misfit. Paper presented at the 103rd Annual Meeting of the American Public Health Assoc., Chicago, Ill.

Immundo, L. V. (1974) Problems associated with managerial mobility, *Personnel Journal*, **53**, 12, 910.

Jackson, E. F. (1962) Status consistency and symptoms of stress, *American Sociological Review*, **27**, 4, 469–480.

Jenkins, C. D. (1971a) Psychologic and social precursors of coronary disease, *New Eng. J. Med.*, **284**, 5, 244–255.

Jenkins, C. D. (1971b) Psychologic and social precursors of coronary disease, *New Eng. J. Med.*, **284**, 6, 307–317.

Kahn, R. L., (1973) Conflict, ambiguity and overload: three elements in job stress, *Occupational Mental Health*, **3**, 1.

Kahn, R. L., Wolfe, D. M., Quinn, R. P., Snoek, J. D., and Rosenthal, R. A. (1964) *Organizational Stress*. New York. Wiley.

Kasl, S. V. (1973) Mental health and the work environment, *J. occup. Med.*, **15**, 6, 509–518.

Kasl, S. V., and Cobb, S. (1967) Effects of parental status incongruence and discrepancy in physical and mental health of adult offspring, *Journal of Personality and Social Psychology*, Monograph 7, Whole no. 642, 1–15.

Kay, E. (1974) Middle management. In O'Toole, J. (ed.), *Work and the Quality of Life.* Cambridge, Mass. The MIT Press.

Kearns, J. L. (1973) *Stress in Industry*. London. Priory Press.

Kornhauser, A. (1965) *Mental Health of the Industrial Worker*. New York. Wiley.

Kreitman, N. (1968) Married couples admitted to mental hospital, *British J. of Psychiatry*, **114**, 699–718.

104

Kritsikis, S. P., Heinemann, A. L., and Eitner, S. (1968) Die angina pectoris im aspekt ihrer korrelation mit biologischer disposition, psychologischen und soziologischen emflussfaktoren, *Deutsch Gasundh*, **23**, 1878–1885.

Lazarus, R. S. (1966) *Psychological Stress and the Coping Process*. New York. McGraw-Hill.

Lebovits, B. Z., Shekelle, R. B., and Ostfeld, A. M. (1967) Prospective and retrospective studies of CHD, *Psychosom. Med.*, **29**, 265–272.

Levinson, H. (1973) Problems that worry our executives. In Marrow, A. J. (ed.), *The failure of Success*. New York. AMACON.

Levy, R. (1973) Relief of the executive headache?, *Duns*, **101**, 101.

McMurray, R. N. (1973) The executive neurosis. In Noland, R. L. (ed.), *Industrial Mental Health and Employee Counselling*. New York. Behavioural Publications.

Marcson, S. (1970) *Automation, Alienation and Anomie*. New York. Harper & Row.

Margolis, B. L., and Kroes, W. H. (1974) Work and the health of man. In O'Toole, J. (ed.), *Work and the Quality of Life*, Cambridge, Mass. MIT Press.

Margolis, B. L., Kroes, W. H., and Quinn, R. P. (1974) Job stress: an unlisted occupational hazard, *J. occup. Med.*, **16**, 10, 654–661.

Mettlin, C., and Woelfel, J. (1974) Interpersonal influence and symptoms of stress, *Journal of Health and Social Behaviour*, **15**, 4, 311–319.

Middle Class Housing Estate Study (1975), Civil Service College, United Kingdom, unpublished paper.

Miller, J. G. (1960) Information input overload and psychopathology, *Amer. J. Psychiat.*, **8**, 116.

Minzberg, H. (1973) *The Nature of Managerial Work*, New York. Harper & Row.

Mordkoff, A. M. and Rand, A. M. (1968) Personality and adaptation to coronary artery disease, *J. consult. clin. Psychol.*, **32**, 648–653.

Morris, J. (1975) Managerial stress and 'the cross of relationships'. In Gowler, D., and Legge, K. (eds), *Managerial Stress*, Epping. Gower Press.

Neff, W. S. (1968) *Work and Human Behaviour*. New York. Atherton Press.

Ostfeld, A. M., Lebovits, B. Z., and Shekelle, R. B. (1964) A prospective study of the relationship between personality and CHD, *J. chron. Dis.*, **17**, 265–276.

Packard, V. (1975) *A Nation of Strangers*, New York. McKay.

Paffenbarger, R. S., Wolf, P. A., and Notkin, J. (1966) Chronic disease in former college students, *Amer. J. Epidemol.*, **83**, 314–328.

Pahl, J. M., and Pahl, R. E. (1971) *Managers and their wives*, London. Allen Lane.

Parsons, T. (1943) The kinship system in contemporary United States of America, *American Anthropology*, **45**, 22–38.

Payne, R. (1975) 'A' type work for 'A' type people?, *Personnel Management*, **7**, 22–24.

Perham, J. C. (1972) Upright executive, *Duns*, **99**, 79–80.

Pierson, G. W. (1972) *The Moving American*, New York. Knopf.

Pincherle, G. (1972) Fitness for work, *Proceedings of the Royal Society of Medicine*, **65**, 4, 321–324.

Porter, L. W., and Lawler, E. E. (1965) Properties of organization structure in relation to job attitudes and job behavior, *Psychol. Bull.*, **64**, 23–51.

Quinlan, C. B., Burrow, J. G., and Hayes, C. G. (1969) The association of risk factors and CHD in Trappist and Benedictine monks. Paper presented to the American Heart Association, New Orleans, Louisiana.

Quinn, R. P., Seashore, S., and Mangione, I. (1971) *Survey of Working Conditions*, US Government Printing Office.

Rosenman, R. H., Friedman, M., and Jenkins, C. D. (1967) Clinically unrecognized myocardial infarction in the Western Collaborative Group Study, *Amer. J. Cardiol.*, **19**, 776–782.

Rosenman, R. H., Friedman, M., and Strauss, R. (1964) A predictive study of CHD, *J. Amer. Med. Assoc.*, **189**, 15–22.

Rosenman, R. H., Friedman, M., and Strauss, R. (1966) CHD in the Western Collaborative Group Study, *J. Amer. Med. Assoc.*, **195**, 86–92.

Russek, H. I., and Zohman, B. L. (1958) Relative significance of hereditary diet, and occupational stress in CHD of young adults, *Amer. J. Med. Sci.*, **235**, 266–275.

Sales, S. M. (1969) *Differences among Individuals in Affective, Behavioural, Biochemical, and Physiological Responses to Variations in Work Load* (Doctoral dissertation, The University of Michigan). Ann Arbor, Mich. University Microfilms, no. 60–18098.

Seidenberg, R. (1973) *Corporate wives—corporate casualties*, American Management Association, New York.

Shekelle, R. B., Ostfeld, A. M., and Paul, O. (1969) Social status and incidence of CHD, *J. chron. Dis.*, **22**, 381–394.

Shepard, J. M. (1971) *Automation and Alienation*. Cambridge, Mass. The MIT Press.

Shirom, A., Eden, D., Silberwasser, S., and Kellerman, J. J. (1973) Job stresses and risk factors in coronary heart disease among occupational categories in kibbutzim, *Soc. Sci. & Med.*, **7**, 875–892.

Sleeper, R. D. (1975) Labour mobility over the life cycle, *British Journal of Industrial Relations*, **13**, 2.

Sofer, C. (1970) *Men in Mid-Career*, Cambridge University Press.

Terhure, W. B. (1963) Emotional problems of executives in time, *Indus. med. Surg.*, **32**, 1–67.

Thomas, C. B., and Ross, D. C. (1967) Observations of some possible precursors of essential hypertension and coronary heart disease. In *Social Stress and Cardiovascular Disease*, Millbank Memorial Fund Quarterly, **45**, 2.

Uris, A. (1972) How managers ease job pressures, *International Management*, 27 June, 45–46.

Vickers, R. (1973) A short measure of the type A personality, *ISR Newsletter*, Michigan, February.

Wan, T. (1971) Status stress and morbidity: a sociological investigation of selected categories of work-limiting chronic conditions, *J. chron. Dis.*, **24**, 453–468.

Wardwell, W. I., Hyman, M., and Bahnson, C. B. (1964) Stress and coronary disease in three field studies, *J. chron. Dis.*, **17**, 73–84.

Wright, H. B. (1967) Institute of Directors Medical Centre in London. In McLean, A. A. (ed.), *To Work is Human: Mental Health and the Business Community*. New York. Rand McNally.

Wright, H. B. (1975a) Health hazards for executives, *J. of General Management*, **2**, 2.

Wright, H. B. (1975b) *Executive Ease and Dis-ease*. Epping. Gower Press.

Zyzanski, S. J., and Jenkins, C. D. (1970) Basic dimension within the coronary-prone behavior pattern, *J. chron. Dis.*, **22**, 781–795.

Chapter 4

The Family:Help or Hindrance?

Charles Handy

London Graduate School of Business Studies

Is the family a source of stress at work, as the placing of this chapter suggests, or a way of alleviating it? Is the family a help or a hindrance? Or, looking at it the other way round, is work a help or a hindrance to the family relationship? Does, for instance, the dominating work role of one partner (often the husband) mean that the other partner has to subordinate his or her true interests?

There is a growing body of writing and research on this relationship between work and family, reflecting perhaps the facts that something like 90% of those who work, work in organizations (Jacques, 1976), that over half of married women today do work outside the home and even more intend to do so (Fogarty *et al.*, 1971), and that the family, so far from declining as a social institution is probably growing in importance even if its forms and norms are changing (Young and Willmott, 1973). A representative list of the recent literature follows this chapter.

At first glance much of this writing and research appears confused, influenced by conflicting value orientations, and it can, in the end, produce rather obvious and perhaps therefore unhelpful conclusions. It is at the same time often absorbing and fascinating research delving as it does into areas and problems which affect so many of us. What we thought was personal to ourselves alone turns out to be common to many. Yet a fund of shared experiences has not yet resulted in agreed conclusions on the proper relationship between work and family. As evidence for the thrust and counterthrust of the argument we might consider these excerpts from some of the literature:

Professionals who were currently married, regardless of whether the marriage was their first or subsequent one, were far more likely to be highly successful than colleagues who were not currently married. Moreover, among professionals who were not currently married, those who were formerly married tended to be more successful than those who had never been married. . . . In brief, marriage per se, but not marital stability is strongly related to occupational success and marital disruption is not a liability, particularly when followed by remarriage. (Marx and Spray, 1976)

Executives who were satisfied with their jobs had wives who were involved with their husbands' work, had a positive attitude towards their husbands working overtime, thought their husbands put their work first and thought their husbands' salary was unimportant.

Executives with a high frequency of stress symptoms had wives who were not involved with their jobs, particularly the content or the social side.

Executives reporting physical symptoms of stress had wives who thought their husbands' salary to be important and disliked their working overtime. (Berger, 1974)

One pattern stands out from all the others: marriages of men whose exclusive or primary emphasis is on their careers to women who themselves place store on integrating their career with their family lives are not very happy. As a matter of fact, the number of couples in this group who describe their marriages as 'very happy' is so low that it is not possible, with the present sample, to investigate the conditions that contribute to or ease the strains of this pattern. It should be mentioned, however, that neither of the two couples of this pattern whose marriages are very happy has children; it should also be said that both husbands are in favour of married women having a career, and both are very satisfied with their own work. It seems then, that under special conditions this pattern can be accompanied by a happy marriage, but the conditions are rare in this sample. (Bailyn, 1970)

There are no clear answers in all of this to that first question—is the family a help or a hindrance? Nor even to the subsidiary questions—is stress inevitable in the family/work situation or can it be avoided? If inevitable, can it be managed? Probably we should not expect clear or universal answers even if the dilemmas are perennial and pervasive. Probably the answers will always be unique to each of us, depending on our values and attitudes, the society in which we live, the stage of life, the job we do or want to do, the number of our children, and the size of our bank balance.

We shall however attempt, in this chapter, to provide a framework for looking at this relationship between work and family. It is a framework based upon a particular piece of research on a particular population but when linked to other research in this area it seems to have a wider and more general application. The framework provides no answers, only a better way of predicting the likely consequences of certain combinations of family and work and their implications for stress. Concealed within the interactions of family and work lies what Gowler and Legge (1975) have called the 'hidden contract'. The framework presented here is a way of making more explicit the quasi-contractual implications for those involved at any particular stage of family or career.

The Sloan research

This research[1] was concerned to investigate the ways in which successful career executives managed to cope with the demands of a managerial job and a growing family. Prototypes of the successful executive in mid-career were available to the researchers as members of the Sloan Programme at the London Business School. This programme was a full-time 9-month management programme for executives who at that time (1972) were usually sponsored by their organizations with the aim of preparing them for a major step upward in the organization. Twenty-three couples were interviewed as part of an exploratory study. Their average age was 34, they were all married, had an average of 2·4 children, worked for large organizations in government, commerce or industry and readily agreed that they fitted the definition of career executive. Although in terms of their age, careers, salaries, etc., they all appeared to be very similar, indeed to be almost stereotype of the successful articulate corporate man, the ways in which they managed their lives turned out to be very different. The research was exploratory and the group far from typical of the total population of managers in this country, let alone all workers, but it may be that the life patterns it threw up have a wider applicability.

As part of a battery of tests and questionnaires the 23 couples completed an attitude test (the Edwards Personal Preference Schedule) which revealed considerable differences between the individuals on certain Attitude Dimensions, particularly Dominance, Achievement, and Affiliation (interestingly, the three needs pinpointed by McClelland in his investigation of motivation). Affiliation was linked with 'Nurturance' or a desire to support as well as to be with (affiliation). We combined these four attitude scores to make two separate dimensions—Achievement/Dominance and Affiliation/Nurturance and plotted the scores of each individual on a matrix with four separate quadrants as shown in Figure 4.1.

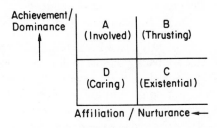

Figure 4.1

The titles for the quadrants were invented by us in an attempt to convey something of the flavour of the attitudes and values of those whose scores located them in each of the quadrants.

Quadrant A we called Involved. These individuals had high needs to achieve and dominate, but also had high social needs. They wanted to belong to and be part of a group or strong relationship. The executives in this were often in staff roles or in the civil service.

Quadrant B we christened Thrusting. This quadrant contained the most visibly successful of the males. They are high achievers with a need for dominance and low scores of Affiliation and Nurturance implying that they are happy to act on their own, with less sensitivity to the group. This group contained the bulk of the executives in our sample.

Quadrant C contains the Existentialists—the loners. They have little desire to control others or to look after others. They are inner directed, not particularly ambitious, but set their own standards for their lives.

Quadrant D are the supportive Caring people who get their satisfactions from looking after others and belonging rather than dominating. Many of the executive wives fell into this quadrant, only two of the men.

The way the group of 46 individuals was distributed across the quadrants was interesting in itself, but more interesting were the differences in the marriage patterns that the matrix threw up. The marriage patterns were arrived at by linking together the individuals in each relationship so that you would have A–A marriages (both in the same 'involved' quadrant), A–B marriages and so on, 16 possible patterns in all. (For convenience we list the male quadrant first, then the female, in defining each pattern.)

In fact only eight of the possible patterns were represented in our sample. B–D was the most common (a thrusting man with a caring wife) with six examples, followed by B–B (two thrusters), A–D (involved husband and caring wife) and A–A (two involved).

The patterns differed:

—in the way roles were defined within the relationship;
—in the priority given to the different activity areas of their lives. These we called 'arenas', the outlets for our attitudes or needs;
—in the ways relationships with others (children, friends, relations) were seen and handled;
—in the way any problems or tensions were handled;
—in the way in which the relationship first started.

During the research we not only asked each couple to fill in various questionnaires, dealing with their own backgrounds, their current way of life, and their perceptions of themselves as well as their general attitudes, but we also visited the family at home and got some impression of how they lived. Although less quantifiable, this impressionistic evidence was often the most meaningful.

Let us look briefly at the principal marriage patterns in turn.

Pattern 1. B–D. A 'thrusting' husband and a 'caring' wife

These patterns, the most frequent in our sample, are role stereotyped. The husband works and the wife minds the home. She wants him and the children to be happy, although achievement and success above a certain point are costly to her. She is concerned with the activity arenas of the husband/wife relationship, the family, and their social network. Roles are clear. The husband may help in the house and must take major policy decisions concerning it but she is operationally in charge, just as he is in charge in the work arena. Their common problems will be in the family arena and may concern money, children or mobility. She is unlikely to want to venture into a work arena herself unless there is a great need for money, in which case she would try to find work which was lucrative without being too demanding on time and energy. The husband would resent her working. Since it would only be done for money it would imply a failure on his part in his work. The wife will be very supportive of her husband in his work although she may not in fact be very interested or involved in its details—it is not a shared arena. One wife in the sample, very supportive, did not in fact know what her husband's job was, although she did know the name of his employers and would have readily moved home if his work demanded it. The husband's need to dominate and achieve is no problem to the caring wife, particularly if he satisfies these needs in the work arena. The wife's task, as she sees it, is to absorb her own problems and not burden her husband. In the family arena his activity will be channelled into his agreed roles and in the husband/wife relationship she expects him to dominate.

The husband, outside his work, will see it as his main duty to maintain a secure and happy home. Within the family arena he will have set times or types of activities with the children, particular duties (buying the drink, servicing the car, house maintenance) and some mini-arena (the vegetable garden, the garage) which are clearly his and not hers. She will often manage the joint social network. These couples often have three social networks, his, hers, and a joint one, which is occasionally confined to relations. His network will meet outside the home, at work or at the golf club.

These couples run a regulated home. There are routines and rules, tidy rooms and disciplined children. There are, in this sample, usually separate roles for separate rooms, a dining-room, a sitting-room, and a kitchen for instance and, if space runs to it, a study for him even though it is rarely used. Conversations within the relationship are more often ritual ('How was the office today?') or logistic ('When is your mother arriving?') than issue raising (politics, religion or philosophy). But while there will be few deep discussions there will be few rows. These couples move *away* from each other under tension. The B type man will act out his tension in a physical ritual. Since there is no appropriate ritual within the home he will take it outside—to sport, the garden or back to his work. The D type wife will not want to impose her tensions on the family and will tend to suffer in silence and solitude. Tension is not talked out, since their conversation rituals do not allow for it.

These relationships have a secure predictability which led us to think of them as *traditional* marriages. They can appear conventional, even dull, to an outsider but a man who is fully involved in a work arena may need this kind of dependable base.

Pattern 2. B–B. The pairing of two 'thrusters'

In these patterns both partners place high value on achievement and dominance. They *both* want an arena where they can hold responsibility and can demonstrate, at least to themselves, that they have achieved something. For the husband the arena is most obviously and frequently his work. If, however, he fails to find full satisfaction for those needs in that arena he may turn to another— his family, a hobby, the community. The wife has equal needs, again most appropriately met by a work arena. In our sample only one of the wives had a full-time, full-commitment job and she was about to give it up since her first baby was due. Part-time work or courses of study were found to be inadequate substitutes by these women. Dominant people need other people. The solitary pursuits of the self-employed or the learner were not therefore fully satisfying.

The B–B marriages can be scenes of considerable discontent. The wife, if children have arrived, finds inadequate outlets for her achievement and dominance needs which she may transfer to the arena of the family, the marriage relationship, putting perhaps unwanted pressure on both, and creating competition rather than support within the home. If both husband and wife are engaged in their independent work arenas the domestic base will tend to be disorganized, even chaotic. Both will find this irritating, but if the husband seeks to blame the wife, forcing her into a caring role, conflict may well develop. Since Thrusting people are aggressive under tension, in this pattern the individuals move *against* each other when they feel tension, clashing in recriminatory arguments.

These then are turbulent relationships which have more chance of survival if they are equal competitions, that is when there are no children and minimal support requirements so that both partners can be thrusting in their own arenas, meeting for companionship and mutual stimulation. It is a pattern frequently encountered among young marrieds where like has married like. It may not easily survive the subsequent stages of child bearing and rearing, or of job plateaux or retirement. We had some suggestions of role separation in these patterns, where both partners find quite separate activities for themselves so that conflict is avoided by not meeting. One couple so arranged their lives, apparently without deliberately meaning to, so that they were very seldom in the house at the same time and had no shared networks. They saw their marriage as stable and contented.

Pattern 3. A–A. The partnership of two 'involved' people

A–A marriages, like B–B marriages, are relationships where two very similar individuals are paired. In our sample A–A and B–B couples typically met at university, were of the same age and shared similar aspirations, but often had dissimilar family backgrounds. This is in contrast to the 'traditional' B–D marriages where the husband was always older than the wife, had more years of formal education but came from similar family background.

The 'involved' people also are dominant and high achievers but these attitudes are tempered or, more often, confused, by the high value they place on 'caring' and 'belonging'. They prefer to share arenas not separate them. In their marriages, therefore, roles frequently overlap. There are few clear duties. Whoever is available or enjoys it may cook the meal, clean the house, put the children to bed. People tend to get higher priority than things. Housework and home maintenance come low on the list. Rooms get used for multiple purposes, and usually reflect it in their decor. Children tend to be full members of the family and can appear 'precocious' or 'undisciplined' to, for instance, a B–D family. Conversations are about issues and values as much as logistics and ritual. Social networks are all shared, and therefore often quite small. Tension is high in these marriages, perhaps because both partners are sensitive. Under tension both partners first withdraw then move *towards* each other, often talking things out for long hours. These are very intense relationships with the potential for a lot of mutual support.

Both the examples A–A patterns in our sample could be described as 'working couples'. In each case, however, they had young children and the wife had only a part-time job. In both cases the husband had a very demanding job and suffered from great tension or stress. Both wives felt that they themselves were under achieving in their work arenas, but were prepared to tolerate this for a time in order to care for their husband and their children. In other words the high value they place on the 'caring' and 'belonging' aspects increased their tolerance for a situation which a purely 'thrusting' wife would have resented more.

Pattern 4. A–D. An 'involved' husband with a 'caring' wife

The A–D marriage is the comfortable equivalent of an A–A. The husband is still ambitious for power and achievement but also values 'caring' and 'belonging'. He is, therefore, if competent, likely to be working very hard and to be feeling under a considerable amount of stress. His wife however will be more willing to support, comfort, and protect him than someone with a more thrusting nature.

Their lives show an interesting mixture of the B–D (traditional) and the A–A (involved). While it is clear that his work is important and her task supportive, the roles are not so clearcut, their lives so predictable or the tension so contained. These relationships are more intense and emotional, more questioning and flexible than the traditional marriages, but less competitive and striving than the involved ones.

Where the wife worked in these marriages it was always a part-time job, but undertaken more to earn money or to provide companionship for herself. The husbands in these patterns usually worked far more intensely and far longer hours than their B type colleagues. As a result the home, for a caring wife, could be a lonely place. In another instance the wife worked as a support to her husband in his work arena—it was done for him more than for her.

Implications and connections

Four attitudes do not define an individual, let alone a marriage. The matrix is an oversimplification to make a point, or rather several points. The central point must be that marriages differ. The factors that produce stress in one situation will be unnoticed in another. The framework of marriage patterns begins to explain why, when some of the other available research is added onto it. The suggestions that spring from the framework and are strengthened by other research are:

(1) That where the activity pattern of a marriage fits that which would normally be required by the underlying *mix of personalities* there will be less 'familial' stress. In other words if an A–A (involved) couple are forced by his success and her children to adopt the traditional B–D life, there will be frustration, tension, and stress which may show up in both family and work.

(2) That our priorities and *central life interests* change as we move through the stages of life. This change in priorities will change the underlying marriage pattern. If the roles, perceptions, and activities of the two partners do not change accordingly there is liable to be stress.

(3) That the nature of one's job or role dictates certain *activity patterns*. If these activity patterns do not fit the marriage pattern which the blend of attitudes would suggest, then either the job or the attitudes or the partners must change if stress and conflict is to be avoided.

The confusion and value conflict noticed earlier in the literature on families and work usually stems from a concentration on one marriage pattern to the exclusion of the others or from a desire to blend them all together into one mould.

(1) We shall first examine the connection between personality mix and activity pattern and link this to other research findings.

We cannot change our personalities as readily as we might sometimes wish and must work and live with that mixture of predelictions, talents, and values which we have inherited and acquired by the time we reach maturity. Young and Wilmott (1973), for instance, devote a chapter of their book on *The Symmetrical Family* to managing directors. They fit clearly into the 'thrusting' quadrant and home is the 'stability zone' (in Toffler's (1973) revealing phrase). They have asymmetrical marriages but not necessarily stressful ones as long as the underlying personalities are also asymmetrical.

We have organized round the necessity of my job. There was a point in our married life when my wife felt that the demands of my job tended to conflict with married life. We managed to sort that out. My wife realised that I couldn't be complete without being absorbed in my work and there would be even greater conflict were this not so.

A B–D marriage. Or again: 'I get no satisfaction from my leisure. I have got a happy family life, and I love my family. But I don't get any real satisfaction out of anything in my life except my work.'

Although Young and Wilmott believe that their managing directors represent a small, and probably diminishing minority, they recognize that many of the middle and lower managers described by the Pahls in their study of *Managers and Their Wives* (1971) fit into the same category. But the 'thrusting' man (or woman) needs a 'caring' counterpart if his marriage is to provide a stability zone and a working life free of imported family stress. In many cases the spouse fits this category. The Pahls say:

A housewife—as most of the women in our study took for granted—is expected to subordinate her own interests to the interests of her husband, children and home. Most do this gladly most of the time, but it makes the problem of taking a job more difficult, when a wife is quite unused, both to taking initiative for herself rather than adapting herself to the daily routines of others, and also to doing things solely because she wants to.

(An example of a 'caring' wife forced by convention to behave like an 'involved' spouse?) Bardwick (1973) describes the wives of the successful men she interviewed in her study:

Their wives are traditional non-career oriented women who, predictably, found identity as wives and as mothers. 7 of the 20 men described their wives as bright and competent and they included the few women who had an achievement competence (i.e. a wife who maintained the financial ledgers; a wife who took on the presidency of an important volunteer organization; a wife who had been a corporate technical salesperson, a costume designer; a sculptor). But those wives were the exceptions and, since no wife worked full-time, the priority of the commitment was clear. Actually, the men usually described their wives very positively and when asked why they felt that way, would describe her as a wonderful wife and mother. Since all of the children were at least in school and the wife's time was freed for large portions of the day, I asked what she did with her time. Pushed, it became increasingly clear that most did nothing important.

But not all 'thrusters' are fortunate enough to have a 'caring' spouse. Bailyn (1970) found considerable unhappiness in her 'conventional' marriages. These marriages in which one partner is career oriented and the other family oriented seem to fit the B–D pattern. Yet happiness in these marriages declines as the number of children increases and as the husband gets more absorbed in his work. It is arguable that the 'caring' element in the attitudes of the wives in these partnerships was insufficient to handle the added amount of role segregation and separate responsibility brought about by a busy husband and several children. A *very* 'thrusting' spouse needs a very 'caring' partner, perhaps. The least happy (and most stressful?) of Bailyn's couples were where an 'integrated' (involved?) wife was married to a 'career-oriented' (thrusting?) husband— a B–A marriage, when only 13% of the couples claimed to have very happy marriages compared with over 50% for all other variations. The 'caring' component of an 'involved' wife is too overlaid by the 'thrusting' component to give the degree of support that a 'thrusting' husband needs to be fully happy.

In the Sloan study the 'thrusting' personalities were noticeably low on the dimension 'order' in the attitude test. It seemed from the interview data that they liked to have others to organize the minutiae of their lives so that they were free to deploy their energies more pro-actively. As one of Young and Wilmott's directors said: 'I am under pressure but I am organized in such a way that I don't feel pressurised. This is because I have a very good secretary and first-class talent around me.' If this order providing facility is removed in the home, there is likely to be real stress for the thruster. As Bardwick says, 'work crises were experienced as a goad to further effort whereas marital crises led to a re-appraisal of the self'. It can happen that the caring wife can change her own attitude priorities after her children have left and when an often absent husband no longer satisfies her affiliation and nurturing needs. If she leaves him, or starts to neglect her caring duties to him the resulting gap in his family situation can start the very stressful process of self-examination.

A–A marriages (of two 'involved' people) are a complex mix of personalities. The Rapoports found that the commonly used character types—neurotic, introverted, dominant, tough minded—did not differentiate dual career partners, presumably because they each had a similar mix of all. The A–A marriage pattern probably co-incides with Bailyn's co-ordinated marriage where both parties look for satisfaction from both work and family. Happiness is highest in these when high income coincides with high ambition in the husband. These are complicated marriages to work logistically, as the Rapoports' descriptions of their dual career couples demonstrate, and a high income does facilitate the situation. Given the mixed orientation to both family and home that is common in the A–A pattern if undue attention has to be paid to the home, then work will suffer. Since, in these patterns, each partner moves *towards* the other's stress, the work problems of the wife can at times absorb the husband's attention (or vice versa) with consequent lack of attention to the work site.

Whereas in the conventional B–D marriages the successful husband may be content to delegate the major interest in his home to his wife and will tolerate the lack of time spent with children or wife, the husband (or wife) in the co-ordinated A–A pattern will resent the growing pressures of work as he becomes successful. Rapoport and Rapoport (1975) point out that there is a correlation between advancement up the managerial ladder and the sacrifice of personal and family leisure in mid-career. The work success of the partner may lead to a greater pressure for the other to take on the domestic management role, forcing him or her down into the caring quadrant in behaviour if not in attitude. This disparity may cause jealousy, friction, and stress in the relationship.

Conversely, however, the A man is more likely to tolerate failure or a levelling off at work, since he will then be able to devote more attention to his family. Bailyn's (1970) data show that over half of her sample of mid-career people place family above the work in a ranking of sources of satisfaction. The 'thruster', frustrated at work, often finds it hard to discover another outlet for his dominance and achievement needs and the resulting vacuum leads to stress at both work and home.

We must conclude that stress will be minimized and satisfaction increased if the activities, responsibilities, and roles of the two partners correspond to their personal dispositions. If their activities fit their natural marriage patterns life will be easier than if they are forced by circumstances or convention to play the part of one marriage pattern while truly belonging to another. Bailyn (1970) has noted that the way in which family orientated people do or do not get linked with career-oriented spouses seems to be haphazard. It is probable, likewise, that love, or convention, or luck and happenstance is a more powerful welder of liaisons at the start than any conscious blend of attitudes. If we are then led by life to forswear our true 'pattern' or if that 'pattern' has changed unconsciously we shall suffer stress and discomfort in both work and family.

(2) The second suggestion was that we need to adapt our marriage patterns to accommodate our needs and interests at different stages of the family cycle. A failure to do this will result in an activity pattern at variance with the personality pattern.

Most studies (e.g. Rapoport and Rapoport, 1975) divide life interest into the three areas of work, family, and leisure. These are some established facts:

—the potential for interest in work increases as the status increases.
—Paradoxically, as competence and status increases the *main* source of satisfaction tends to shift to family or leisure.
—Women generally find family the source of principal satisfaction but over 50% of men in most studies also view the family as the central life interest.
—The areas of interest are not constant, their mix for each individual changes over time.

In a study of graduates Fogarty *et al.* (1971) found that career was the central life interest for 53% of single men but that this gave way to the family (59%) when they were married and had children, with career declining to 29%. For women the difference was even more marked. Forty-two per cent of single women preferred career and 43% 'other' but 82% of the mothers put family first.

Alice Rossi has differentiated four phases in what she terms the role cycle of families—the anticipatory or preparatory phase, the honeymoon phase, the plateau stage, and the disengagement phase. The plateau stage in particular, involving children and the management of a household, is one into which people often get catapulted by convention with little awareness of, or preparation for, the implications. It is in the plateau stage that the money needs of the family are highest while at the same time (25 to 40 years of age) the demands of work are often at their most intense.

There have been no true longitudinal studies of families living through all the stages. What data there is over time is usually culled from personal recollections. Other evidence rests on asking similar questions to apparently similar people at different stages in their lives. The suggestions that follow are therefore very speculative.

From the evidence of Fogarty's graduates it looks as if there is a shift from career to family orientation after marriage and child bearing, particularly for the women. This suggests a cycle of men moving from quadrant B (thrusting) to A (involved) and perhaps on to C (caring) in some cases, with a minority (less than a third) sticking in B. Women, who start their working lives in B or A, move predominantly in the plateau stage to C. It is probably no accident that half the marriages in the Sloan study were B–D marriages *at that point* in the family life cycle. The problem arises for that minority of wives who do not shift their priorities to fit the D (caring) quadrant, or, in some cases, for the man who does not want the B (thrusting) characteristics which a role as head of the house or breadwinner thrusts upon him.

The suggestion behind the idea of the symmetrical family (Young and Wilmott, 1973) is that of an A–A pattern. This is what Young and Wilmott term the stage 3 position. Society, however, is still largely geared to their more traditional stage 2, male dominated, role segregated family (the B–D pattern, or Bailyn's conventional marriage) except in such societies as the countries of the Communist Bloc. Fashion, education, and personal inclination may decree that the symmetrical marriage of the A–A pattern with two roles for each is desirable, but until society is re-organized particularly the work of the organizations in which 90% of us work, and until some old diehard norms disappear, it will remain a hard model to implement. As Bardwick (1973) discovered, the achievement oriented wives of the 'thrusting' husbands confined their work roles to a part-time commitment and Fogarty found that many of his working wives worked only 'as long as' they were not required at home. The true dual career marriages remain a marginal part of Western society, confined to the successful, where money lubricates the logistics, or to the poor where sheer need obliterates other family obligations.

It is likely then that we shall find many A type women in D type roles. Bailyn's finding that satisfaction decreased as husband got more successful and children increased would then be explained as an A type wife feeling drowned in her D type world. Since she would then be inadequate D type support to a B or even an A husband we might find instances of family troubles distracting the husband from his work. It is a common accusation that fashion in the form of women's liberation has made many women uncomfortable in their traditional roles. We would translate this into our model as a pressure on D type women to emulate A or even B models. If, by force of circumstances, they cannot act our their claimed desires, frustration and stress is likely to follow.

Another source of stress is likely to occur at the disengagement phase. Here the role for a D (caring) wife is diminished as children leave home; the home needs little maintenance or management while the husband is still engaged in his work commitment. Alternatively, a woman may have tolerated her caring role, subordinating her achievement and dominance instincts in order to fulfil her obligations to husband and children. Obligations satisfied, her instincts to achieve will surface once again, pushing her up into the A or even the B (thrusting) quadrant. If her husband is not attuned and sympathetic to this shift of priorities in his wife he may feel unloved, uncared-for, and neglected. The new discordance in their priorities can lead to stress. From the husband's point of view, the day when his children leave home can signal the end of his 20 years of obligation. If this moment coincides with a plateau in his career, or a time of sudden disinterest in his accustomed work, it can release a surge of experimentalism. There are plenty of recorded stories of husbands physically leaving home at this period of release from obligation to make us suspect that there must be many more who long for release from the thrusting role that obligations and youth's ambitions thrust upon them. In terms of attitudes and values this release can mean a shift into the C or 'existentialist' box—a wish to do one's own thing without ambition or involvement or the desire to dominate. To a caring wife the new behaviour can seem very strange, threatening—and stressful.

There seems to be good circumstantial evidence that priorities and values change at the junctions between honeymoon, plateau, and disengagement phases in the family cycles of many of us. One man, introduced to the matrix of four quadrants, explained that his marriage had moved from A–A to B–D, to C–C at which stage they were arranging to separate by mutual agreement. Unless the partners can adapt to the changed roles, perspectives, and priorities that a change in pattern involves there is likely to be stress. Even if this stress is mainly expressed in the family situation it is bound to affect in some degree the behaviour at work. To be a help, there has to be an appropriate, and accepted, marriage pattern at work in the family.

(3) The kind of work and job that each of us does is bound to affect our family life—if indeed one is possible at all. It is not possible to discuss marriage patterns without taking account of the nature of the work.

The Rapoports (1965) point out that work assumes its maximum personal meaning for individuals:

when the occupational role is highly individualized, notably among the professions. Other high-status occupations, e.g. executives in large corporations, demand a similar primacy of commitment, with perhaps somewhat less scope for individualized participation than the 'free' professions, but with other incentives for a high degree of involvement. Where especially gratifying incentives do not exist, as in the lower-status occupations, work has less salience, or it may take on negative significance, with different kinds of repercussions on family life.

A shift worker, a pilot, a sailor, and a travelling salesman all have jobs which remove them from home for substantial periods when other people could be interacting with their families. This way of life will tend to demand a B–D pattern from the marriage if there are children and they are to be brought up in any kind of security or continuity.

It could be argued that the dual career marriages studies by the Rapoports (1971) are relationships of high-achieving individuals who have control over the pattern of their days. These, the prototypical A–A couples, could not each share in the achievement, dominance, and affiliation which each requires without a high degree of control over their time. At the other extreme dual careers are possible where time is not controlled but is totally predictable. Young and Wilmott (1973) describe one accountant who could *guarantee* leaving the office between 5.30 and 5. 35 every day of his life. In the Sloan study there was another such man whose hour of arriving home was so precisely predictable that his wife could plan to pass him at the garden gate on her way out to her work, leaving him to assume the home responsibility (they were both 'C'—'existential'). Many factory and office workers have work lines of such predictability, a predictability which allows their partners much more scope for an independent life—should they want it.

Individuals who have very little control over their time at work will often find that they have also little scope for exercising their desires for achievement or domination (if they have such desires). They will therefore often seek to find outlets for these needs in their family or leisure lives. This is heteromorphism (different behaviour at work and at home) observed, among others, by Dubin (1956) and the Rapoports (1965) who quote C. Wright Mills's comment 'each day men sell little pieces of themselves in order to try to buy them back each night and weekend with little pieces of fun'.

While predictable work hours do make it possible for more variations of marriage pattern at home (e.g. a thrusting wife and a caring husband) the need for the man (or the woman) to compensate for lack of individuality at work may lead to a distorted and forced pattern which can cause stress. 'Involved' (A) characters, for instance, who are forced by the nature of their jobs to be solitary thrusters (actors, astronauts, racing car drivers) may overcompensate for the lacking affiliative element in their work by wanting to adopt the caring role in the family, much to the confusion of the spouse accustomed to the public thrusting image of her partner.

It is generally agreed that complementarity is the usual order of the day—we try to satisfy different needs at work and at home—and that this is particularly true where there is some degree of alienation in the work place. This should be an added argument to encourage wives to do some work or activity away from the home as a way of providing an outlet for those needs unsatisfied at home. The difficulty, however, can be to decide which area (home or work) is the residual. If the work provides all that an 'involved' woman needs there may be no 'caring' element left over for the home. If the garden or the darts team meets the man's needs for achievement, he will not be a 'thruster' at work. The switch recorded by Fogarty et al. (1973) between orientations to career and family as men and women become fathers and mothers suggests that we would like work to become more and more the residual as we move out of the honeymoon phase. Unfortunately, for many, this inclination coincides with the need to earn money and to establish oneself in one's work or career. This 'residual' conflict can easily spill over into the family with the wife resenting the man's work (his substitute 'mistress'), disliking the residual marriage pattern forced upon her and the husband agreeing with her at heart but unable in reality to do anything about it if he is to keep, and succeed at, his job.

In summary, Young and Wilmott's ideal of the symmetrical marriage, or the Rapoports' notion of dual careers, must remain a minority fact, even if a universal dream, as long as the work place dictates the family pattern. Parsons and Bales, among others, have pointed out that the tendency is nearly universal for families, and societies, to assign 'instrumental' activities to men and 'affective' activities to women. The sexual revolution has a long way to go to reduce this prevailing norm. The re-design of jobs to allow shared roles, the reduction in the working week and shorter working lives may all be steps to reducing the dominance of the work place. On the other hand the emphasis on putting more scope for individuality into work (the quality of working life), increasing labour productivity, and the general professionalization of all work roles are factors working in the opposite direction.

We must conclude that the necessary shape of the marriage pattern is going to be determined for a long time for most people by the type of work that we do and by the relative importance of that work in our lives. It is also probable that at least during the plateau child rearing stage of peak money needs the man will be pushed towards a thrusting role and the woman towards a caring posture. For some it may be possible, with careful management of their time, to maintain a joint A–A (involved) pattern. For those without children the twin 'existential' (C–C) pattern is possible, although not always long lasting. For the rest, unless the pattern forced on them by circumstances is accepted, at least for a time and for a part of their lives, there will be frustration, aggression, misunderstanding—stress.

The conclusions of all this are inevitably banal. The family should be, and can be, a complementary relationship to those of work, a place where other needs are satisfied, other behaviours welcomed, which go to make up the whole person. It should, and can be, a resting place, a place to regain any flagging strength or purpose. It should and can be the mainspring of the children's growth and future, where they acquire their values, priorities, and models of behaviour.

Conversely, if the family relationship is not right it must affect the other variables—work, the whole person, the children. The family can be both a help and a hindrance. This chapter has suggested that where the marriage pattern fits the requirement of circumstances (work and stage of life) *and* the underlying personal priorities of the individuals at that point in time, *then* the family is likely to be a help. Where the pattern is out of line with the true priorities of the partners (circumstances have priority) or where they are behaving according to their beliefs without regard to the demands of job or of family (personalities have priority), *then* the family is a hindrance, to them or to those associated with them.

In a world where most men change their jobs twice in their lives, sometimes their careers as well, move home every 8 years, where 49% of married women now work, where people grow up, marry, and have children earlier, where one in eight people (many more in California) will change partners in their marriages at some time, is it ever likely that we shall find that three-way fit between personalities, type of work, stage of life which we have argued is the recipe for the family to be a help? Are there actions that could be taken by society, by organizations or by individuals themselves which might make things easier?

To start with, it would ease the problem if there were more understanding of the nature and extent of the problem. Marriage is perhaps too private an institution, particularly in these days of the nuclear family. Individuals who have a genuine respect and affection for each other can still find that marriage is, at times, a traumatic and oppressive relationship. This chapter is an attempt to explain why this might be so. Yet so little are the problems understood that the trauma and oppression of the marriage are seen as personal failings, to be concealed from the world, gnawed upon in one's heart with anguish, or unleashed on an unwitting world in various forms of catharsis. If the processes of marriage were more talked about, made more mundane, then we might have more realistic expectations of it. No one expects one's relationship with one's siblings to be for ever rosy. There are stages to be lived through. So it can be with marriages and families. To understand all is to forgive much. A man with a pain in his stomach is much relieved to learn that it is only indigestion not cancer. The pain is no less but the anguish is.

Where should this understanding start? In *schools*, perhaps, where the education might reasonably include some preparation for life in small groups of all sorts and for the maintenance of interpersonal relationships. Why are these lessons, arguably the most crucial in our lives, the ones which we learn wholly from experience? In the media and in literature where, again, family life could be more than the source of comedy, romance or adultery, and more of an example of living in a small community. In the churches, whose intolerance of failure in a relationship of extreme difficulty, can only increase the guilt and the anxiety. In organizations, who can use the supposed privacy of the relationship as an excuse for not getting involved—but often they are involved, maybe through no fault of their own. In better provision for confidential private counselling—some organizations retain outside counsellors for the private benefit of their staff—more flexible leave and salary arrangements (the cafeteria approach to benefits in which the individual adjusts the package to his needs), more advanced notice of moves and career changes.

Then there are institutional measures which might be taken to help—women particularly. Not all married women want to work, although 49% do at present. Perhaps most do not want a full-time commitment when their children are small. But the provision of crèches and nursery schools, the understanding by employers that school holidays are difficult times, more opportunities for part-time work or for jobs shared by husband and wife, would all make it easier for the mother who did want to work to avoid becoming completely trapped in her caring (D) role. And why should not more men have the opportunity of a D role, with part-time work, or work to be done at home? There must be more opportunities for take-out work in our organizations, or for flexitime on a great scale. Any such arrangements would, by creating more flexibility around the family, make it possible for either husbands or wives to readjust their marriage patterns to suit themselves rather than their jobs or roles.

Finally of course we can help to prepare our own children to understand better the dilemmas of a relationship which we may ourselves have mishandled. In a time when so many of our institutions are under almost unbearable strain it would be a pity if this, the most ancient of them all, did not survive, if it could not be a help rather than a hindrance.

Note

1. P. Berger and C. B. Handy, *Work and Family*. Unpublished research at the London Business School.

References

Bailyn, L. (1970) Career and family orientations, *Human Relations*, **23**, 97–113.

Barker, D. C., and Allen, S. (1970) Dependence and exploitation in work and marriage, *Human Relations*, **23**, 2.

Bell, C., and Newby, H. (1976) *Husbands and Wives: the Dynamics of the Deferential Dialect*. London. Longman.

Berger, P. (1974) *Executive Job Satisfaction*. Unpublished report, London Business School.

Christenson, L. (1971) *The Christian Family*. London. Fountain Trial.

Dahlstrom, E. (1962) *The Changing Roles of Men and Women*. New York. Beacon Press.

Dubin, R. (1956) Industrial workers' worlds, *Social Problems*, January issue.

Fogarty, M. P., Rapoport, R., and Rapoport, R. N. (1971) *Sex Career and Family*. London. Allen Unwin.

Gowler, D., and Legge, K. (1971) *Managerial Stress*. Epping. Gower Press.

Jaques, E. (1976) *A General Theory of Bureaucracy*. London. Heinemann.

Marx, J. H., and Spray, S. L. (1976) Marital status and occupational success among mental health professionals, *Journal of Marriage and the Family*, February issue.

Pahl, J. M., and Pahl, R. E. (1971) *Managers and Their Wives*. London. Allen Lane.

Rapoport, R., and Rapoport, R. (1965) Work and family in contemporary society, *American Sociological Review*, **30**.

Rapoport, R., and Rapoport, R. (1971) *Dual Career Families*. London. Penguin.

Rapoport, R., and Rapoport, R. (1975) *Leisure and the Family Life-Cycle*. London. Routledge Kegan Paul.

Toffler, A. (1973) *Future Shock*. London. Panther.

Young, M., and Willmott, D. (1973) *The Symmetrical Family*. London. Routledge Kegan Paul.

PART III

Factors in the Person

Chapter 5

Personality, Behavioural, and Situational Modifiers of Work Stressors

Anthony J. McMichael

Commonwealth Scientific and Industrial
Research Organization, Adelaide

I think the simple-minded invocation of the word stress . . . has done as much to retard research in this area as did the concepts of the miasmas at the time of the discovery of microorganisms. (Cassel, 1976)

Introduction

The human mind is readily seduced by simple formulations, simple models. 'Stress', in the past, has often been viewed as an external agent, capable of inducing in the human organism a response commensurate with the amount of exogenous stress. By analogy to earlier, turn-of-the-century causal models of acute infectious disease, the role of stress, as an external and direct cause of disease, was inevitably appealing. Further, this exogenous stress was usually held to be somewhat specific in its disease producing effects. A mixture of empirical observation and intuitive reasoning led the early psychosomaticists to posit 'stress diseases' such as ulcers, hypertension, and mental disturbance as the usual specific outcomes of stressful human experience.

Ironically, Selye and Wolff, as original proponents of the concept of 'stress', envisaged it as a bodily state, and not an external component of the environment. Thus Wolff states: 'I have used the word stress in biology to indicate that state within a living creature which results from the interaction of the organism with noxious stimuli or circumstances' (quoted in Hinkle, 1973). Despite this careful formulation, many subsequent investigators have tended to apply the term 'stress' to these external noxious stimuli or circumstances. As Cassel (1976) has pointed out, this simplification of the cause–effect model with respect to external 'stress' and consequent disease, has—by analogy to the specific relationship between a particular micro-organism and its trademark disease—the corollary that there will be etiologic specificity. That is, the presumption emerges that a specific type of external stress (i.e. 'stressor') will lead to a specific 'stress disease', and that there will be a dose-response relationship (the greater the stressor, the more the likelihood of disease).

More recently, however, the prevailing formulations of the relationship of stress to disease have again become more subtle—and, inevitably, more complex. Stress is now widely viewed, not merely as something exogenous, but as the product of a dynamic mismatch between the individual and his/her physical or social environment. This interactive view of stress holds that situations are not inherently stressful; rather, it is the combination of the particular situation and an individual, with his specific personality, behavioural pattern, and life-situation circumstances, that results in a stress producing imbalance.

A related, but not identical, view of the stress producing interplay between objective environmental conditions and the psychosocial characteristics of the individual worker has been formalized in the 'person–environment fit' model—discussed in detail in chapter 7. In their comprehensive presentation of person–environment fit theory, French, Rogers, and Cobb (1974) emphasized two kinds of fit between the individual and his job environment. One kind of fit is the extent to which the person's skills and abilities match the demands and requirements of the job. For example, the goodness of fit between a particular aspect of work environment and the person might be measured by determining how much work load an individual worker has. The same individual is then asked to indicate his preference for this work characteristic; for example, 'How much work load would you like to have?' By subtracting the amount preferred by the person from the amount in the job environment, a quantitative score of person–environment fit is produced. Another kind of fit is the extent to which the needs of the person are supplied in the job environment. The basic assumption of the theory is that when person–environment misfit of either kind threatens an individual's well-being, stress will occur and manifestations such as job dissatisfaction, anxiety, depression, and physiological problems will follow.

At the 'outcome' end of this elaborated model of stress and disease, there is a growing recognition of the wide range of biological consequences of stress. While the available information still indicates that some diseases are more obviously stress related than others, it now seems probable that most, if not all, disease processes are influenced by bodily response to stress (see, for example, Cassel, 1976). This influence acts via disturbance of the body's neuroendocrinal, immunological, or other homeostatic system. A growing body of research suggests that the risk of developing a wide range of diseases, as different as cancer and chronic respiratory disease, is increased in the presence of stress.

Ironically, again, this perspective of non-specificity was embodied in Selye's (1956) formulations on stress. He envisaged a wide variety of environmental agents (or 'stressors') as all producing a common, specific pattern of bodily reaction. He postulated an initial lowering of bodily resistance, followed by an activation of bodily defence mechanisms characterized by arousal of the autonomic nervous system (with adrenaline discharge; increased heart rate, blood pressure, and muscle tone; and increased digestive secretion). If prolonged, this bodily state of persistent stimulation of the hypothalamic-hypophyseal-adrenocortical axis and generalized adrenergic responses results in a wide range of what Selye termed 'diseases of adaptation' (e.g. cardiovascular-renal diseases, rheumatism, arthritis, ulcers, inflammatory and allergic diseases, etc.)—that is, diseases caused by the body's own attempts to adapt to stress, rather than by any external agent directly. More recently, Selye (1976) has described the diseases of adaptation as those that 'depend primarily upon as excessive or inappropriate response to indirect pathogens'.

Wolff, too, wrote of the non-specific and indirect effect of stressors upon health status, reflecting their capacity to act as signals or symbols, likely to be perceived differently by each individual. Cassel (1976), in discussing how these potential stressors act by altering the neuroendocrinal balance thereby increasing the body's susceptibility to direct noxious stimuli (or 'disease agents'), reminds us that their effect is not invariant between individuals—'what is one man's meat is another's poison'. Stressors within an individual's life situation, acting as signals or symbols, trigger responses in terms of the information they are perceived to contain. Since this perception depends upon the differing personalities and the salience of the experience to different individuals, it follows that the stressfulness of any particular life situation is very much determined by these personal 'conditioning variables'.

These two basic conceptual developments in stress theory (i.e. stress resulting from interactive imbalance between individual and environment, and the etiologic non-specificity of stress) might be seen more clearly by analogy to a similar progression of research thinking in the area of cigarette smoking and lung cancer. The original question, in the 1950s, was relatively simple: 'Does smoking increase the risk of lung cancer?' Comparative follow-up study of populations of smokers and non-smokers enabled epidemiologists to answer, statistically, 'Yes'. But then a more subtle question arose: 'So, why do only a minority of all smokers actually get lung cancer?' This question has prompted a search for a particular high-risk combination—the individual who is inherently more susceptible (perhaps because he possesses a particular configuration of respiratory tract enzymes) to the potentially carcinogenic effect of exogenous cigarette smoke. Simultaneously, cigarette smoking has been implicated in an increasing number of diseases—for example, cancer of the urinary bladder, coronary artery disease, and low birth weight. As with stress, the modes of action, and the biological consequences, of cigarette smoke are now known to be more subtle, more complex, and more diverse than was previously thought. It has taken several decades of research to shrug off, and more beyond, the simple cause–effect models of nineteenth century infectious disease research.

Stress research, however, has been hampered by more than the distracting legacy of earlier models. There has also been a tendency to regard it as a less fruitful source of explanation of human disease than the study of more palpable infectious or noxious physicochemical agents. As witnesses to the human condition, we are all too readily conditioned, imprisoned, by the boundaries of our own cultural experience; accordingly, we underestimate the extent to which the stresses of life and work, within our culture, can impose demands on the human organism that are different from and, perhaps, greater than those that prevailed during the millenia of human evolution. The pressures, priorities, and conflicts arising from latter-day human social organization have often gone largely unrecognized as potent contributors to tipping the balance of health towards disease. Now, however, that recognition is becoming well established; and, increasingly, these demands of daily existence are understood as substantial, although not sole, determinants of stressful human experience and a wide range of consequent diseases.

One final remark will help introduce this discussion of the ways in which an individual's characteristics interact with his work environmental circumstances, in the genesis of stress. To paraphrase John Donne, no man exists in a social vacuum. While personality and behavioural attributes, at a single point in time, can perhaps be comfortably construed as the exclusive property of the individual, nevertheless his response to a potentially stressful work environment is also influenced by an assortment of life-situational factors—factors that constitute his social environment. The discussion that follows will therefore consider, on the one hand, personality and behavioural traits, and, on the other, social environmental characteristics as related but distinct factors that influence the experiencing and perception of stress at work.

Conceptual model

There are many potentially stressful circumstances (stressors) within the work environment—some predominantly 'objective' and quantifiable (e.g. fast machine paced assembly line work, heavy work load), and some rather more qualitative (e.g. work role ambiguity, unsympathetic or inaccessible superiors). However, not all people will experience a given job situation as stressful, nor will a given individual experience all job situations as equally stressful. Rather, stress occurs when the abilities of the person are incongruent with the demands of the job environment, or where clear obstacles exist to fulfilling strong needs or values. In such situations, there is a bad 'fit' between the individual and his environment. It thus becomes crucial to consider what, and how, aspects of personality, behaviour, and social circumstance influence an individual's response to potential stressors.

As indicated above, the fundamental premise underlying the following discussion is that different individuals will react differently to the same work environmental conditions—some finding them comfortable and rewarding, others experiencing them as quite stressful. For example, one person finds a job working with people very satisfying, while another finds it a source of stress or dissatisfaction because of a lower need for interpersonal affiliation. House (1974a) emphasizes that the experiencing of stress is a subjective response which results from a combination of particular objective conditions of work and particular personal characteristics (e.g. abilities or needs). Characteristics of social situations (e.g. highly competitive peers) may also combine with conditions of work (e.g. heavy work load) to produce stress. The likely outcomes of given work environment stressors can therefore be predicted much more accurately if we also know other relevant individual and/or social situational characteristics.

Further, even if a number of people report the same amount of subjective stress in their work, seldom do they all incur the same type or degree of psycho-physiological response, or ultimately, illness. How the person responds to the stressful situation is of crucial importance. In the face of a heavy work load one person may successfully reorganize his style of work, or gain new skills, or successfully call on others for help; while another flounders along, unable to alleviate the stress, and may ultimately incur a heart attack. To predict whether a person copes well or poorly under stress requires additional know-ledge of individual and social situational characteristics which determine what a person can do (or is likely to do) in response, and how successful he will be.

In reviewing recent stress research theory, House (1974b) has identified and integrated five classes of variables into a proposed comprehensive paradigm of stress research: (1) objective social conditions conducive to stress; (2) individual perceptions of stress; (3) individual responses (physiological, affective, and behavioural) to perceived stress; (4) more enduring outcomes of perceived stress and responses thereto; and (5) individual and situational conditioning variables that influence (or 'specify') the relationships among the first four sets of factors. Figure 5.1, as synthesized by House, presents a model relating these five classes of variables. The arrows between boxes indicate hypothesized causal relationships, while the arrows descending from the box labelled 'conditioning variables' indicate that these individual and social variables 'condition' the nature of these relationships. (Notice that the term 'conditioning' is used in stress research not only in the Pavlovian sense, but also to designate those factors that can influence the individual's mental or physical receptivity to a stressor.) Similar models have been proposed by other investigators (e.g. French, 1963; Caplan et al., 1975), but, importantly, all incorporate the notion of conditioning variables, both personal and situational.

This chapter is primarily concerned with the nature and operation of these conditioning variables, as they influence the impact of potential stressors within the work environment. In House's words, 'we must be attuned to when and why potentially stressful situations are, or are not, perceived as stressful by the persons involved'. We are therefore concerned, as another example, to understand why two different employees, each with his differing temperament, abilities, training, and social circumstances, will react differently to the same objective levels of work supervisory responsibility—one may find it a pleasant challenge, while the other may experience it as more than he can handle.

Despite the heuristic nature of the model proposed in Figure 5.1, in seeking to integrate the five interdependent classes of variables that permeate current stress research theory, the primary purpose of this chapter is to consider the relationship between classes 1, 2, and 5 (i.e. objective circumstances, subjective perception, and intervening conditioning variables). However, it will obviously be necessary to consider how some of these 'conditioning' variables not only

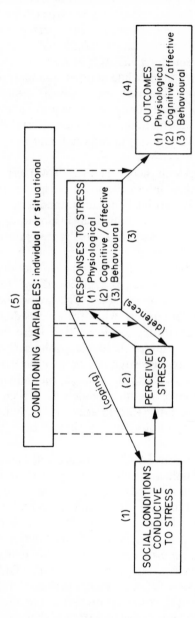

Figure 5.1 A paradigm of stress research

Note: Solid arrows between boxes indicate presumed causal relationships among variables. Dotted arrows from box(5) intersect solid arrows, indicating an interaction between the conditioning variables and the variables in boxes (1), (2) and (3) in predicting variables in box (4). Reproduced from House (1974b), by permission of American Sociological Association determine the extent to which the work environment is actually perceived and experienced as stressful, but how they also then influence both the psychophysiological response to stress, and the effect of that response in producing disease states.

Nearly all of the information gleaned about the relationships between these classes of variables, in human workers, has necessarily been gathered from non-experimental epidemiologic studies of work environment, stress response, and health outcomes. While one major strength of this approach is its being earthed in the reality of complex human experience, an inevitable disadvantage is the inability to determine, in classic experimental mode, the specific, unbiased effect of each particular relevant psychosocial variable. Ethical constraints normally preclude the random allocation of individual workers into two or more work environments, identical in every respect except for the one, or perhaps several, variable(s) of interest. For this reason, the 'proof of existence' of these stress conditioning phenomena depends heavily on, first, the replication of findings in diverse study settings where valid measurements of variables have been made and where the chronology of human experience is apparent, and, second, the psychophysiological plausibility of the inferred phenomena.

Personality and behavioural factors

Perhaps the most widely discussed personal characteristic contributing to stress at work, in recent years, has been the Type A versus Type B differentiation. Particularly, it has been associated with an increased risk of heart disease. It will therefore be accorded primacy in this section.

By far the most frequent cause of death in Western society today is coronary heart disease, or 'heart attack'. Myocardial ischemia, causing symptoms known as angina pectoris, and often progressing to life threatening myocardial infarction, has attained epidemic proportions within the adult population aged over 40. This disease, as is well known, has long been regarded as one of the pre-eminent 'stress diseases'. The 'epidemic proportions' of heart disease and related circulatory disorders in modern societies have made them the central focus of those interested in the effects of work stress upon health.

In 1900, cardiovascular diseases accounted for less than a quarter of deaths in the Western world, but for the past 20 years they have accounted for over half of all deaths. The elimination of cardiovascular diseases as causes of death would increase life expectancy by approximately 10 years—more than four times the gain that would be achieved by elimination of any other cause of death. Coronary heart disease accounts for one-third of all deaths (i.e. the majority of cardiovascular disease deaths). The problem is particularly serious among younger males, with coronary heart disease being the leading cause of death among males from age 35 on. The second leading cause of mortality from cardiovascular disease is cerebrovascular disease ('stroke'), accounting for just over one-tenth of all deaths. In general, there are many similarities in the biomedical factors (e.g. high blood pressure, smoking, cholesterol) predisposing people to both coronary heart disease and 'stroke'.

During the past 25 years, extensive epidemiologic and clinical research has documented and sought to quantify the now well recognized coronary heart disease risk factors—obesity, blood pressure, serum lipids, cigarette smoking, age, exercise pattern, and family history. More recently, attention has been paid to the question: is there a pattern or style of behaviour that, like these other risk factors, permits prospective identification of persons at higher risk of coronary heart disease?

Cumulative epidemiologic evidence suggests there is a positive answer to this question. Scientists in the United States, the Netherlands, Australia, and Israel have independently reported empirical studies of coronary heart disease patients and control groups indicating that patients with coronary disease strive more diligently towards achievement, are more perfectionist, tense and unable to relax, put forth more effort and commitment to job or profession, and are more active and energetic than their corresponding comparison groups (Jenkins, 1971). These four traits are compatible with one another and, considered as a single syndrome, they approximate the 'coronary-prone behaviour pattern' (Type A) as formulated by Friedman and Rosenman, who also included the important ingredients of aggressiveness and time urgency as essential parts of the behaviour pattern (Rosenman et al., 1964; Friedman, 1969).

It must be recognized that 'Type A' does not describe a static personality trait, nor is it a stress reaction; rather, it is a style of behaviour with which some persons habitually respond to circumstances that arouse them. It follows readily, then, that this behaviour predisposition may be a potent conditioning variable, likely to render work environment stressors into obvious stressful experience with severe disease enhancing consequences. Research since 1970, at many research centres, has demonstrated repeatedly that the Type A pattern can be reliably rated and is a deeply ingrained, enduring trait. A comprehensive and up-to-date review of this recent research has been compiled by Jenkins (1976).

A central example of the epidemiologic research carried out on the role of Type A behaviour in increasing the risk of coronary heart disease is the Western Collaborative Group Study (WCGS), carried out prospectively in the United States over an 8·5-year period (Rosenman et al., 1964, 1970, 1975). All members of the study population underwent a structured interview, at the onset of the period of follow-up, specifically designed to measure the coronary-prone behaviour pattern. The incidence rates of clinical coronary heart disease after 4·5, 6·5, and 8·5 years of follow-up have shown that men judged as Type A at intake had 1·7 to 4·5 times the risk of new coronary heart disease as men judged as Type B (i.e. relaxed and easy-going). The behaviour pattern was judged 'blind', without knowledge of the presence or absence of other cardiovascular disease risk factors, and subsequent diagnosis of disease was made without knowledge of behaviour type or risk factors. More recently, multivariate predictive data analysis of the WCGS data by Brand et al. (1976) has reconfirmed the independent risk status of the Type A behaviour pattern in coronary heart disease.

Of course, the description of the Type A style—intense striving for achievement, competitiveness, easily provoked impatience, time urgency, abruptness of gesture and speech, overcommitment to vocation or profession, and excessive drive and hostility—strikes ready chords of recognition in most of us, as indeed does the converse, easy-going behaviour pattern, Type B. Although Friedman and Rosenman have systematically studied, packaged, and labelled this behaviour pattern, it was clearly anticipated by Dunbar (1943). She studied an uncontrolled series of coronary patients, and characterized them thus: 'compulsive striving; urge to get on top through hard work, self-discipline, and mastery of others . . . they are strongly governed by their principles, and their sense of propriety . . . they attempted to subdue or surpass authority and dislike sharing responsibility'.

Beyond that accumulated, and compelling, evidence for the existence of an identifiable coronary-prone behaviour pattern, Type A, the question arises within the work context: how does the Type A disposition act, as a conditioning variable, to increase the perception and experiencing of stress at work? Alternatively, perhaps it acts directly rather than as a 'conditioner'. Sales, however, implying that this trait might not act as a simple conditioning variable, has suggested that the Type A person possesses personality traits (e.g. impatience, ambition, competitiveness, aggressiveness) that cause self-selection into jobs that entail greater exposure to stressors (Sales, 1969)—rather like the proverbial warhorse, relishing the smell of battle. Similarly, House (1972) suggested that a central psychological trait of the Type A is his 'desire for social achievement' (reflected in ambition, competitiveness, aggressiveness, etc.), a trait apparently analogous to what others term 'status seeking' or extrinsic motivation for working (i.e. desire for money, status, recognition) as opposed to intrinsic motivation (i.e. desire for interesting, self-satisfying work).

In a wide ranging study of job demands and worker health in the United States (Caplan et al., 1975), 23 jobs were selected to represent a diversity of job stressors, care being taken to include jobs known to have high rates of illness (e.g. air traffic controllers and train dispatchers). A questionnaire was administered to 2010 men employed in these jobs, and physiological data were collected from 390 of these men in eight of the 23 jobs. The questionnaire measured 20 types of job stressors, 17 types of 'strain' (i.e. stressful experience), and a variety of demographic and personality variables, including Type A/B disposition.

The investigators recognized that different group experiences of job stress, between the 23 job groups, might reflect, at least partially, differences in the type of person within that job. Self-selection, selection by employers, and changes in personality traits as a result of socialization by the job may all produce such differences. If so, this would be consistent with Sales' hypothesis (Sales, 1969—see also above) that persons with particular personality and behaviour characteristics tend to seek out certain types of work environment.

Caplan and his co-workers found that, with respect to the Type A behaviour pattern, administrative professors and family physicians scored highest. This finding on administrative professors is consistent with earlier studies of professors and administrators in academic settings (e.g. French *et al.*, 1965) in which the administrators had higher scores on measures of achievement orientation than did the professors (predominantly non-administrative). Although there appear to be no previous published studies of Type A among the medical profession, Russek (1960) reports that general practitioners, such as family physicians, have a much greater risk of coronary heart disease than medical specialists. Among the blue collar workers studied, the occupation with the highest Type A score was tool and die making, while the lowest score was for the assemblers on machine paced lines and the continuous flow monitors. The score difference entailed more than a two-fold variation.

Similar differences were found for the Personality Flexibility score, with professors, scientists, computer programmers, engineers, and physicians scoring high, and many of the blue collar groups scoring low (forklift drivers and train dispatchers had the lowest score—i.e. they were assessed to be the least flexible, the most rigid). This pattern of flexibility scores suggests, generally, good compatibility between mind and job—in other words, good person-environment fit. Academics live in a world of uncertainty, a world where 'yes' and 'no' answers to problems are rare. The endless quest, through scientific research, for knowledge is very dependent on the ability to seek and intellectually exploit contradictions and ambiguities. For the physician, too, great flexibility is required—no prescription is ever a certain cure, no diagnosis is ever a certain truth. The rigid person, on the other hand, tends to agree with such questionnaire items as: 'Our thinking would be a lot better off if we could just forget words like "probably", "approximately", and "perhaps".' Such persons should fit best in jobs where clear rules and obvious criteria exist for making decisions. So it seems likely that selective processes are at least partly responsible for the inter-occupation differences in flexibility—although, of course, education (itself highly correlated with flexibility) is also a basic criterion in selection into different occupations.

Another approach, perhaps with more immediate intuitive appeal, to the meaning of the Type A behaviour pattern holds that, under potentially stressful objective conditions, Type A persons are more prone to perceive stress, maybe in quite exaggerated fashion. It is easy to envisage such a person, enmeshed in his inexorable torrent of life, creating harsh but unnecessary self-imposed deadlines and work standards; making a mountain of urgency and perfection out of a molehill of moderate work demands. Caplan (1971) found support for this contention in his research on professionals in the US National Aeronautics and Space Administration. He proposed that the dramatic and consistent results derived from the Friedman–Rosenman programme of research may have been due to the fact that the classification of a person as Type A indicates that he both possesses certain behavioural traits, and experiences greater situational pressures. Reviewing Caplan's study, House (1974b) concluded that the role of personality and behaviour in leading men into situations of stress and/or in accentuating the effects of such situations will only be clarified by further research. In the meantime, there is clear empirical evidence that the Type A person both experiences more stress at work, and experiences more coronary heart disease, with the latter apparently partially due to the former.

Despite the recent prominence of the Type A research hypothesis, other facets of personality and behaviour have also been studied in the context of job stress. The extent to which role conflict at work, as a source of 'tension', is conditioned by psychosocial factors has been studied by Kahn and co-workers (1964). They selected 53 people from major American corporations, to represent the full range of jobs from first-level supervisor to corporate officer. Data were collected by interview, written questionnaire, and personality test from each of the 53. Interviews were also conducted with 381 other persons who had been identified as members of the role sets of the 53 'focal persons'. These 381 people held jobs that made them functionally interdependent with the 53 focal persons, and hence their expectations and demands defined the roles of the 53. The degree of conflict or harmony, ambiguity or clarity, in the role requirements confronting the focal 53 persons was thus determined, as was the type and degree of resultant stress.

Kahn found that the responses of individuals to role conflict were not uniform, but were mediated or 'conditioned' by the personality of the focal person and by the quality of his interpersonal relations. Under high-conflict conditions, people who generally tended to be anxiety-prone experienced the conflict as more intense, and reacted to it with greater tension than people who were not anxiety-prone. Similarly, introverts reacted more negatively to role conflict than did extroverts; they suffered more tension and reported more deteriorated interpersonal relations. The personality dimension of flexibility–rigidity mediated still more strongly the relationship between role conflict and tension, with the flexible people accounting for almost the entire tension producing effect of role conflict, and the rigid people reporting virtually no greater tension in the high-conflict situation than in the low.

With respect to the conditioning effect of on-the-job interpersonal relations, Kahn found that the more frequent the communication between role senders and focal person, the greater the functional dependence of the focal person on the role set—and the more the signs of stress he showed when role conflict occurred.

In another industrial epidemiologic study in the United States, Christenson and Hinkle (1961) found that managers in a company who, by virtue of their family background, socio-economic status, and educational experience, were least well prepared for the demands and expectations of industrial manage-ment, were at greater risk of disease than age matched managers who were better prepared. They found that this increase in disease risk included all diseases, major as well as minor, physical as well as mental, and long term as well as short term.

In a study of the relationship of work load to stressful experience (as reflected by job dissatisfaction), Harrison (1975) has analysed questionnaire data gathered from four occupational groups—administrators, policemen, scientists, and assembly line workers—themselves a sample of the larger study described above (Caplan *et al.*, 1975). The relationship between work underload and job dissatisfaction changes from one occupation to another. Work underload seems to have little effect on the job dissatisfaction of assembly line workers and policemen. Work underload increases job dissatisfaction for administrators, and tends to increase job dissatisfaction for scientists, though the relationship is less clear than for administrators.

Why should the relationship between work load and job satisfaction vary across these occupations? Harrison suggests an explanation concerning intrinsic gratification in various occupations. Professionals such as scientists and administrators have been found to want a high level of intrinsic satisfaction in their jobs. Work underload can reduce the availability of intrinsic satisfaction and thus increase overall job dissatisfaction. Assembly line workers have been found to be less concerned about intrinsic satisfaction in their jobs. Work underload would therefore not be expected to increase their job dissatisfaction. This explanation may possibly apply to policemen as well.

Of course, not only can personal variables act as modifiers of the stress inducing effect of work environment stressors, but those stressors can themselves vary from day to day. Work stress can thus acquire a type of 'seasonality', in which the interplay between altered levels of both stressor and conditioning variable becomes more complex. For example, in a fascinating earlier study, Friedman *et al.* (1957) reported observing marked increases in serum cholesterol in American tax accountants as the 15 April deadline for filing Federal income tax returns approached. Similarly, other studies have found significantly higher levels of cholesterol in students on the day before exams as compared with times when they were not facing exams. It is plausible that these changes are attributable to increased work load under the pressure of tax deadlines or examinations. They also appear to highlight what it is about work overload, as opposed to sheer work load, that makes it stressful—the feeling that one does not have enough time or ability and hence may fail.

Now, whereas individual personality and behaviour can be construed as aspects of the worker as person, there are equally important aspects of his life situation, his social circumstances, that modify his perception and experience of stress at work. These are discussed in the following section.

Social situational factors

Cassel (1976), discussing how psychosocial factors can alter the susceptibility of an individual to external stressors, emphasizes that a more explicitly fullsome, 'two dimensional' approach is needed. Not only can psychosocial conditioning variables increase the experiencing of stress (and subsequent disease), but they can also act beneficially, as protective buffers. In Cassel's words, they might be 'envisioned as the protective factors buffering or cushioning the individual from the physiologic or psychologic consequences of exposure to the stressor situation'.

Kaplan *et al.* (1973) have suggested that a characteristic common to most social environmental stressor situations is the inability of the individual to obtain meaningful information which indicates that his actions are leading to desired consequences. For example, such circumstances would pertain in most situations—at work or elsewhere—of role conflict, role ambiguity, blocked aspirations and cultural discontinuity. In these situations, they believe that the protective factors are largely a function of the nature, strength, and availability of social supports.

The question then arises as to how, psychobiologically, this stressor-conditioning effect of social–situational variables operates. The mechanisms or processes through which such interpersonal relationships may function have been predominantly a matter of speculation. Theories have been advanced, however, at both the biological and the psychosocial level. Bovard (1962) has suggested an attractive biological theory, whereby stressful stimuli are mediated through the posterior and medial hypothalamus leading, via the release of a chemotransmitter of the anterior pituitary, to a general protein catabolic effect (i.e. breakdown of protein). He further suggests that a second centre, located in the anterior and lateral hypothalamus, when stimulated by an appropriate social stimulus (e.g. the availability of a supportive relationship) induces in the organism a 'competing response' which inhibits, masks or screens the stress stimulus such that the latter has a minimal effect. While these mechanisms have been reasonably well documented in animal research, and afford a clearly plausible explanation for many of the experimental findings, there is no certainty that such processes function in this manner in humans.

Both animal and human studies have provided evidence supporting the beneficial effects of social support mechanisms. For example, Conger *et al.* (1958) have shown that the occurrence of peptic ulcers in rats, following an unanticipated series of electric shocks, is markedly influenced by whether the animals are shocked in isolation (high ulcer rates) or in the presence of litter mates (low ulcer rates). Henry and Cassel (1969) produced persistent hypertension in mice by placing them in intercommunicating boxes all linked to a common feeding place, thereby developing a state of territorial conflict. Hypertension only occurred, however, when the mice were 'strangers'. Populating the system with litter mates did not produce these effects.

The evidence from human epidemiologic studies, inevitably non-experimental in this context, is less consistent and compelling. This may be largely due to lack of awareness by many investigators that social supports are likely to be protective against adverse health consequences only in the presence of stressors. But overall, the findings have been in the same direction as those of the animal experimental studies. In particular, a number of occupational epidemiologic studies have given support to the hypothesis that supportive social relations can protect a worker from the detrimental effects of occupational stressors.

An early study in this area was located in the mountains of Appalachia (eastern United States), where the population had been isolated from developing civilization for about 150 years (Cassel and Tyroler, 1961). In the early 1900s a factory was established in one of the mountain coves, and over the ensuing 50–60 years recruited its labour force from the surrounding mountain cove communities. By 1960, the factory was populated by about 3000 workers living in the company town, eating similar diets, and doing the same work for the same pay. In the course of the study, two categories of workers were distinguishable: those who were the first of their family to leave behind their life in the traditional mountain community for a new and strange life in the factory town (where relationships, rights, and obligations were no longer determined by kinship, and where personal identity and worth did not depend on the family one came from), and those whose fathers had worked in the same factory before them. The company, as would be expected, made no distinction whatever between these two groups, and the only way they could be identified was by examining the company records to find out whether a particular worker had had a relative of the same name there before him.

The investigators hypothesized that the second group, by virtue of previous family experience in the industrial setting, would be better prepared for the expectations and demands of industrial living than the first group, and should therefore be healthier. Using components of a widely used and validated health questionnaire (the Cornel Medical Index) to assess health status, this prediction held true. The better health of the 'second generation' workers was evident at all ages of study subjects, and was deemed to indicate that the better attuned family support of the second generation workers acted as a buffer against the otherwise unsettling and stressful experiences of a major subcultural dislocation.

Other more recent studies have reported similar findings with respect to the beneficial effects of social support in reducing the impact of work environment stressors. Caplan (1971) reported that, for a sample of US National Aeronautical and Space Administration scientists, administrators, and engineers, good work relations, particularly with one's subordinates, served as a buffer between a variety of environmental stressors (especially ambiguities within work related role sets) and resultant psychophysiological stress. It may be that peers and supervisors are perceived as the sources of the ambiguities, and are thus unlikely candidates to be called upon for support. Caplan suggests that relations with subordinates show such strong effects because the person expects that they will help him to remedy the situation. Role ambiguity was likely to lead to elevated levels of serum cortisol only if the worker experienced poor interpersonal relations with his or her subordinates. Similarly, a positive relationship existed between work load and serum glucose and blood pressure only among those having poor relations with their supervisor, coworkers, and subordinates.

Gore (quoted in Quinn, 1975) studied the reactions over a 2-year period of middle-aged, blue collar men who had lost their jobs because of plant closings. For most of her indicators of stress she concluded that 'the individuals most at risk were those who both experienced considerable unemployment and were inadequately supported'. Under similar objective conditions of stress, the socially supported men within this population were protected from harmful consequences in terms of cholesterol levels, days with illness complaints, and incidence of peptic ulcer. Investigating the effects of role ambiguity upon workers in five employing establishments, Beehr (quoted in Quinn, 1975) reported that 'people who perceive their supervisor as supportive are less likely to experience role strain in ambiguous work roles than people who do not'. While this difference was in the direction just stated with regard to five of Beehr's seven measures of stress (life dissatisfaction, low self-esteem, depressed mood, work related illnesses and injuries, and somatic complaints), none of the differences was statistically significant.

With regard to the function of social support, the laboratory work of Schachter (1959) provides a useful point of departure. He studied the effects of experimentally induced states of anxiety on the desire to be with people, i.e. 'the affiliative tendency'. His results may be interpreted to suggest that affiliative tendencies are the manifestation of 'needs for anxiety reduction and needs for self-evaluation'. Ambiguous situations or feelings lead to a desire to be with others as a means of socially evaluating and determining the 'appropriate and proper reaction'.

In a recent cross-sectional survey of the American work force, Hite (1975) studied the correlates of not being adequately challenged by one's work. He found that lack of challenge was most closely associated with low self-esteem and depressed mood where workers reported receiving inadequate support from their supervisors and co-workers.

In an ongoing epidemiologic study among a population of 1809 white male American rubber workers (blue collar workers), Wells (1977) has examined the conditioning effect of perceived social support upon the relationship between perceived work stress and health. Data were gathered with a mail questionnaire, to which a 70% response rate was attained. The three items that measured social support asked the worker to indicate how much support he perceived as originating from each of four separate sources: his supervisor, wife, co-workers, and friends and relatives. The correlation among these four reported levels of social support was not great. The measures of perceived stress included job satisfaction, work self-esteem, and five measures derived from principal components analysis of a number of job pressure items (job versus non-job conflict, role conflict, concern for quality, responsibility, and work load). The five health outcomes were self-reported symptoms or angina pectoris (myocardial ischemic pain), ulcers, skin itch and/or rash, persistent cough and phlegm, and neurotic symptoms. Intercorrelations among these five health outcomes were generally low.

The pattern of results reported by Wells indicated that the socio-emotional support of wives and supervisors was much more effective in mitigating the effects of perceived stress on health than was the support of co-workers and friends and relatives, that this support particularly protected workers against developing ulcers in response to perceived stress, and that this support was more effective in alleviating the effects of feelings of deprivation or lack of rewards (such as satisfaction and self-esteem) than in mitigating the effects of pressures or job demands which exceeded the worker's capabilities. This pattern has obvious plausibility, since emotional support can help to de-emphasize the importance of these feelings ('don't worry about it, it's not important'), or to modify workers' goals or motivations ('don't expect so much from yourself/your job'). In this regard, a worker's supervisor is best placed to help him deal with feelings of personal inadequacy at work, while wives can suggest that negative feelings about the job are unimportant along-side non-work rewards (family life, leisure, etc.).

Notice that this study highlights the importance of considering the source of social support. The much greater importance of support from supervisor than from co-worker suggests that organizational and hierarchical factors may be critical in this context. With respect to support from outside the work place, wife support is more important in conditioning work stress than is friend and relative support. These findings call into question theories which emphasize strong peer group and kinship relations and a firm division between the sexes as characteristic of the blue collar workforce.

Clearly, research in this area is bedevilled by methodologic pitfalls, such as ensuring valid measures of actual perception or experience, obtaining, in addition, measures of the objective (as opposed to perceived) presence of work environment stressors and social support, and determining the chronology of events (e.g. does perceived stress precede illness, or vice versa?). In contrast to the general tenor of the above mentioned studies, Pinneau (see Quinn, 1975) analysed social support among men selected from 23 occupations, and concluded that 'evidence . . . that social support reduced physiological strains, or that it buffered against any type of strain, was quite weak. In the many tests for interactions between support and job stresses in producing psychological strains, results were inconsistent. The significant results equally supported and opposed the buffering hypothesis and may be attributable to chance'.

These various studies, and their inconsistencies, argue against advocating social support as an all-purpose buffer against occupational stress. Indeed, this is one of the major points emphasized by Wells. Locating an all-purpose social support buffer may prove just as elusive as identifying the stress resistant individual. What is more likely to emerge from future research is a more detailed specification of the circumstances under which social support does and does not ameliorate the perception and effects of stress at work. Quinn (1975), arguing in favour of a refinement of research in this area, a specifying of more detailed research questions, writes:

While these questions may seem to treat one concept—social support—too exquisitely, answers to them seem necessary if solutions are to be adequately tuned to the requirements of stress situations and to the people who are subjected to them. Otherwise, we may be lead to propose solutions that are prematurely intended as panaceas but turn out to have more limited effectiveness. As a result, the solutions may be entirely discarded when they should in fact only be applied more selectively. Research is obliged to suggest to practitioners both what solutions should be applied and the circumstances under which they will be most effective.

Conclusion

In the world of work, with rows of assembly line, blue collar workers and corridors of neatly pigeon holed, white collar workers, it is easy to underestimate, even ignore, the individuality of each worker. Workers of all shades of collar colour are, after all, people—not personnel. Given this ever present, marked human variability, it follows that an individual's response to his work environment will be idiosyncratic; tempered by his past experiences, his current attitudes and aptitudes, and all the psychosocial subtleties of his life situation. Work environment stressors, therefore, induce different types and amounts of stress in different workers.

The social psychologists have refined this general idea, and have offered it to us as Symbolic Interaction Theory. Yet the essence of this grand sounding theory differs little from the essence of the preceding discussion—namely, that an individual perceives and interprets his environment on his own terms. The objective reality that surrounds an individual at work translates into personal symbols and signals; situations that are perceived as burdensome, threatening, ambiguous, or boring are likely to induce stress.

The growing awareness, and documentation, of how an individual worker's response to environmental stressors is conditioned by personal and life situational variables accords with a similar growing awareness in other areas of biomedical research. And, ultimately, all such awareness is, implicitly, a recognition of how the process of natural selection necessarily operates.

The evolution of species depends upon a relentless screening, by trial-and-error, of interactions between individual organisms and their environment. Genetically determined variability between individual members of a species is a prerequisite for the evolutionary process, and such variability is therefore a fundamental fact of human existence. It follows, then, that individual workers, with genetically determined differences supplemented by socioculturally determined differences, when exposed to a given micro-environment at work, will experience it and respond to it differently. Those workers who are most compatible with that environment will 'survive' best or longest. Those less compatible will either move away from that environment, or will function (in a psychophysiological sense) poorly in it.

Recently, human variability in susceptibility to the effect of exogenous physicochemical agents has commanded an increasing attention from biomedical researchers. Within the occupational setting, this perspective is gradually overshadowing a tendency to regard individual members of a given group of workers, exposed to some noxious agent, as being at uniformly increased risk. Recognition that there must be unseen determinants of why an exposed individual either does or does not succumb to the potential adverse effects, and that, given improved research technology, these determinants may now be identifiable and measurable, opens up the possibility of important new biological insights—and improved occupational preventive medicine programmes.

Occupational respiratory disease affords several ready examples of 'conditioned' susceptibility to industrial exposure agents. Epidemiologic studies have consistently revealed an increased risk of mesothelioma (a rare type of lung cancer) in asbestos workers. However, with uniform asbestos exposure experience, the individual risk nevertheless varies markedly depending on whether or not the individual is a cigarette smoker. Non-smokers are at only negligibly increased risk of mesothelioma, whereas smokers are at greatly increased risk (Hammond and Selikoff, 1972). Thus, the consequence of inhaling asbestos fibres is modified, or conditioned, quite crucially by the presence or absence of cigarette smoking. Similarly, the risk of developing chronic respiratory disease from prolonged exposure to dusts is altered dramatically by the presence or absence of an enzyme, alpha-antitrypsin, in the mucosa of the respiratory tract (Mittman et al., 1973). This enzyme, whose level of activity is genetically determined, is thus a major determinant of the actual impact of the exogenous factor, dust.

Despite differences in terminology (epidemiologists would usually refer to the above two respiratory examples as 'synergistic interaction' or 'effect modification', while sociologists may refer to stressor modification as 'conditioning') the phenomena are essentially identical. Indeed, it would be quite in accord with Selye's original formulations (see Introduction) to refer to all such noxious physicochemical agents as 'stressors'.

In striving to illuminate the psychosocial phenomena involved in the experiencing of, and responding to, occupational stress, different investigators have proposed models of varying elaboration and complexity. Given that models are not themselves reality, but are merely stylized, and necessarily simplified, representations of an inferred reality, the risks of overly elaborate models should be borne in mind. A good model must, among other things, communicate and inform—by capturing the essential ideas, without distracting by the inclusion of unwarranted detail. For example, the proposed addition (Caplan et al., 1975) of the 'person–environment fit' as a separate and distinct entity within their model, impinging in supplemental fashion upon the five entities represented in Figure 5.1, appears to introduce an unnecessary level of statistical abstraction. It could be argued that it merely represents an approach towards analysing and labelling the data, and does not introduce a new and distinct conceptual entity. After all, the notion of person–environment fit is already implicit in simpler models, of which Figure 5.1 is representative—tension between boxes 1 and 5, when job conditions and personal resources are incongruent, is, by commonsense definition, person–environment misfit.

However, models aside, the recent emphasis upon the phenomenon of individual idiosyncratic conditioning of stressor impact has greatly advanced our insights into the nature of 'stress at work'. As our knowledge grows in this area, so we will better understand that it is not possible to build, physically, an inherently stress-free working environment. Manipulation of the assembly line or of office layout, while usually desirable, is not enough—it must necessarily be supplemented with an enlightened flexibility regarding the demands made by management, supervisors, or their equivalent of the individual worker. Recent widely publicized experiments by the Volvo Company, in Sweden, dismantling the tyranny of the assembly line, and allowing greater production autonomy among workers building cars, are a step in the right direction.

One final and increasingly relevant sidelight on this issue relates to stress *after* work, rather than stress *at* work. With the steady reduction in the retirement age, and the gradual increase in life expectancy, the issue of a happy, healthy life after retirement assumes increasing social significance. Retirement, as a major life change, is associated with a number of potential stressors— loss of income, loss of social identity, and removal from peer group—and is likely to prove stressful for some categories of persons. Research findings in this as yet relatively neglected area have been recently reviewed by Haynes *et al.* (1977), including their own findings in production workers undergoing retirement from the American rubber tyre industry. They found, for example, that in the so-called 'disenchantment phase' (3–5 years after compulsory retirement), those workers who had held high-status jobs were at greatest risk of dying.

The field of stress research, perennially replete with competing terminologies and conceptual models, is itself a rich source of intellectual stressors. (Indeed, it would be surprising if this book did not reflect some of these disagreements!) However, the key point to be gleaned from this chapter, and one that is now generally accepted by stress researchers, is that stress—whether at work or elsewhere—is not an exogenous entity. Rather, to paraphrase a time honoured aphorism, stress is in the eye of the beholder.

References

Bovard, E. W. (1962) The balance between negative and positive brain system activity, *Perspectives of Biology and Medicine*, **6**, 116–127.

Brand, R. J., Rosenman, R. H., Sholtz, R. I., *et al.* (1976) Multivariate prediction of coronary heart disease in the Western Collaborative Group Study compared to the findings of the Framingham Study, *Circulation*, **53**, 348–355.

Caplan, R. (1971) Organizational stress and individual strain: a social–psychological study of risk factors in coronary heart disease among administrators, engineers, and scientists. Ann Arbor, Mich. Research Center for Group Dynamics.

Caplan, R. D., Cobb, S., French, J. R. P., Harison, R. V., and Pinneau, S. R. (1975) *Job Demands and Worker Health*, US Department of Health, Education, and Welfare, publication no. (NIOSH) 75–160.

Cassel, J. C. (1976) The contribution of the social environment to host resistance, *American Journal of Epidemiology*, **104**, 107–123.

Cassel, J. C., and Tyroler, H. A. (1961) Epidemiological studies of culture change: I.

146

Health status and recency of industrialization, *Archives of Environmental Health*, **3**, 25–33.

Christenson, W. N., and Hinkle, L. E. (1961) Differences in illness and prognostic signs in two groups of young men, *Journal of the American Medical Association*, **177**, 247–253.

Conger, J. J., Sawrey, W., and Turrell, E. S. (1958) The role of social experience in the production of gastric ulcers in hooded rats placed in a conflict situation, *Journal of Abnormal Psychology*, **57**, 214–220.

Dunbar, F. (1943) *Psychosomatic Medicine*, New York. Hoeber.

French, J. R. P. (1963) The social environment and mental health, *Journal of Social Issues*, **19**, 39–56.

French, J. R. P., Rogers, W. and Cobb, S. (1974) Adjustment as person–environment fit. In Coelko, G. V., Hamburg, D. A., and Adams, J. E. (eds), *Coping and Adaptation*, New York. Basic Books.

French, J. R. P., Tupper, C. J., and Mueller, E. F. (1965) *Work Load of University Professors*. Co-operative Research Project no. 2171, US Office of Education, Ann Arbor. The University of Michigan.

Friedman, M. (1969) *Pathogenesis of Coronary Artery Disease*, New York. McGraw-Hill, pp. 75–135.

Friedman, M., Rosenman, R. H., and Carroll, V. (1957) Changes in the serum cholesterol and blood clotting time of men subject to cyclic variation of occupational stress, *Circulation*, **17**, 852–861.

Hammond, E. C., and Selikoff, I. J. (1972) Relation of cigarette smoking to risk of death of asbestos-associated disease among insulation workers in the U.S., *Proceedings: Working Group to Assess Biological Effects of Asbestos*, International Agency for Research on Cancer, Lyon, France.

Harrison, R. V. (1975) Job stress and worker health: person–environment misfit, Paper presented to the American Public Health Association Convention, Chicago, Ill.

Haynes, S. G., McMichael, A. J., and Tyroler, H. A. (1977) The relationship of normal involuntary retirement to early mortality amongst rubber workers, *Social Science and Medicine*, **11**, 105–114.

Henry, J. P., and Cassel, J. C. (1969) Psychosocial factors in essential hypertension: Recent epidemiologic and animal experimental evidence, *American Journal of Epidemiology*, **90**, 171–200.

Hinkle, L. E. (1973) The concept of 'stress' in the biological and social sciences, *Science of Medicine and Man*, **1**, 31–48.

Hite, A. (1975) *Some Characteristics of Work Roles and the Relationships to Self-esteem and Depression*. Ph.D. dissertation, The University of Michigan (quoted in Quinn, 1975).

House, J. S. (1972) *The Relationship of Intrinsic and Extrinsic Work Motivations to Occupational Stress and Coronary Heart Disease Risk*. Ph.D. thesis, The University of Michigan.

House, J. S. (1974a) in James O'Toole (ed.) *Work and the Quality of Life: Resource Papers for Work in America*, Cambridge, Mass. The MIT Press, 145–170.

House, J. S. (1974b) Occupational stress and coronary heart disease: a review and theoretical integration, *Journal of Health and Social Behaviour*, **15**, 12–27.

Jenkins, C. D. (1971) Psychologic and social precursors of coronary disease, *New England Journal of Medicine*, **284**, 244–255.

Jenkins, C. D. (1976) Recent evidence supporting psychologic and social risk factors for coronary disease, *New England Journal of Medicine*, **294**, 1033–1038.

Kahn, R. L., Wolfe, D. M., Quinn, R. P., Snoek, J. D., and Rosenthal, R. A. (1964) *Organizational Stress: Studies in Role Conflicts and Ambiguity*, New York. Wiley.

Kaplan, B. H., Cassel, J. C., and Gore, S. (1973) Social support and health. Paper presented to the American Public Health Association Convention. San Francisco. Calif.

Mittman, C., Barbela, T., and Leiberman, J. (1973) Alpha-1-antitrypsin deficiency as an index of susceptibility to pulmonary disease, *Journal of Occupational Medicine*, **15**, 33–38.

Quinn, R. P. (1975) Job characteristics and mental health. Paper presented to the American Public Health Association Convention, Chicago, Ill.

Rosenman, R. H., Brand, R. J., Jenkins, C. D., Friedman, M., Strauss, R., and Wurm, M. (1975) Coronary heart disease in the Western Collaborative Group Study: final follow-up experience of $8\frac{1}{2}$ years, *Journal of the American Medical Association*, **233**, 872–877.

Rosenman, R. H., Friedman, M., Straus, R., Wurm, M., Kositchek, R., Hahn, W., and Werthessen, N. T. (1964) A predictive study of coronary heart disease: the Western Collaborative Group Study, *Journal of the American Medical Association*, **189**, 15–22.

Rosenman, R. H., Friedman, M., Straus, R., *et al.* (1970) Coronary heart disease in the Western Collaborative Group Study: a follow-up experience of $4\frac{1}{2}$ years, *Journal of Chronic Disease*, **23**, 173–190.

Russek, H. I. (1960) Emotional stress and coronary heart disease in American physicians, *American Journal of the Medical Sciences*, **240**, 711–721.

Sales, S. M. (1969) *Differences among Individuals in Affective, Behavioural, Biochemical, and Physiological Responses to Variations in Work Load.* Ph.D. thesis, The University of Michigan.

Schachter, S. (1959) *Psychology of Affiliation.* Palo Alto. California, Stanford University Press.

Selye, H. (1956) *The Stress of Life.* New York. McGraw-Hill.

Selye, H. (1976) Forty years of stress research: principal remaining problems and misconceptions, *Canadian Medical Association Journal*, **115**, 53–56.

Wells, J. A. (1977) *Differences in Sources of Social Support in Conditioning the Effect of Perceived Stress on Health.* Paper presented to 1977 Annual Meeting of Southern Sociological Association, Atlanta, Georgia, U.S.A.

Chapter 6

Learning: Cause and Cure

H. R. Beech

Withington Hospital, University of Manchester

There are, broadly speaking, two explanations offered to account for malfunctioning as a result of factors associated with one's occupation. On the one hand, it is well known that certain physical hazards accrue from working in the asbestos industry, handling radioactive materials, and so on, and, hence, it is thought that the resulting illness may have little to do with the individual, save that he or she had the misfortune to choose badly, respecting occupation. On the other hand, it is believed that there are more psychological conditions affecting employment (work overload, adverse work relationships, uncertainty of tenure, etc.) which can produce disorders of either a physical or psychological kind. The evidence for these latter effects is less satisfactory than, say, that which associates respiratory disorders to the inhalation of coal dust, but it is claimed that evidence for stress reactions to the psychological work environments is accumulating (Kahn and Quinn, 1970; Margolis *et al.*, 1974; Kornhauser, 1965).

However, it is abundantly clear that far from all individuals who are exposed to the same work conditions develop abnormalities, either of a physical or a psychological character. Most, fortunately, seem to manage reasonably well. Hence, while data is available to show that events or circumstances at home or at work are associated with dysfunction, it is evident that we are dealing with an interactional process in which the particular organism may be seen as either more or less at risk.

Recent evidence in respect of breast cancer, for example (Wheeler and Caldwell, 1955), suggests the importance of the individual's psychological make-up as a determinant of whether or not tumours develop. Indeed, on the basis of steadily accumulating evidence, it has been suggested (Schmale and Iker, 1966) that the psychobiological state of the organism, particularly as related to a sense of hopelessness, may provide the appropriate internal environment for cancer to develop. Or, again, it has been suggested (Jenkins, 1971a, 1971b) that the appearance of coronary heart disease is related to the presence of certain personality characteristics. By and large, these studies are correlational in character, showing associations but not necessarily revealing causative influence, and so are not entirely satisfactory.

It may be, for example, that coronary attacks are found statistically more frequently among those who are impatient, ambitious, and competitive, but it does not necessarily follow that such characteristics *cause* or contrive in the occurrence of such attacks. Correlational evidence of this kind does not establish causality, and the literature is replete with accounts of the painful consequences of making errors of this kind. Indeed, it may well be that the notion of the so-called Type A characteristics (competitive, striving, etc.) being related to coronary risk is quite erroneous; Friedman (1976) in his re-examination of relevant data and hypothesis, suggests that the evidence indicates that the greater risk attaches to the phlegmatic individual with low self-esteem. However, the general hypothesis is certainly plausible and, in the area of laboratory investigation, more direct evidence linking the individual organism and susceptibility to breakdown or malfunctioning is available.

A recent example of this has been provided by Seligman (1975) who places his observations in the context of what he terms 'learned helplessness'. The basic observation which he made was that, given certain types of experimental conditions, largely to do with the repeated presentation of inescapable painful stimulation, an animal may cease to behave in a wildly uncontrolled way (as it is prone to do, at first) and becomes inert and unresponsive, even when opportunities to escape noxious stimulation are readily available. Some animals clearly take the first chance of escape which is offered to them, but others need considerable inducement before abandoning the 'helpless' state. So far as one can tell such differences in reaction are not the product of different experiences or learning but, rather, reflect some innate property or properties of the organisms themselves. Similar observations have been made by Pavlov (1927) and Masserman (1943), among others.

Of course, it is possible that different life experiences could of themselves render an organism more or less susceptible to stresses, i.e. such experiences could have a 'weakening', or sensitizing influence. Indeed, there is relatively little specific evidence for the direct link between the organism's qualities and stress reactions, although recent experiments by Asso and Beech (1975) and Vila and Beech (1977) point to such connections, and suggest the possibility that adverse reactions can be acquired as the outcome of combining external stress with a particular internal state of the organism.

Briefly, these experiments were based upon the argument that it is not only the severity of the stress or the multiplicity of stresses acting upon the individual which may occasion breakdown, but the state of the organism at the time when stress is imposed, which is important. This is not to say that we are lacking evidence relating the imposition of stress and adverse reactions; far from it, for there is ample evidence from so-called Experimental Neurosis studies which establishes this relationship beyond doubt. However, such evidence is often used simply to reinforce the notion that the environment is solely responsible for the resulting dysfunction, and little or no attention is paid to the nature of organism itself as an important determinant of outcome.

Perhaps a brief account of the Experimental Neurosis literature will clarify the point.

While it is true that early studies (see Pavlov, 1927) indicated the complex nature of the relationship between the organism and its environment in producing stress reactions, later studies tended to focus rather narrowly upon the mere manipulation of environmental circumstances. No doubt such emphasis reflected the viewpoint that, while one may be relatively unable to alter the basic substance of the organism, modification of the environment offered the brighter prospect. Whether or not such pessimism characterized investigators, it is certainly the case that intensive application to studying the effects of changes in the external world was the rule. Wolpe (1958) was a comparatively late example of such investigation, in studying the effects of inescapable electric shock upon cats, and arguing from these results to the problems of the human neurotic condition. He held the somewhat simplistic view that electric shock produces anxiety, which then becomes attached to other cues which happen to be present at that point in time, so that, in his experiments, the animals would come to fear the cage in which they had received the shock, and would evince signs of disturbance even when brought into the room where the cage was kept. The key to the disturbance—which is now 'irrational', since no further shocks are administered—is a piece of simple associative learning. The same process, it is argued, could produce impotence in the man who fails to make love to his wife in the hotel room which has a wallpaper motif associated with a past anxiety making event.

Interestingly enough, Masserman (1943) had already conducted a series of rather similar experiments, and made rather similar observations, to Wolpe's, but had been at pains to point out that not all his experimental animals reacted adversely. Some of Masserman's cats would apparently rather starve to death than eat in a situation where, previously, they had been given electric shocks or suffered some other noxious stimulation; others were able to overcome any reluctance to feed with comparative ease.

The question, it seems, is not so much whether we are concerned with both the organism *and* the environment, but with the degree of importance to attach to the former, the mechanisms to which the organism's sensitivity is responsive, and the degree of control we might come to have over such states. Posing such questions—to which there are, as yet, no very satisfactory answers—should not be construed as an attempt to dispose of the external environment as an important influence. It is merely that one must examine and account for all elements which contribute to psychological breakdown and dysfunction.

Perhaps to briefly describe our own recent research data will help to clarify the need for caution. Reference has been made to work by Asso and Beech (1975), and Vila and Beech (1977), which sought to examine the role of the organism's state in the acquisition of symptoms. In these investigations, samples of normal women, as well as those suffering from psychiatric disorders, were provided with an opportunity to learn an aversive reaction to an unpleasant noise. Should the general proposition be true that the sensitivity of the organism to respond to noxious stimulation is important, then we would expect the psychiatric population to show more speedy acquisition of some new learning which depends upon that sensitivity. This, in fact, was confirmed, but in some ways a more interesting finding was that a temporary state of the organism could also alter capacity to learn an unadaptive and unwanted response.

The latter was investigated by examining the women for their vulnerability to acquiring unwanted reactions at certain points in the menstrual cycle. Briefly, women exposed to noxious stimulation in the few days prior to menstruation showed a significantly enhanced tendency to exhibit 'jumpiness' to an innocuous blue light when that stimulus had been associated *only once before* with an unpleasant noise. This facility to learn what could be called a nervous reaction, was almost entirely absent in similar groups examined outside the period of time in question.

These findings raise many important questions, including those concerned with the problem of whether women are more at risk in stressful conditions by reason of the alterations in state associated with the menstrual cycle. At least it could be considered that the apparently increased vulnerability of women which these findings suggest could account for the disproportionately large number of phobic reactions observed among the female population.

There seems little doubt that one must take seriously the state of the organism, whether this is temporary or long term, as an important determinant of reactivity to stress. But the other major consideration, very clearly, is that the organism's reactions are partly attributable to a learning process, and it seems appropriate to pay some attention to the mechanisms of learning involved so that, if necessary, some 'unlearning' may be arranged.

So far as the former influence is concerned, it may be that only limited action is possible, among which may be the elimination of 'high-risk', exceptionally vulnerable individuals, dampening down of the more obvious signs of distress with medication, and so on. It could be argued that to consider more fundamental changes as possible (e.g. the transformation of a neurotic constitution to one which epitomizes positive qualities) is wishful thinking. Such evidence as is available indicates that neurotic tendencies are relatively permanent characteristics, perhaps inclining to show fluctuations from time to time, but always placing the individual at greater risk to breakdown.

Perhaps one more thing should be said in this vein which should affect our approach to the problems of stress at work and its treatment. There is now some quite useful evidence relating temperament to choice of occupation, some of which suggests that certain high-risk individuals seek out opportunities to test themselves in stressful environments, and eschew opportunities to find more sheltered work where their weaknesses may be less obviously exposed. Effective treatment in such cases could well involve advice to find less exacting employment, although one recognizes that certain personality demands may make such a decision difficult for the individual concerned.

Let me now turn to the conditioning/learning model of psychological dysfunction and the treatment implications which this carries. In doing so it is important to state that the model has been confined to the more obviously psychological reactions (e.g. anxiety, tension, headaches, depression, and so on) rather than to the role which the mechanisms of learning might have in the obviously physical disorders resulting from exposure to noxious substances, such as asbestosis and cancer.

The basic assumption which the model makes is that the symptoms of stress are acquired in much the same way as are other pieces of learning. While the mechanisms involved can be very complex (and this aspect need not concern us here) it is argued that certain relatively simple concepts and operations are implicated, which can be illustrated by reference to laboratory studies.

One of these, for example, is described by Pavlov (1927) in which a dog is taught to discriminate between a circle and an ellipse. Gradually the ellipse is made to appear more and more circular in appearance until the experimental animal, no longer able to discriminate, shows evidence of considerable psychological disturbance. Similarly, Liddell (1944) contrived a situation in which sheep were forced to make (for them) difficult discriminations between signals which heralded electric shock and those which did not. The result again was considerable emotional and behavioural instability which persisted in time. Yet another example, and a more interesting one since it involved a human subject, is Watson's and Rayner's (1920) study of Little Albert. In this experiment Albert, a stolid, healthy, 9-month-old child was first shown a number of stimuli (a white rat, a rabbit, a dog, fur, etc.) in order to establish any trace of fear, which in fact he did not show. However, it could easily be established that Albert showed the kind of distress typical of young infants to a sudden, loud, and unpleasant noise. The object of the experiment was to transfer the fear from the 'natural' stimulus to those which, hitherto, were neutral or even attractive to Albert. The means by which this was achieved were dramatically simple—whenever Little Albert reached out to take the white rat, a startling noise sounded which the child quickly came to associate with the animal. By this means, Watson created what he considered to be a conditioned emotional reaction of fear to take the place of whatever previous feelings Albert had entertained.

As those subscribing to this model of fear acquisition are quick to maintain, Little Albert's fear was found to have spread to other objects or stimuli which bore some resemblance to the white rat, e.g. a ball of cotton wool or a piece of fur, while dissimilar objects, such as building blocks, were not affected.

Furthermore, the fear showed persistence over time, even though Albert was not again exposed to the 'training' procedure. Such findings have very considerable appeal for anyone wanting to account for psychological reactions of an abnormal kind. They suggest that simple accidental associations might be sufficient to produce such reactions, that there can be extensive generalization or spreading of the reaction, and that persistence of the abnormality can be expected. All these points are very relevant to a good theory of neurosis. Such a model is obviously applicable to rather different situations than that in which Little Albert found himself. A good example of this is Rachman's (1966) attempt to teach a 'sexual fetish' to otherwise sexually healthy individuals. Here the investigator wanted to examine the possibility that sexual arousal could be transferred from appropriate to inappropriate stimuli by a simple arrangement of the conditions for learning. Having first shown that young male students would become sexually aroused (experiencing penile erections) by looking at slides of an erotic nature, Rachman set out to teach his subjects to respond similarly to various pictures of boots. This in fact was fairly readily accomplished by arranging the presentation of the pictorial material so that each exposure of a 'boot' picture was followed by one depicting a pretty, naked female.

These are, of course, merely analogue studies; they indicate the *plausibility* of the conditioning/learning models as explanations of how individuals might come to acquire abnormal reactions, maladjustment, or unadaptive ways of dealing with their environments, but they do not establish that neurotic or 'stress' reactions *are* acquired through the action of such mechanisms. Perhaps one other example of an analogue study is pertinent, especially as the investigation to be quoted has been the subject of considerable debate in a 'work' context. Brady (1958) and his colleagues, in their investigations of the emotional reactions of monkeys, reported that 'stress brought about dramatic alterations in the hormone content of the animals' blood, but a more extensive study of 19 monkeys was brought to a halt when many of them died'. The latter problem was traced to a procedure in which monkeys had had to learn to avoid an electric shock by pressing a lever.

Such animals were deemed to have exercised 'executive' responsibility, and it was they who reacted to stress rather than 'yoked' control animals who got the same number of electric shocks but for whom the lever provided had no effect on what happened.

This frequently quoted study, however, has been shown to have major faults, and urges caution in accepting the results of analogue studies. In particular, Brady chose the four 'executive' monkeys from the group of eight by taking those who first started pressing the lever in an 'executive' situation. In short, it is likely that these were the more emotional monkeys (more hyper-responsive) to begin with. Furthermore, when the study was repeated, with a more appropriate design (this time using rats) by Weiss (1968) the results were in line with the executive animal showing *reduced* anxiety.

Indeed, as Seligman has indicated (1975), there is a good deal of evidence that a crucial factor in the appearance of abnormality under conditions of stress is whether or not the animal can exert some degree of control over events. Masserman (1943) also found that even partial control over the environment seemed to encourage more adaptive behaviours in experimental animals, and Seligman's own work endorses this view, suggesting the form which treatment might take for 'helpless' and unadaptive reactions to stress. Of course, for the most part, the kind of unadaptive behaviours described so far can be seen as examples of faulty acquisition, i.e. the accumulation of superfluous, unwanted behaviours. The problem here, naturally, would be to remove such behaviours from the individual's repertoire since they would stand in the way of satisfactory adjustment. On the other hand, there are obvious examples of *failure to acquire* modes of response which would facilitate adjustment or capacity to cope with the stresses and strains of life. Good examples of this which occur clinically are the failure to acquire those social skills which enable an individual to function well in personal relations, a failure to acquire a sufficient degree of assertiveness to be able to represent views adequately, and a failure to match the desire to achieve with what he can actually accomplish.

Clearly, the latter examples represent quite a different category of problem for which it is necessary to consider building up new learning as opposed to eliminating 'old' superfluous responses. The implication for prophylaxis is very evident, since it points directly to the identification of existing categories of response deficiency and the setting up of programmes in which these deficiencies are made good.

Such a viewpoint has been expressed by L. Burns (1976) who has indicated the merits of a behavioural approach to such problems. This attitude is one which I would also endorse and have some commitment to in the shape of a research project which is being conducted by D. Burns (1977).

The latter study had, as its starting point, the identification of those coping skills which characterize individuals who consider themselves to be relatively immune from stress, and which were not possessed by those thinking of themselves as more vulnerable. The next stage of such an enquiry, logically, would be the training of hypothetically vulnerable individuals in the skills which they may appear to lack.

At this point at least two major possibilities would be encountered. In the first place, it may be the case that the lack of coping skills is merely another way—using other labels—for expressing a basic emotional instability or neuroticism. In such a case, one might find that little or no benefit might accrue from instruction—the problem being one of a constitutional disposition to find life hard-going, rather than a deficiency of habits amenable to improvement.

A second major difficulty might be that, even though one might find that response deficiencies were indeed the cause of stress experiences, these may turn out to be specific rather than general. If this were the case, then it might be somewhat difficult to establish a general prophylactic programme which would afford protection for the idiosyncrasies of maladjustment or stress experience which could be manifested.

Whether or not it is possible to identify common coping skills which could be taught as a means of avoiding stress experience is a matter of fact rather than of opinion. It is certainly a seductive idea that such skills might be involved, and the apparent 'good sense' of such an idea could lead us to assume that it is also a valid one. But the literature in the field of work stress is already well stocked with opinion (one might reasonably feel that the substitution of attractive idea for hard evidence has been often elevated to an art form in this field), and a more scientific approach to the problem is clearly necessary.

The difficulty with which one must contend here is that, since we have very little knowledge or experience of prophylaxis in dealing with work stress, it is often only possible to offer opinions. It seems to me that, in these circumstances, it is doubly important to stay as close to the facts as possible and, hence, suggestions concerning prophylaxis and remedial action should at least come from a body of evidence of established theoretical and empirical value. More often, it seems, such advice is based upon areas where there is a notorious weakness in these respects, and it is therefore entirely appropriate that one should address oneself to the possible implications of behavioural methods. While there are very obvious shortcomings in this approach it is undoubtedly true that, both in theoretical and empirical (treatment) terms, such a claim is probably greater than that of other available alternatives. Indeed, in applying such models and strategies, deriving as they do from extensive research in the laboratory and the natural environment, one is getting closest to the utilization of scientific psychological principles to the problem areas.

In making a beginning to the business of applying behavioural strategies to work stress, it may be appropriate to say that we would need to differentiate between existing aberrant reactions and prophylactic measures. Where the latter are concerned we are on more difficult ground, since this is the least well developed aspect of any psychological approach, and it is very obviously rather more difficult to establish that something *does not* happen as a result of one's efforts, than that some clearly defined thing *does* happen. Much easier is to apply the behavioural approach and technique to the existing experience of stress, and to examine the ways in which unadaptive reactions may be eliminated in favour of useful and constructive approaches to stressful conditions. Perhaps it is appropriate here to point out that there is really no pressing need to assume that the unadaptive reaction should be strong before meriting attention; indeed, there is good evidence that the weaker the 'habit' the more amenable to correction it will be. By and large, one would not expect the problems of work stress to have assumed the dimensions which may lead to psychiatric hospital admission, nor would one have in mind reactions conforming in strength and severity to those which are witnessed in major neurotic breakdown. Such considerations would encourage one to feel that the task of applying a behavioural approach would, if anything, be easier than usual.

But perhaps it is important here to emphasize the particular reasons why the behavioural approach could be argued not only to be a useful adjunct to existing methods, but also that having the greatest potential in the area of work stress. It is, as I have tried to show, firmly grounded in experimental observation and the scientific tradition, both of which are much needed qualities not always present in psychological enquiry. Furthermore, it clearly represents directness of observation, measurement, and 'operationism', with active avoidance of the inferences, explanatory fiction, and reifications which are so commonplace in psychological theorizing. In short, such an approach comes closest to securing the degree of scientific rigour upon which useful knowledge is so dependent. Finally, and perhaps most crucial to the purpose at hand, is the substantial accumulation of empirical data concerning the successful strategies which have been applied.

The following account of how one might utilize existing knowledge and strategies from behavioural psychology is, of course, only an outline. It is certainly far from exhaustive in terms of recounting the techniques which are available, and it is not comprehensive with reference to the range of reactions which could be discussed. Clearly, more definitive accounts are needed and, in particular, the task of relating the behavioural approach to work stress will require the pains-taking collection of data relevant to the theoretical model involved.

However, one might begin by suggesting three types of intervention which could, hypothetically, be required. First, assuming that work stress (or the experience of such stress) leads to alterations in feeling state, such as anxiety, depression, anger, would invite us to examine behavioural techniques designed to dissociate certain cues from such feelings. Second, it is reasonable to assume that certain unadaptive cognitions or behaviours which have been acquired as a result of stress or previous learning, simply persist as 'bad habits' which lead to maladjustment at work and perhaps in other contexts. Third, it is conceivable that stress, or the experience of stress, occurs as a function of the absence of appropriate adaptive reactions and that behavioural techniques should be aimed at developing such responses. Let us begin with the first of these categories.

Unwanted emotional reactions

A concern with the problems of superfluous anxiety was central to behaviour therapy in the 1950s and 1960s, this focus of attention probably deriving from the findings of experimental neurosis studies. Indeed, the first systematic attempt to provide a substantive theoretical model and technique for behavioural treatment (Wolpe, 1958) assumed anxiety to be the prerequisite of unadaptive behaviour. Appropriately, the aim was to detach the emotional reactivity from the innocuous cues to which it had become associated.

Wolpe's own experimental work, as well as that of others, led him to the conclusion that the elimination of such anxiety was best accomplished by arranging for the progressive and gradual exposure of the subject to the anxiety stimuli, and for the systematic inhibition of the emotional reaction. Evidence had suggested that, while it might be impossible to deal with anxiety generated in large amounts, it became a distinct possibility to suppress such feelings when experienced in lesser degrees. Hence, the technique of systematic desensitization required the construction of an hierarchy—a set of conditions which were all related to the object of the fear, but which evoked different amounts of anxiety. At each step in the hierarchy, according to Wolpe, it would be necessary to permanently inhibit the experience of anxiety, so that the cues associated with that state were no longer capable of activating adverse emotion. In this way, it is argued, the next step in the hierarchy could be confidently taken, since some anxiety had already been extinguished. Stage by stage, the subject would, therefore, be exposed to cues to anxiety which would be dealt with in turn until no further unfavourable reaction was forthcoming. In animal subjects, where superfluous anxiety had been deliberately created by administering repeated noxious stimulation, this regime appeared to work very well. Clinical trials with human subjects also bore out the value of this approach, both with non-psychiatric subjects (Wolpe, 1958) and then with psychiatric patients (Lazarus, 1963). The basic differences between these groups was generally thought to involve only the intensity of anxiety experienced and the spread or range of behaviours affected.

In short, it seems that there was clear evidence that superfluous emotional reactions could be traced to specific learning experiences, and that the mechanisms and procedures for *unlearning* had been identified. In practice, the process of constructing a relevant anxiety hierarchy, and of inhibiting the unwanted emotional reaction at each stage, were gradually refined into a standard procedure which could readily be utilized in the clinical setting. This was called imaginal systematic desensitization (Wolpe, 1969). The unlearning involved first teaching the individual muscle relaxation which, it was assumed, would effectively inhibit the experience of anxiety, and the presentation of cues to emotional reaction as 'scenes' depicted by the therapist, while the patient was relaxed. Step by step, the treatment would advance by the presentation of scenes from the anxiety hierarchy, at each stage care being taken to extinguish all traces of emotional reactivity before moving on. Evidence suggested strongly that this technique was extraordinarily effective in the elimination of unwanted anxiety, not only in the 'imagined' situations utilized, but also in actual life circumstances (Beech, 1969).

It is easy to see how such a method could have value in cases of work stress, and the model itself would be plausible enough given the assumption that anxiety can be generated by certain work situations which, fortuitously, has become attached to innocuous cues. The treatment of basically stable individuals who suffer unwanted emotional reactivity to what are really 'neutral' stimuli, could perhaps be accomplished in relatively few sessions. But even such brief training might be out of the question if the problem occurred on a substantial scale and, for this reason, the treatment of groups of individuals by these methods was developed. Naturally, it is important that these individuals can be grouped in terms of the object of their disturbance. One could imagine, for example, that such commonly experienced anxieties might appear in situations where important decision making is involved, where particularly delicate business negotiations are being undertaken, where industrial accidents have produced nervous reactions to the circumstances where they have occurred, or one might think of bomb disposal as an extreme case where the model and technique would apply.

It will be appreciated here that, in these cases, anxiety could be reasonably expected to be present to some degree and, especially in the last example given, might be seen as entirely appropriate to the circumstances. We have, therefore, two conceptually separate problems with which to deal, the first being the anxiety generated by the specific stresses represented in the nature of the circumstances themselves, the second being the tendency for anxiety to be transferred from appropriate stimuli to entirely innocent cues which happened to be present at the time.

The attitude one might take in these two cases requires careful thought. On the one hand, we would need to recognize that a certain amount of anxiety could be of considerable value as a drive state impelling action, while on the other hand too much or inappropriate anxiety has been shown to incapacitate and render the organism ineffectual. The aim, presumably, should be to eliminate all inappropriate anxiety (that which is generated by purely neutral stimuli as a result of learning), and to reduce 'appropriate' anxiety to that level which allows the individual to act with greatest efficiency.

One could, of course, think of circumstances in which one might wish to actually *increase* anxiety to produce an hypothetical optimal drive state (e.g. in athletes, footballers, etc.). I have, for example, over several years, attempted to examine the way in which increases in drive level can be used to increase performance effectiveness, or in which reduction of certain drives can act upon the level of some other drive (anxiety).

Systematic desensitization has been probably the best documented and most successful method of dealing with problems of unwanted anxiety. It has still very considerable value, and the gradual approach which it involves could be argued to have enjoyed a long history, with a certain 'natural' appeal, as Jersild and Holmes (1935) discovered, as a means of eliminating fear.

On the other hand, what appears to be quite the opposite kind of training has a certain basic attraction, where the individual possessing morbid anxiety is, as it were, thrown in at the deep end. Early investigations of this alternative were not at all promising (e.g. Jones, 1924) but, later, the strategy under the titles of 'flooding' and 'implosion' was seen to have some potential (Wolpe, 1969; Stampfl and Levis, 1967).

Very probably, there is much more to discover about the way in which this method works, as well as with whom and in what circumstances. At this point in time suggestions have been made that it is of greatest value when desensitization has failed, where more intense anxiety is being experienced, and where an element of 'reality testing' is needed. The latter point is best seen in the context of individuals who may have constructed elaborate expectations about the nature of their anxieties and may need to gain reassurance from experience that these expectations are wholly unrealistic.

In practice, I believe that most therapists have recourse to a mixture of these two approaches, finding it unnecessary to plod tediously and meticulously through all the steps of a hierarchy, finding it unnecessary to extinguish all traces of anxiety at each stage before proceeding, but finding that the patient may balk if the going is too tough at any particular time, so that the pace of progress must be geared to what can be tolerated.

These methods, of course, have been elaborated and extended, and numerous sub-techniques (such as aversion-relief) have been directed to the problem of removing unwanted anxiety. The choice must obviously be related to the type of problem and other relevant variables.

One of the more immediately useful ways of dealing with problems of those feeling states which disorganize and render action ineffectual or inefficient, is to make use of relaxation alone. Indeed, there is a substantial amount of evidence that the state of muscle relaxation is incompatible with raised anxiety, elevated blood pressure, and other indications of stress reaction, and there is good reason to think that training in muscle relaxation has beneficial effects. Briefly, the individual is taught to assume a degree of control over muscle tension and, whenever stress is experienced, a degree of relaxation is put into operation so that, in this way, the individual may be able to reduce or eliminate anxiety, or the physical reactions to unpleasant experience. There are at least two important advantages which this technique offers: the rapidity with which the skill can be acquired by most people, and the fact that the individual can acquire the mastery of relaxation largely through his own unsupervised practice.

It can be pointed out, of course, that anxiety or other unwanted feeling states may occur *without* the presence of exaggerated muscle tension, so that training in the control of muscles could be unhelpful. More recent evidence has, fortunately, provided what appear to be useful alternatives to relaxation, in the form of training in electrodermal responses and in the control of hand temperature. Since the latter procedure will be referred to in a later section, a detailed description need not be given here. However, what one might say is that changes in the resistance or potential of the skin surface, as well as body temperature, appear to be related to autonomic functioning. Alteration in the individual's 'feeling' state is reflected in changes on these measures and it has become apparent that a reciprocal relationship may hold, at least partially. In short, training the individual to lower his skin resistance (a surprisingly easy task) or to raise his hand temperature (again much easier than one might suppose) might enable that individual to assert some control over his autonomic nervous system.

The basis for choosing between these control methods is, at this time, inadequately delineated, but it seems likely that such choice will be ultimately related to the special characteristics of the individual as much as to extraneous factors, such as training time involved, portability of apparatus, ease of use, and so on.

It is interesting to note that portable devices for accomplishing these effects have become well developed, and there is now available a desk top model which allows the busy executive to self-train in skin resistance.

Finally, in this section, it is pertinent to observe again that anxiety is by no means the only feeling state associated with the imposition of stress. Indeed, depression is a state which is so familiar that we may readily agree to call it 'the common cold of psychopathology' (Seligman, 1975).

Behavioural psychologists have, however, only recently turned their attention to explaining and treating depressive reactions, the hallmarks of which (in the mild degree with which we are concerned here) are a characteristic mood, impairment of motivation, and the general fall-off in responsiveness. Several behavioural models are available from which to choose, all of which have a good deal in common, but of special interest is that propounded by Seligman.

He sees depression as an example of learned helplessness which is the result of exposure to uncontrollable events. In the modern working environment, characterized by bureaucratic controls and other sources of pressure over which it is difficult or impossible to exert influence, it would be hardly surprising to find that depression is a common experience, and that feelings of helplessness are widely experienced.

Experimental work, as I have indicated earlier in this chapter, suggests that, once the organism has succumbed to these conditions, it may be difficult or impossible for the individual to escape from the inert state.

Behavioural psychologists have made some important contributions to the understanding and treatment of such reactions, the latter being mainly concerned with getting the individual to produce behaviours which *do* alter his environment.

Essentially the therapist's task is to arrange situations in such a way that the individual is tempted, or forced, to produce *any* response which is successful, and then to progressively increase task requirements until the individual functions normally again. These methods are, as yet, promising but not well developed.

Persistence of unwanted habits of thought and action

There is little doubt that certain patterns of behaviour, which interfere with efficient functioning, may do so without any accompanying disturbance of feeling. Furthermore, there are reasons for believing that certain changes in behaviour can only be effectively achieved when the most intense emotional reactions have abated (see Beech, 1975). In any event, it is not essential that an individual has insight into the faulty behaviours and, quite often, these only become apparent to him under special circumstances, such as videotape playbacks. There are any number of good examples of such lack of awareness. For example, the writer was asked recently to treat an individual for stuttering who exhibited gross motor activity and facial grimaces of which he was almost totally unaware. Mere mention of this problem produced denials from the patient, and it was only after showing videotape of the contortions which accompanied speech activity that the patient could concede that there was something more to treat. Here the motor spasms had no apparent emotional significance, but had probably developed as methods (albeit failing) to assist speech production, and could be treated as simple, persistent, frequently occurring habits.

Tics quite often seem to fall into this category, too, showing a kind of functional autonomy, and their appearance may be independent of the feeling state of the individual concerned. However, such behaviours are not particularly significant in the context of work stress reactions.

More pertinent to the issues with which this contribution is concerned are examples of inadequate and inappropriate behaviours which are related to cues arising in the context of work functions. Here one may have in mind the unadaptive modes of thought and action which, perhaps having been found to be satisfactory in one context, are preserved as general responses to situations and conditions, with or without accompanying emotionality.

A homely example might be that an individual, who has discovered a means of exerting authority in a domestic situation, continues to employ this strategy in relation to work situations where he perceives the need for control; clearly, the need might be appropriate, but the method could be quite unsuited to the latter situation. The idea that intelligent and otherwise sophisticated individuals might, without awareness, adopt behaviours which conspire to produce effects opposite to those intended, often seems implausible. But one has only to examine any segment of human interaction to see how inefficient we can be in achieving goals.

In cases of marital disharmony, for example, it is readily apparent that the 'feedback' which the partners provide for each other falls well short of that needed to sustain good relations, primarily in respect of failing to strike a proper balance of positive and negative reinforcers—roughly corresponding to rewards and punishments.

There is now incontravertible evidence for the influence of consequences in altering the appearance of behaviours, and we all subscribe to this law to some extent, offering prizes for 'good' behaviour and punishments for that deemed to be 'bad'. There are, of course, many less obvious examples of the action of 'reinforcers', and there is much to be learned concerning the relationships between reinforcer type, behaviour type, personality, and so on, but the deliberate and calculated control of behavioural consequences (operant control), and the way in which this changes and shapes behaviour is now well documented.

This can be illustrated by returning to the example of marital disharmony. Whenever the affected couple are seen together it is very evident that they have to some extent become the unwitting purveyors of negative reinforcers. Even when they are trying (one supposes) to show understanding and tolerance, the words used seem to be ill-chosen and evoke the wrong response from the partner. Teaching people to emit positive reinforcements is reasonably easy, if those concerned are motivated to change. In the example given, the first step is to create awareness of the communication problem, and simply tape-recording their exchanges on any topic area is usually sufficient for this purpose, when accompanied by evaluative comments from the therapist. Thereafter, major changes can be effected in the character of verbalizations by arranging a simple game in which the partners are each equipped with counters, and learn to reward (give a counter) or punish (take away a counter) their partner according to whether a positive or negative verbal reinforcer has been uttered. This apparently facile game in fact greatly increases awareness of the offending behaviours used, and the increased use of words which have greater appeal begins to influence attitudes and behaviours.

Learning to use language effectively (i.e. so that the behaviour of others is influenced in a way of which one approves) is an important skill. Naturally, there are more considerations than words in human interactions, but these additional considerations would also be potentially amenable to the same operant procedures. It is not difficult to see how an important source of stress at work may simply arise out of problems of communication, and that an important contribution of behavioural psychology might be to reduce the stress occasioned in this way by the application of operant control.

A whole range of external behaviours amenable to operant training has been described in the literature, but the difficulty of influencing what might be termed 'internal functioning' seems, at first sight, a considerably greater problem. Indeed, since a good 90% of behaviour is 'internal' (i.e. generally not observed) it is clearly important to see whether one can apply the same principles of positive and negative reinforcement to this relatively uncharted area.

In doing so, of course, one may be working within a more basically 'causal' framework since, in the case of external behaviours, one may be only hopeful that any changes effected could alter cognitive components (ideas, fantasies, intentions, reasoning, etc.). It is often thought more plausible to regard the 'natural' relationship as being that of ideas being the mainspring of external behaviours. By directly working upon the 'operants' of the mind (Homme, 1965), one might argue, it should be possible to control the external appearance of behaviours.

But the relation between internal and external behaviours is still far from clear, although there is at least some evidence that both are amenable to the same basic mechanisms. It may be, therefore, that it is irrelevant to ask whether it is better to alter internal behaviour (say, attitudes) in order to change external behaviour (say, football hooliganism), than to shape actions in order to alter attitudes; perhaps the more appropriate question might be the convenience which attaches to each possibility, the speed and efficiency at which changes should take place, the durability of changes produced, and so on. It may be useful to quote two simple examples of what might be thought to represent each possibility.

In an experiment by Krasner *et al.* (1964) an attempt was made first to use simple reinforcement contingencies to effect a change in those verbal behaviours representing attitudes to the medical profession. Here, the experimenter merely rewarded any endorsement of statements favourable to the medical profession, noting that the willingness to agree with such statements increased under these conditions. The 'reward', or positive reinforcement, was the approval of the experimenter. In the next part of the experiment a 'representative' of 'medical science' sought the co-operation of subjects who had been subjected to such conditioning, and others who had not, in pulling as hard as possible on a dynamometer (measuring strength of grip). It was found that individuals whose attitudes had been changed in the direction of being more favourable to the medical profession (as measured), showed significantly higher scores on the dynamometer, in this way showing how external behaviour had conformed to the internal changes produced.

In another study, with my colleague, Mrs Asirdas (1975), we were able to show that a new form of conditioning treatment for sexual dysfunction led to a general shift towards more favourable attitudes towards the partner. This result clearly illustrated how changes in external behaviours (strictly, physical/ sexual functioning) began to exert an influence upon internal states (attitudes).

Since I know of no examples relating such methods to the specific area of work stress, I can do no more than point to the very obvious implications of the principles and methods involved.

There is no reason to doubt that stress at work may result in the build-up of attitudes or external behaviours which are aberrant, and which would be amenable to the methods described. Indeed, it is apparent that faulty behaviours, both external and internal, may either merely reflect persistent habits related to a remotely historical cause or, at least, superfluous forms of unadaptive behaviour which actively impede the acquisition of useful means of coping with stress.

It is appropriate here to point to one or two further examples of the way in which one might approach the problems to be found in this area, and here one might refer to the potential importance of 'self-control' methods which have begun to assume importance in behavioural psychology.

One of the early suggestions relating the principles of operant training to mental functioning, with the contingency manager being the self, is found in Homme's (1965) paper. He argued that ideas might be strengthened in much the same way as had been shown in the case of externalized behaviours, if they are followed by some reward (positive reinforcements). If one wished, for example, to increase the obtrusiveness of anti-smoking ideas (coverants), then one could deliberately rehearse these notions and reward them by eating chocolate, reading a preferred piece of literature, listening to some favourite music, having a drink, or engaging in any other 'rewarding' consequence.

Controversy still surrounds the issue of whether or not one can accomplish all that is needed here—particularly, if it is possible to produce the desired behaviour at will and to reward oneself for doing so, and still achieve the same result as if external control agencies were involved. Whether or not the technique has validity, behavioural 'tips' for increasing self-control have been shown to have some value, and brief reference to them is appropriate.

However, it is important to point out that these techniques have been less well authenticated in theoretical than in practical terms although, even in the latter cases, there is still some room for dissatisfaction. In recounting some of these methods it will be apparent that they are often in accord with common-sense and common practice, and this should provide a measure of reassurance. What is distinctive about self-control procedures is that they represent a systematic and intensive application to the problem of learning, which stands in sharp contrast to the more often encountered *tentative* effort to change which is part of human experience. It may well be that the methods succeed to some extent simply because of the dedicated weight of effort brought to bear, rather than because there is anything intrinsically important in the methods themselves. What is clear, I believe, is that in attempting to change and redirect behaviour we tend to pass up opportunities to introduce modification, and an important beginning to self-control may be the motivation to change, which may be generated internally, or come from some external source or stress.

The methods of self-control may be very simply outlined in the following way:

(1) Introducing changes in the stimulus situation

Here, the subject deliberately sets out to so alter the cues to the unwanted behaviour that it becomes less troublesome. Putting a box of chocolates out of sight to avoid eating them might appear to be a trivial gesture, but if chocolate consumption is dependent upon visual cues being present, it could be a very useful piece of self-control to exercise. Clearly, there are many much more complex situations which would demand considerably greater ingenuity in devising the type of stimulus control required.

(2) Using aversive stimulation

In this category the individual is attempting to control behaviours by providing his own noxious contingencies for the behaviours to be eliminated. There are any number of possibilities here for the use of personally administered unpleasant stimulations, of both a psychological or a physical kind. Again, much is going to depend upon the circumstances in deciding in what way and under what conditions this method is employed. The making of public declarations may be cited as an example of a self-arranged contingency in this category if, for example, it involved arranging to do something which would lead to embarrassment if we failed to carry out the task.

(3) Rehearsing alternative responses

Naturally, the exercise of self-control methods requires an acute and detailed awareness of the to-be-controlled behaviour and its antecedents. Awareness of biting (or wanting to bite) one's nails cannot always be assumed, for example, and it is essential that such awareness is conferred before effective control can take place—in this case, perhaps, by engaging in some other pre-arranged activity of an innocuous and socially acceptable kind. In this context, it is interesting to note the value of this method in dealing with the compulsions of severely disturbed psychiatric patients (Beech, 1975) who find it possible to learn to recognize a growing tendency towards compulsive action and to divert this impulse in the way described.

But we may often find it impossible to exercise the degree of restraint necessary to change our habits when temptation is strongest. The glutton may find that, once seated at the table, knife and fork in hand, and faced with the most succulent food, the temptation to guzzle is irresistible. In order to make some degree of control possible it may be necessary to select a point at some considerable remove from the most compelling situation and, at this point, exercise and develop self-control by switching into alternative activities. It is often the case that 'bad habits' have a long chain of antecedent behaviours which, with practice, can be identified, one link of which can be chosen as being sufficiently weak to allow the substitution of a competing alternative behaviour.

This causal chain is readily recognizable in compulsive states, and the strategy of directing the patient into acceptable rather than pathological behaviours is a useful adjunct to other treatments. The strategy especially works well when the competing activity is attractive to the person concerned, as well as being one which requires a good deal of concentration and attention.

The implications for unadaptive behaviours prompted by the cues to work stress are obvious although, again, not worked out for these situations. It is not difficult to imagine that stress at work may sometimes be amenable to the same analysis, and that unadaptive behaviours occasioned by stress might be dealt with by training in substitute behaviours of an adaptive kind.

(4) Positive self-reinforcement

While we are quite used to the idea of dispensing rewards, we tend to think more of such practices as the culmination of, or end point in, a behavioural chain—the prize being given at the end of the race, so to speak. In short, we are less well geared to examining closely the relationship between reward and the satisfactory build-up of useful or desirable behaviours, although it is quite likely that such a process often occurs quite naturally. In short, it is necessary to recognize the importance which might attach to the systematic and thoughtful application of self-administered rewards in order to secure progression towards certain defined behavioural goals. Perhaps this point may be illustrated by the following examples. The 'reward' for criminal behaviour is imprisonment, and that for successful examination results the diploma, but these are end points in what is usually a long sequence of events in which the behaviours relevant to the goals (prison or diploma) have been maintained in some way. Diplomas are not gained without study, and prison sentences may occur after a string of successful burglaries; what is required in order to change or sustain certain behaviours which are deemed 'desirable' and 'appropriate' is the arrangement of relevant contingencies so that achievement of goals is more likely. Stage by stage the shaping and control of sub-behaviours essential to the achievement of the final goal can be built up, each separate step being consolidated by the positively reinforcing contingency.

Of course, some internal behaviours, such as raised blood pressure, may only come to attention when the condition has reached critical levels, and where treatment by medication would be essential to preserve life. However, biofeedback procedures hold considerable promise, the essence of which approach is the provision of immediate information about some change in physical function, such as heart rate, blood pressure, body temperature, electrical activity of the brain or muscles, and so on. This information, when provided for the individual, enables him to apply conscious control to the function in question. By this means an unexpected degree of influence has proved possible over what have been traditionally regarded as quite involuntary functions and, as might be expected, a number of pathological conditions related to these 'involuntary' processes have been also brought under control (Kamiya, 1969; Schwartz, 1976; Sheffield, 1977). In a number of such cases, such as essential hypertension and cardiac conditions, the disorder seems to be, at least in part, related to the experience of stress.

The report by Reading and Mohr (1976) on the use of biofeedback in the treatment of migraine patients is particularly interesting, since the patients taking part in this study were all seriously handicapped by their disorder, and none had improved as a result of the medication they had received. Here, patients were presented with the task of learning to control hand temperature, and the acquisition of this skill was paralleled by increased capacity to control migraine attacks. Similarly, Sheffield (1976) has found encouraging results from the application of muscle tension feedback to the control of hypertension in cases drawn from an industrial management population.

There is little doubt that these methods have provided us with two important conclusions: first, that the degree of control over 'involuntary' functions can sometimes be surprisingly great; and, second, that such control can have important implications for disorders related to work stress as much as for the effects of stress in general.

Dealing with response deficiencies

It is easier to see clearly the way in which superfluous responses arise in the context of stress imposition, than it is to see the way in which a dearth of adequate responses—an absence of effective and appropriate behaviours—can create stress. Of course, in most cases, both problems are present to some degree, and the individual not only produces responses (feelings and behaviours) which are unadaptive, but also tends to have no repertoire of *appropriate* behaviours to produce. These latter response deficiencies alone, however, create stress, as can be seen in the example of nocturnal enuresis.

It was thought, until a few years ago, that bedwetting was simply the symptom of some underlying maladjustment, and that the removal of this 'habit' could lead only to the development of other pathological manifestations. This could well be true if indeed the symptoms were subserved by some deep-seated cause or 'complex'. Protagonists of this point of view could point to the disharmony which tended to be present in the family of the bedwetting child as evidence of the validity of such a theory. On the other hand, one might take the view that the bedwetting child is one characterized by a deficiency of response—he has simply not learned to wake up when he has a full bladder, or to inhibit the release of urine while asleep. To the extent to which this notion is tenable, then it should be found that teaching the missing skills will not only eliminate bedwetting, but might also be found to produce improvement in family relationships, since an unpleasant source of irritation has been removed. In short, bedwetting would be the cause of discontent in families, rather than the *symptom* of it.

These twin benefits have in fact accrued through the use of conditioning techniques, and such evidence is widely regarded as an important test case of the rival merits of the behavioural and psychodynamic approaches to dysfunction. But this is only one example of many which testify to the important theoretical and empirical advantages of the behavioural approach (Beech, 1969).

One other useful example of how response deficiencies can lead to psychological disturbance, and of how a straightforward application of behavioural techniques can achieve a great deal, is found in the area of social skills. Anxiety attaching to social situations, or a failure to become effective in such conditions, can often be traced to never having acquired the appropriate skills, although it could also be the case that specific traumatic experiences could have produced this state of affairs. Plainly, however, there are many individuals who have never acquired a reasonable degree of social dexterity, and such lack of skill is understandably capable of producing a degree of stress. The problem may well be modest in proportion, or even slight in itself, such as not being able to maintain a suitable amount of eye-contact, being unable to terminate a conversation effectively, or being clumsy and gauche in social interactions, but the outcome may go well beyond the trivial. Lack of social skills can promote unwelcome attitudes and unwanted responses from others, which in turn makes the life of the socially inept individual more stressful and unpleasant. Besides which, he is also less able to attain the rewards which society provides in abundance for those possessing ample skill, such as promotional opportunity.

Basically, two processes are necessary to the acquisition of useful levels of social skill. First, one must recognize that one's problem arises from this source, and become more aware in a detailed way of the less desirable behaviours which are being emitted, and those of importance which are lacking. Second, one must acquire appropriate responses through the rehearsal of these latter behaviours in a variety of prepared social situations (often through role playing) together with feedback of performance. In addition, the most appropriate behaviours to exhibit in certain situations are demonstrated (modelled) for the learner to copy.

For the most part, life's circumstances have determined or allowed for the development of a reasonable level of social skill. But it is manifestly the case that individual experiences have afforded different opportunities for learning, resulting in varying levels of acquisition of relevant behaviours. Furthermore, job requirements now often demand a particularly high level of social competence, and a familiarity and ease with social roles which may be very different from one's own. There is little doubt, therefore, that training in social skills would serve the useful function of assisting in the reduction of specific work stress, as well as in promoting a general level of confidence and resistance to the effects of stress.

There is, however, another important area of enquiry which could produce important benefits for the individual exposed to stressful working environments. At the moment we know relatively little about the basic differences between those who react to stress and those who appear not to do so, save for the appearance of the reaction itself, or its absence. It was argued earlier in this chapter that a basic difference might lie in the emotional stability of the individual concerned, so that constitutionally robust individuals survive well, while others fare rather badly. It seems likely that there is considerable substance to this notion, although there is some reluctance to accept a proposition which might only enable one to eliminate the 'reactors' from appointment to high-stress positions. This course may have something to be said for it but, since those vulnerable to stress are just as likely to possess important and useful qualities as those who are more robust, then we would wish to examine the possibility of providing a protective coating for the former type of individual. In any event, the situation merits a more positive approach.

It could be that such a possibility is more viable than may at first sight appear, and the plausibility of effective intervention may be found in the following example.

In the investigation of individuals suffering from sexual problems, such as impotence in males or orgasmic failure in women, Asirdas and Beech (1975) examined the value of a suggestion made by Beech et al. (1971) that positive conditioning may offer a speedy, easily applied, and successful resolution of the problem. The technique proved to be extremely beneficial in the cases selected by Asirdas and Beech, but it seems at least possible that the results may have been attributable to mechanisms other than conditioning. The alternative explanation to that originally thought to be implied is that the differences between healthy individuals and sexually dysfunctional patients is due to their differential use of fantasies.

Evidence from various lines of enquiry indicates that fantasies play an important role in normal sexual functioning, a finding somewhat at variance with the tendency to regard such activity as the product of a disturbed imagination. Asirdas and Beech have suggested that such fantasies may serve the useful purpose of acting as a moderator of sexual impulses, being 'switched on' to heighten sexual interest, but remaining in abeyance when sexual drive is adequate. In effect this would mean that normal, sexually adjusted, individuals may make deliberate use of erotic imagery as a means of making good a temporary or more permanent decline in experienced sexual drive. The point here is that the richness and character of mental functioning may have an important bearing upon psychological and behavioural adjustment.

There is no doubt that mental mechanisms operate to advantage (and sometimes to disadvantage) in other contexts than in sexual functioning, and, as we have seen in an earlier section, unwanted anxiety can be dealt with by arranging the mental rehearsal of an hierarchical presentation of relevant scenes, which leads us to examine the role which imaginal rehearsals may have in those able to cope with stress. In the case of sexually dysfunctional individuals, I would suggest that one may discover an inability to make use of relevant fantasy as part of the clinical picture, and a therapeutic programme might include training in producing such imagery, as required. By the same token it is self-evident that most people, anticipating some difficult situation with which they must deal, go over it in their minds, perhaps in a variety of different ways. Although we have no direct experimental evidence of this, it is not too implausible to suggest that such rehearsals—which would have the appearance of worrying—might serve the vital purpose of allowing an opportunity to *adapt to the threatening situation*, and to inhibit the anxiety we feel.

Obviously, some individuals who are incapacitated by anxiety spend a great deal too much time on such rehearsals, and may find that the mental pictures formed are always of the most gloomy kind. Such rehearsals, rather than diminishing negative emotion, only serve to heighten these feelings. In other words, the differences between individuals in their susceptibility to stress could have a great deal to do with the organization of mental functioning in anticipation of stressful experiences. It could also be that under-rehearsal of the anticipated problem leaves the individual badly prepared, just as much as over-rehearsal of negative consequences may do. Perhaps fantasies involving successful outcome are associated with stress resistance, while pessimistic imagery is the hallmark of the vulnerable.

These differences in what one might think of as 'coping skills' remain hidden or only partially revealed at this point in time, and detailed experimental enquiry would be needed to expose them.

Clearly, if the above suggestions as to differences in mental preparation are shown to be true, then training programmes of prophylactic significance could be embarked upon with benefit.

In conclusion

I have tried to indicate the importance of bringing the behavioural philosophy, methodology, and technique to bear upon the special problem of stress at work. In my view the adaptations necessary are minimal, and I have tried to indicate the broad lines along which one might proceed.

In certain areas, such as systematic desensitization, self-control, social skills training, and so on, the case of the behavioural approach has obvious appeal. In certain other areas, as has been shown, there is greater uncertainty about both the mechanism involved and the relevance of application to work stress.

It is important, however, to conclude by pointing out that the behavioural approach is only as helpful as the people who make use of it. The essential value of this approach is that of being guided by the facts and evidence, rather than by fashion and whim, and the characteristic virtue has been a close adherence to scientific methodology and an experimental approach to understanding. It is, one feels, only too easy to focus narrowly upon technique, applying an apparently successful practice from one area of functioning to another, without due consideration and proper enquiry, and there are many extant examples of this failing.

References

Asirdas, S., and Beech, H. R. (1975) The behavioural treatment of sexual inadequacy, *J. Psychosom. Res.*, **19**, 345–353.

Asso, D., and Beech, H. R. (1975) Susceptibility to the acquisition of a conditioned response in relation to the menstrual cycle, *J. Psychosom. Res.*, **19**, 337–344.

Beech, H. R. (1969) *Changing Man's Behaviour*. Harmondsworth. Pelican.

Beech, H. R. (ed.) (1975) *Obsessional States*. London. Methuen.

Beech, H. R., Watts, F., and Poole, A. D. (1971) Classical conditioning of a sexual deviation: a preliminary note. *Behav. Ther.*, **2**, 400–402.

Brady, J. V. (1958) Ulcers in executive monkeys. *Scientific American*, **199**, 95–100.

Burns, D. (1977) Unpublished data to be submitted in partial fulfilment of Ph.D. requirements, University of Manchester.

Burns, L. (1976) The Management of Stress. Course organized under auspices of Extramural Department, University of Manchester, and presented at University of Bangor.

Friedman, E. H. (1976) Psychosocial factors in coronary care and rehabilitation. In *Psychosocial Approaches to the Rehabilitation of Coronary Patients*. New York. Springer.

Hariton, E. B., and Singer, J. L. (1974) Women's fantasies during sexual intercourse. *J. Consult. Clin. Psychol.*, **3**, 313–322.

Homme, L. E. (1965) Perspectives in psychology: XXIV. Control of coverants, the operants of the mind, *Psychol. Record*, **15**, 501–511.

Jenkins, C. D. (1971a) Psychologic and social precursors of coronary disease, *New Eng. J. Med.*, **284**, 244–255.

Jenkins, C. D. (1971b) Psychologic and social precursors of coronary disease, *New Eng. J. Med.*, **284**, 307–317.

Jersild, A. T., and Holmes, F. B. (1935) Methods of overcoming children's fears, *J. Psychol.*, **1**, 25–83.

Jones, M. C. (1924) The elimination of children's fears, *J. Exp. Psychol.*, **7**, 383–390.

Kahn, R. L., and Quinn, R. P. (1970) Role stress. In McLean, A. (ed.), *Mental Health and Work Organization*. Chicago. Rand McNally, pp. 50–115.

Kamiya, J. (1969) Operant control of the EEG alpha rhythm and some of its reported effects on consciousness. In Tart, C. T. (ed.), *Altered States of Consciousness*. Wiley. New York, 507–517.

Kornhauser, A. (1965) *Mental Health of the Industrial Worker*. New York. Wiley.

Krasner, L., Ullman, L. P., and Fisher, D. (1964) Changes in performance as related to verbal conditioning of attitudes toward the examiner, *Percep. Motor Skills*, **19**, 811–816.

Lazarus, A. A. (1963) The results of behaviour therapy in 126 cases of severe neurosis, *Behav. Res. Ther.*, **1**, 65–78.

Liddell, H. (1944) Conditioned reflex method and experimental neurosis. In Hunt, J. McV. (ed.), *Personality and the Behaviour Disorders*. New York. Ronald Press.

Mahoney, M. J. (1974) *Cognition and Behavior Modification*. Cambridge, Mass. Ballinger.

Margolis, B. L., Kroes, W. H., and Quinn, R. P. (1974) Job stress: an unlisted occupational hazard, *J. Occup. Med.*, **16**, 654–661.

Masserman, J. H. (1943) *Behaviour and Neurosis*. University of Chicago Press.

Pavlov, I. P. (1927) *Conditioned Reflexes*. Oxford University Press.

Rachman, S. (1966) Sexual fetishism: an experimental analogue, *Psychol. Record*, **16**, 293–296.

Reading, C., and Mohr, P. D. (1976) Biofeedback control of migraine: a pilot study, *Br. J. Soc. Clin. Psychol.*, **15**, 429–433.

Schmale, A., and Iker, H. (1966) The psychological setting of uterine cervical cancer, *Annals of the New York Acad. of Science*, **125**, 807–813.

Schwartz, G. E. (1976) Self-regulation of response patterning, *Bio-feedback & Self-reg.*, **1**, 1, 7–30.

Seligman, M. E. P. (1975) *Helplessness*. San Fransisco, Caly. W. H. Freeman.

Sheffield, B. F. (1977) Personal communication based upon research findings from an industrial management population.

Stampfl, T., and Levis, D. J. (1967) Essentials of implosive therapy: a learning-theory-based psychodynamic behavioural therapy. *J. of Abnormal Psychology*, **72**, 496–503.

Vila, J., and Beech, H. R. (1977) Vulnerability and conditioning in relation to the human menstrual cycle, *Br. J. Soc. Clin. Psychol.*, **16**.

Watson, J. B., and Rayner, R. (1920) Conditioned emotional reactions, *J. Exp. Psychol*, **3**, 1–14.

Weiss, J. M. (1968) Effects of coping response on stress, *J. Comp. Physiol. Psychol.*, **65**, 251–260.

Wheeler, J. L., and Caldwell, B. M. (1955) Psychological evaluation of women with cancer of the breast and of the cervix, *Psychosom. Med.*, **17**, 256–262.

Wolpe, J. (1958) *Psychotherapy and Reciprocal Inhibition*. Standford University Press.

Wolpe, J. (1969) *The Practice of Behaviour Therapy*. Oxford. Pergamon.

PART IV

The Person in the Work Environment

Chapter 7

Person–Environment Fit and Job Stress

R. Van Harrison

The University of Michigan

Pervin (1968, p. 65) points out that: 'In one way or another, the history of psychology reflects systems based upon an exaggerated emphasis on the individual or the environment—McDougall (1908) and Ross (1908), psychoanalysis and S–R theory, introspection and behaviorism, need theory and role theory, the nature versus nurture controversy.' These emphases can also be found in the job stress literature. Some researchers have chosen to study the effects of job characteristics such as technology or standard performance levels. Other researchers have emphasized effects of characteristics of the person such as social status or personality type. Human behaviour, however, is not understood in terms of either the environment or the person alone, but in terms of the interrelationship between the two. This chapter presents a theory of stress which describes the interrelationship of the person and the environment in terms of their 'fit' or 'congruence' with each other.

The first section of the chapter presents a general theory of the interrelationship between the person and the environment. The process of adaptation is described within this framework. The second section presents a more detailed consideration of the relationship between stress and the degree of fit between the person and the environment. The theory is used to predict relationships between strain and person–environment (P–E) fit. The third section presents data relevant to the theoretical predictions and the findings are used to evaluate the usefulness of the theory. The fourth section presents suggestions for reducing job stress which follow from the theory. The chapter concludes with some suggestions concerning future research and development of the theory.

A model of person–environment fit

Over several years members of the Social Environment and Mental Health research programme at the Institute for Social Research, The University of Michigan, have elaborated a general model of theoretical relationships between job stress and health (Campbell, 1974; Caplan, 1972; French and Kahn, 1962; French *et al.*, 1974; Harrison, 1976; House, 1972; Pinneau, 1976). The theory is based on descriptions of motivational processes by Lewin (1951) and Murray (1959). Two kinds of fit between the individual and the environment are considered. One kind of fit is the extent to which the person's skills and abilities match the demands and requirements of the job. Another kind of fit is the extent to which the job environment provides supplies to meet the individual's needs. When misfit of either kind threatens the individual's well-being, various health strains will result.

The theory is presented in Figure 7.1. A basic distinction represented in the figure is the differentiation of the person from the environment which surrounds the person. A second basic distinction is made between objects and events as they exist independently of the person's perception of them and objects and events as they are perceived by the person (i.e. subjectively).

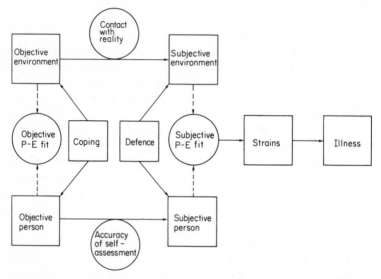

Figure 7.1 A model describing the effects of psychosocial stress in terms of fit between the person and the environment. Concepts within circles are discrepancies between the two adjoining concepts. Solid lines indicate causal effects. Broken lines indicate contributions to interaction effects

The *objective environment* refers to the environment as it exists independently of the person's perception of it. The objective environment includes objects which do not come into contact with the individual as well as those which do: the physical environment, the family environment, and other aspects of the physical and social worlds which exist independently of the person's perception of them. The present discussion focuses on the psychosocial environment of the work places as the objective environment of major interest.

The objective environment is causally related to the person's *subjective environment* (see Figure 7.1). The subjective environment represents the person's perceptions of his objective environment, i.e. it is the person's psychological construction of the world in which he lives. This includes his perception of the various kinds of supplies available to meet his needs and the demands for him to perform in certain ways before the supplies will be made available to him.

The *objective person* refers to the person as he really is. This includes his needs, values, abilities, and other attributes which are more or less enduring. The *subjective person* represents the individual's perception of objective self, i.e. the self-concept or the self-identity of the person. Thus, the subjective person includes the individual's perceptions of his needs, values, abilities, and other attributes. As with the objective and subjective environments, the present discussion is chiefly concerned with those parts of the objective and subjective person which deal with his needs, values, abilities, and other characteristics which are relevant to the work place.

French *et al.* (1974) point out that the objective environment, the objective person, the subjective environment, and the subjective person can be used to define the four additional concepts which are represented within circles in Figure 7.1. Two concepts represent inaccuracies in the individual's subjective perception of the objective world. The individual's *contact with reality* is defined as the discrepancy between the objective environment and the individual's perception of it. The individual's *accuracy of self-assessment* is defined as the discrepancy between the objective person and the individual's subjective perception of self. Since these two types of discrepancy represent inaccuracy of perception, they are placed in Figure 7.1 next to the arrows which represent the perception of the objective environment and the objective person.

Two additional discrepancies describe the degree of compatibility or fit between the characteristics of the environment and those of the individual. A good fit occurs when the job environment can provide the supplies wanted by the person (e.g. money, social involvement, opportunity to achieve) while the person can provide the abilities required by the job environment (e.g. manual dexterity, computer programming ability, good physical health). The degree of P–E fit can be determined objectively or subjectively. *Objective P–E fit* refers to the fit between the objective person and the objective environment, i.e. fit independent of the individual's perceptions of it. *Subjective P–E fit* refers to the fit between the subjective person and the subjective environment, i.e. the individual's perceptions of his P–E fit. P–E fit represents the interaction of the person and the environment rather than an outcome which each causes. The broken lines in Figure 7.1 represent this interaction process.

French *et al.* (1974) point out that the four types of discrepancy can be measured only if the objective environment, the subjective environment, the objective person, and the subjective person are measured on the same conceptual dimension. For example, typing speed could be used as a dimension. A secretary who thinks she is able to type 55 words per minute (subjective person) may in actuality only type 40 words per minute (objective person). The secretary's boss may expect her to type at a rate of 70 words per minute (objective environment), while the secretary thinks the boss expects her to type about 60 words per minute (subjective environment). The secretary's objective P–E fit, subjective P–E fit, contact with reality, and accessibility to self can all be determined with respect to typing speed because this same conceptual dimension was used to measure the objective and subjective environment and the objective and subjective person.

Each of the four discrepancies described in Figure 7.1 represents an important measure of mental health. Good mental health is represented by no discrepancy or low discrepancy for each of the four comparisons.

P–E fit can be used to define job stress. A job is stressful to the extent that it does not provide supplies to meet the individual's motives and to the extent that the abilities of the individual fall below demands of the job which are prerequisite to receiving supplies. In both cases, the individual's needs and values will not be met by supplies in the job environment.

Job stress (i.e. poor fit in the job environment) can lead to several types of *strain* or deviation from normal responses in the person (see Figure 7.1). Psychological strains include job dissatisfaction, anxiety, or complaints of insomnia and restlessness. Physiological strains include high blood pressure or elevated serum cholesterol. Behavioural symptoms of strain include smoking more, over-eating, or frequent trips for medical help. Any such strains can occur singly or in combination with other strains as the level of job stress increases.

As the individual experiences various job related strains over a period of time, their effects may culminate in various kinds of *illness* (see Figure 7.1). Such illnesses can include both mental health (e.g. chronic depression) and physical health (e.g. coronary heart disease, peptic ulcer). Generally, the incidence of morbidity, mortality, and accidents should increase as job related strain increases.

Although Figure 7.1 emphasizes the negative outcomes of poor P–E fit, good P–E fit can also produce positive health outcomes. Morse (1975) suggests that the continued experience of good fit enhances the individual's sense of competence, self-worth, or 'feeling of efficacy' (White, 1963). The continuously enhanced and increased sense of self-competence at work contributes to the individual's total personality growth. This outcome is a positive mental health benefit in its own right. Indirect positive effects on health may also result from good P–E fit. To the extent that increased self-worth motivates health maintenance behaviour, the individual's physical health will also be improved (cf. Becker *et al.*, 1974; Caplan *et al.*, 1976).

Feedback relationships are necessary to describe the functioning of the model over time. As the experience of poor P–E fit results in strain and illness, the individual may seek to improve the fit between himself and the job through coping or defence (see Figure 7.1). *Coping* refers to activities of the individual directed to changing the objective environment or changing the objective person in ways to improve the fit between the two (Kroeler, 1963). For example, an individual unable to keep up with the current work load may ask a supervisor to reduce the work demands (change the objective environment) or the individual may seek training to improve his abilities to handle the work load (change the objective person). French *et al.* (1974) define coping by changing the objective environment as *environmental mastery* and coping by changing the objective person as *adaptation*. Successful coping of either type results in improved objective fit. When the change in the person and/or the environment is perceived, subjective fit is also improved.

Defences are mental processes which distort the person's perception of the objective environment and the objective self. The defences are unconscious mental processes (e.g. repression, projection) which enable the ego to use distortions to reach compromise solutions which reduce strain associated with the situation (Freud, 1966). For example, an individual unable to keep up with the work load may distort the perception of the work load to a lower level than is actually present in the objective environment (change in subjective environment). A person may also distort the perception of his abilities to higher levels than he is actually capable of performing (change in subjective person). Defences can also be used to distort the individual's perception of P–E fit or to deny the experience of strain. To simplify Figure 7.1, these additional possible effects of defences have not been represented. While defences do not improve the objective fit between the individual and the environment, distorted perceptions of the individual and the environment result in improved subjective P–E fit. Although the improvement in subjective P–E fit lowers the level of stress and/or strain which is experienced, defences decrease the individual's contact with reality and accuracy of self-assessment (cf. Binder *et al.*, 1974).

A number of factors in addition to coping and defence may affect P–E fit over a period of time. Strain and illness may produce changes in the person which intensify misfit. For example, a worker who is unable to keep up with the work load may begin to experience a great deal of anxiety. If the anxiety decreases the person's ability to handle the work load, a vicious circle will begin and result in increasingly poorer P–E fit. Other factors which may affect the person's abilities and motives include a decrease in some physical abilities as he ages and changes in values with marriage and parenthood. The work environment will change as modifications are made in the present job or as the individual moves into a new job. As changes occur they can be described in terms of the concepts represented in Figure 7.1. The resulting effects on P–E fit can then be used to determine whether the change will increase or decrease health strains and illness.

The subjective environment, the subjective person, and strain

Subjective P–E fit is a critical juncture in the model presented in Figure 7.1. This construct links the subjective environment, the subjective person, and strain. The relationship between these four parts of the model will be considered in more detail. An elaborated representation of these relationships is presented in Figure 7.2.

Job stress and P–E fit

What is the basis for the relationship between the job, the individual, and strain? Researchers in the 'stress' field (e.g. Basowitz, Persky, Korchin, and Grinker,

180

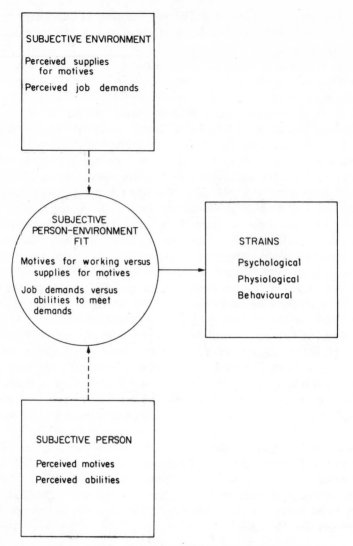

Figure 7.2 A model of the relationship between the subjective
environment, the subjective person, and strain

1955; Lazarus, 1966; Mason, 1975; Miller and Worchel, 1956; Wolff, 1953)
tend to agree that motive arousal is the mediating factor leading to psychological
and physiological responses which constitute health strain. Lewin (1951)
and Murray (1938) emphasize the motivational basis of relationships between
the person and the environment. A motivational theory typically identifies
goals or states which the individual strives to attain. The goals include requirements for the individual's continued subsistence as well as objectives which

the individual has learned to value through socialization. The attainment of goals is generally associated with the maintenance or the enhancement of the well-being of the individual. To the extent that goals are not attained, the well-being of the individual is limited or impaired. The notion of 'fit', 'matching', or 'congruence' between the individual and the environment is implicit in these concepts relating motivational forces within the individual to specific goals concerning the environment.

Several authors (e.g. Atkinson, 1964; Feather, 1975; Lazarus, 1966) point out that the *expectation* of inadequate supplies for goals will result in motive arousal similar to that produced by the *actual* condition of insufficient supplies. Man's cognitive abilities are central to this process. An individual predicts future events on the basis of present circumstances and past experiences. The 'stress' on an individual can be conceived as the sustained tension which occurs when the environment either does not provide or threatens not to provide the goals which the individual seeks.

Job stress can be defined in terms of motive arousal without specifying the particular motives involved. In the terms used by Campbell *et al.* (1970), P–E fit theory is a 'mechanical or process' theory. The theory attempts to conceptualize relationships between forces acting on the individual. These relationships apply to forces resulting from any of a number of motives which may be considered (e.g. physical needs, achievement motive, a need for consistency in one's cognitive view of the world, cf. Lawler, 1973; Pervin, 1968).

In Figure 7.2 the individual's motives and the individual's abilities are identified separately. A parallel distinction is made between the demands of the job environment and the supplies in the job environment. The foregoing discussion has indicated that an individual's experience of job stress is reflected in discrepancies between the individual's motives and the supplies in the job environment. Misfit between the person and the environment may also be described on dimensions describing the job demands and the individual's abilities (French, 1971; House, 1972; Lofquist and Dawis, 1969). Such dimensions reflect the requirements of the job (e.g. typing speed, market knowledge, leadership) and the degree to which the individual can meet these demands. Discrepancies between job demands and individual abilities will be related to strain when they result in insufficient environmental supplies for the individual's goals. Fit on a demand–ability dimension may reflect the level of supplies for motives in two ways: (1) when access to supplies is contingent on meeting the demand and (2) when the demand has been internalized as a value.

When access to supplies (e.g. pay, esteem from others) is contingent on meeting role demands, the individual's behaviour is extrinsically motivated. The motives which instigate the attempts to meet the demands are not directly satisfied by meeting the demand, but by other events which will occur once the demand has been met (cf. House, 1972). Those individuals with 'reward power' (the power to provide or withhold supplies) establish the specific role demands on which supplies are contingent (cf. French and Kahn, 1962).

The second relationship between role demands and motives occurs through the process of acquiring values. French and Kahn (1962) point out that both needs and values can motivate behaviour. Needs are described as innate behavioural predispositions, while values are learned. Values develop from internalized role demands through the process of socialization (Becker, 1969; Feather, 1975; Levinson, 1970). When norms for role behaviour are accepted by the individual as values which he should seek to exemplify, the role demand acquires motivational properties. In meeting the role demand the individual not only wins the approval of others who share the same value, the individual's own self-esteem and sense of positive self-identity are enhanced. Failure to meet the internalized role demands can result in the individual having feelings of guilt and of shame (cf. French and Kahn, 1962). The satisfaction of the motivating force associated with the internalized role demand occurs immediately when the internalized demand is met. An individual's behaviour in trying to meet internalized role demands (i.e. values) is therefore characterized as intrinsically motivated (cf. House, 1972; Katz and Kahn, 1966). With the internationalization of role demands, those abilities of the individual which are required by the role demands become supplies to satisfy the goals of the internalized motive. The individual's preferences concerning the level of a role demand may therefore reflect the desire to use abilities relevant to valued role demands.

Motive–supply and ability–demand dimensions are intimately related. Job demands can act as both positive and negative incentives for motives. Several job demands may be incentives for one motive. For example, contacts with superiors, co-workers, and subordinates may all provide opportunities for social interaction and thereby meet affiliation needs. Similarly, one job demand may have incentive value for several motives. For example, accomplishing a challenging task may directly fulfil a need for personal growth, while recognition of the accomplishment by the employer and others fulfils needs for esteem and security. In effect, motive dimensions of fit and job demand dimensions of fit may describe the same reality from two perspectives.

Ideally, a study or a series of studies would measure the environment and the person on dimensions reflecting both motives and job demands and clarify their interrelationship. Going to this effort, however, is probably not necessary for many investigators. Demonstrated or assumed relationships between these two perspectives are available in existing literature (e.g. Hackman and Lawler, 1971). Additionally, the issues which an investigator wishes to study may naturally lead the investigator to pay more attention to one of the two types of dimensions. A researcher interested in the different levels of strain experienced by individuals on the same job may prefer to measure their fit on motive dimensions. A researcher interested in why some particular occupations tend to be differently associated with strain may prefer to measure P–E fit on job demand dimensions.

P–E fit and strain

Health strain refers to the deviation from normal responses in the person (Caplan *et al.*, 1975). As Figure 7.2 indicates, these deviations may be.(1) psychological responses such as job dissatisfaction, depression, low self-esteem, and unsolved problems; (2) physiological responses such as high blood pressure, change in blood eosinophils, and elevated serum cholesterol; and (3) behavioural responses such as heavy smoking, stuttering, and dispensary visits (Appley and Trumbull, 1967; Caplan *et al.*, 1975).

Some authors use P–E fit measures to represent strain rather than to predict it. For example, Porter (1961) and Slocum and Strawser (1973) operationalize job satisfaction as the extent to which the job environment provided opportunities to meet the individual's higher order needs. The larger the discrepancy, the more dissatisfied the individual is defined to be. Hulin and Blood (1968) point out, however, that the theoretical distinction should be maintained between an individual's perception of self in relation to the environment and the resulting affective response to these circumstances. Moss (1973) also points out that most theories about stress distinguish between person–environment situations and responses to those situations. Most studies using P–E fit measures have followed the view that poor P–E fit causes strain rather than represents it (cf. Kulka, 1976).

P–E fit theory as developed by French *et al.* (1974) emphasizes the theoretical necessity of the causal link between P–E fit and strain. Though the necessity of the causal link is widely recognized, the exact content and processes of that link remain unclear. Factors determining which type of strain(s) will occur in response to P–E fit include: (1) motive(s) which are not being met; (2) genetic and social background of the individual; (3) defence and coping predispositions of the individual; and (4) situational constraints on particular responses. At least partial attempts to develop theories to define and interrelate these strain determining factors have been made by Caudill (1958), Lazarus (1966), Mechanic (1968), Moss (1973), and Scott and Howard (1970).

Predictions of which strain will occur in an individual experiencing person–environment misfit require information concerning each of the four areas considered above. P–E fit theory predicts only that some form of strain occurs with misfit and that the magnitude of the strain will be proportional to the degree of misfit. The prediction is based on the direct relationship assumed between sustained motive arousal (or tension) and strain responses. The four factors presented above transform the sustained motive arousal into specific strain responses, but do not alter the direct relationship: *strain should increase as P–E fit dimensions reflect increased insufficiency of goal supplies for motives.*

French *et al.* (1974) and Caplan *et al.* (1975) use the likely occurrence of insufficient goal supplies for motives to identify three differently shaped relationships between various P–E fit dimensions and strains. These relationships are illustrated in Figure 7.3. The horizontal axis of the figure represents a scale of person–environment fit. The numbers on the scale represent discrepancies between person and environment scores on commensurate dimensions. The zero at the centre of the scale represents perfect fit where the person score and environment score are equal. The negative scores to the left of perfect fit represent increasing deficiency where the person score is increasingly larger than the environment score. The positive scores represent increasing excess where the environment scores are increasingly larger than the person scores. In addition to these definitions, it must be assumed that the P–E fit scale is an equal interval scale. The vertical axis in Figure 7.3 represents any strain which may result from sustained motive arousal.

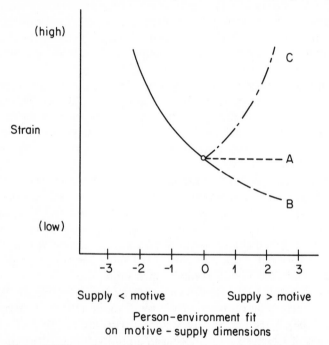

Figure 7.3 Three hypothetical shapes of the relationship between P–E fit on motive–supply dimensions and strains

The distinction between commensurate P–E fit on motive–supply dimensions and on ability–demand dimensions was pointed out in the preceding discussion. General relationships between fit on motive–supply dimensions will be discussed first. Then the application of these relationships to ability–demand dimensions will be considered.

The solid line in Figure 7.3 illustrates the monotonic decrease in strain associated with the increase in environmental supplies to the point of matching the motive levels. This monotonic relationship applies to all motive–supply dimensions where supplies are not sufficient to meet motive levels. Insufficient food, money, love, opportunities for growth, or any other supply will produce strain.

The relationship between fit and strain becomes complex when the effects of supplies in excess of motive strength are considered. Excess supplies may result in no change in the level of strain, decreased strain, or increased strain, depending on the implications which excess supplies for the motive have for supplies for other motives. The possibilities are explained and illustrated below.

House (1972) points out that fit should have an asymptotic relationship with strain (described by the solid line and line A in Figure 7.3) when excess supplies for one motive are not exchangeable for supplies for other motives. For example, a hungry man eats until he is full and then does not eat additional food even if it is offered to him. Similarly, the dimension of fit on opportunities for personal growth and development should be asymptotically related to strain. As the individual is presented with more opportunities than he wants or can use, the motive arousal for personal growth should remain low. Additionally, the unused opportunities are not likely to be transformed into supplies for other motives. Surplus opportunities for growth should therefore not affect strain levels.

The monotonic relationship represented by the solid line and curve B in Figure 7.3 will occur when excess supplies for one motive can be used directly as supplies for other motives. One of the most common uses for excess amounts of *preservable* supplies is to store them in case the availability of the supplies should be reduced in the future. The accumulation of preservable supplies for various motives is in itself a goal of security motives. Coch and French (1948) note an example where workers were given tickets for every piece produced and the individual's pay was determined by the number of tickets turned in at the end of a day. Many workers held on to a few tickets so that they could be turned in on days when they were not able to meet their quota. To the extent that the future availability of supplies is uncertain, accumulating excess supplies which are preservable should increase the individual's security and therefore reduce strain below its level at perfect fit between the present motive level and supplies for it.

House (1972) suggests the monotonic relationships represented by the solid line and curve B in Figure 7.3 will also occur when excess supplies for one motive can be *exchanged* for supplies for other motives. For example, if a person receives less money than he desires, he may not be able to live according to his needs and values, and strain should be high. On the other hand, additional money can be used to purchase comforts beyond those he would normally expect. By satisfying other motives, strain is reduced below its level at perfect fit on income.

The reader should note that a monotonic relationship may occur between certain measures of fit and strain which is not the same as curve B. This occurs for situations where the supplies do not exceed the level of motive strength. The fit scores fall only along the solid line in Figure 7.4. For example, Evans (1969), Porter (1961), Wall and Payne (1973), and Wanous and Lawler (1972) point out that most people report that their jobs do not offer sufficient supplies for their higher order needs. Therefore only deficiency scores were found on the fit dimension. These authors report linear relationships between these deficiency scores and job dissatisfaction similar to the solid line in Figure 7.3.

The final relationship between P–E fit and strain has the U-shape illustrated by the solid line and curve C in Figure 7.3. French *et al.* (1974) suggest that the presence of excess supplies for one motive may result in deficient supplies for another motive. Consider, for example, P–E fit on the dimension of privacy. Strain should be high when the individual has less privacy than is wanted, with strain decreasing as the opportunities for privacy increase towards the desired level. As the individual experiences more privacy than is wanted, supplies for affiliation motives may be reduced, thereby increasing strain. (The quality of the specific strain response may differ from one side of perfect fit to the other.) Katzell (1964) and Locke (1969) also explicitly recognize the theoretical operation of an excess on one motive producing a deficiency on another, resulting in the U-shaped relationship between fit and strain.

The relationships between fit on ability–demand dimensions and strain are similar to those between fit on motive–supply dimensions and strain since both sets of relations are based on the extent to which motives may be satisfied. As Figure 7.4 indicates, the only difference between these two sets of relationships is the reversed meaning of the P–E fit dimension when P–E fit continues to be defined as the person score subtracted from the environment score (P–E fit = E − P). For motive–supply dimensions, negative fit scores (E < P) represent insufficient environmental supplies for motives and positive fit scores (E > P) represent excess supplies. For ability–demand dimensions,

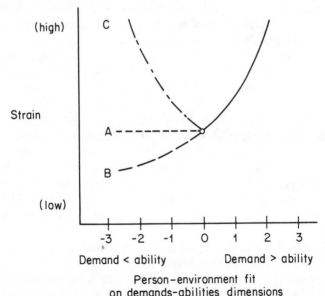

Figure 7.4 Three hypothetical shapes of the relationships between P–E fit on ability–demand dimensions and strains

however, positive fit scores (E > P) represent situations where environmental demands exceed worker abilities, resulting in insufficient supplies for the worker. Negative fit scores (E < P) represent situations where worker abilities exceed job demands and the worker may have excess supplies.

The solid line in Figure 7.4 represents the relationship between strain and ability–demand fit when demands exceed abilities. Strain increases monotonically as job demands increase beyond worker ability. When individual abilities (e.g. typing speed, work pace, leadership) are insufficient to meet job demands, job provided supplies (e.g. pay, seniority, self-esteem, opportunities for intrinsically satisfying work) are threatened and strain increases.

The possible effects of excess abilities on strain parallel the possible effects of excess supplies on strain. When excess abilities are present they may have no relationship with motive supplies and therefore not affect strain (curve A). For example, having a knowledge of mathematics somewhat beyond that required by the job may have little effect on supplies for other motives. Excess abilities may provide supplies for motives other than those threatened by insufficient abilities (curve B). For example, being able to easily handle the work load required may allow time for socializing, reading, or other activities which satisfy other motives. Excess abilities may reflect insufficient supplies for other motives and produce increased strain (curve C). For example, an individual with abilities to handle a much more complex job may have internalized higher levels of role demands as values. The inability to use his abilities could result in lowered self-esteem and other strains.

P–E fit theory is appealing because it clarifies and extends ideas which many researchers have used at an intuitive level. While the elegance of the formal definition of several constructs makes the theory conceptually attractive, the usefulness of the theory in predicting strain must be evaluated.

The utility of P–E fit theory

An evaluation of the usefulness of P–E fit theory necessarily entails the question, 'Can the variation in strain predicted by P–E fit be accounted for more simply in terms of the component E and P measures?' Cronbach (e.g. Cronbach, 1958; Cronbach and Furby, 1970) has consistently pointed out that a more complicated measure should only be used when it demonstrates a significant improvement in the prediction of data over linear predictions based on the component scores separately or together. P–E fit theory attributes meaning to the discrepancy between E and P measures as well as to the E and P measures themselves. If strain can be predicted equally well from simple (i.e. linear) relationships to E and P measures as from P–E fit measures, then the simpler explanation using only the E and P measures is to be preferred. The justification for the use of P–E fit measures must depend on their demonstrating a significant improvement in the prediction of strain over linear predictions from E and P measures.

The discussion in the previous section noted that P–E fit theory predicts both linear and curvilinear relationships between fit and strain. The prediction of curvilinear relationships is a potential advantage over stress theories which predict a linear relationship (or at least a monotonic relationship) between strain and the level of some environmental characteristic or of some attribute of the person. The fulfilment theory of job satisfaction is an example of this simple linear approach. Fulfilment theory proposes that job satisfaction varies directly with the extent to which a characteristic is present in the job (cf. Lawler, 1973). Job satisfaction increases as the amount of the characteristic (or group of characteristics) increases. Job dissatisfaction decreases as the amount of the characteristic decreases.

Figures 7.3 and 7.4 illustrated the three shapes of relationships with strain predicted by P–E theory: linear, asymptotic, and U-shaped. The differentiation of these three shapes evolved from the recognition that the point at which environmental supplies match the person's preferences is a potential turning point in the relationship between fit and strain. The patterns of strain represented by asymptotic and U-shaped relationships with P–E fit cannot be predicted by separate measures of the environment and the person or by an additive combination of them. If these curvilinear relationships are found, the use of P–E fit theory and measures can be justified.

Curvilinear relationships between P–E fit and strain

To determine whether or not a relationship between strain and a measure of person–environment fit is curvilinear, it is necessary to have a distribution of fit scores on both sides of the point of perfect fit. Unfortunately, a great number of the studies which relate P–E fit to strain do not present evidence concerning the curvilinearity of the relationship since the fit scores represented only insufficient supplies for goals (e.g. Evans, 1969; Porter, 1961; Wall and Payne, 1973; Wanous and Lawler, 1972). Studies using measures of fit between the demands of the job and preferences of the individual have been more likely to obtain scores on both sides of the point of perfect fit (e.g. Caplan, 1972; Kulka, 1976; Locke, 1969). Even when a full distribution of the fit scores is reported, however, a curvilinear relationship between fit and strain is not always expected. Only when excess supplies and abilities are not relevant to the individual's goals (asymptotic curve) or when excess supplies or abilities hinder the accomplishment of some goal or goals (U-shaped curve) will the relationship be curvilinear.

Several studies with full distributions of scores on one or more fit dimensions report instances of the expected asymptotic and U-shaped relationships between fit and strain (e.g. House, 1972; Kulka, 1976; Locke, 1969). A good example of the U-shaped relationship is presented by Caplan *et al.* (1975). Workers in 23 occupations were included in the study. One dimension on which person–environment fit was measured was the complexity (qualitative demands) of the job. A multiple item measure of job complexity was used which included items concerning the absence of a work routine, handling of several tasks at once, and dealing with a variety of people at the job. A worker was asked to rate the complexity of the job (subjective environment) and the level of complexity preferred by the individual (subjective person). Reports of several kinds of strains (e.g. job dissatisfaction, depression, anxiety) were also obtained from the workers. These strains were also measured using multiple item scales. The depression measure, for example, included the items, 'I feel sad, I feel depressed, I feel blue', and had been clinically validated in previous research (Zung, 1965). The relationship found between job complexity and depression is presented in Figures 7.5 and 7.6. In Figure 7.5 the solid line illustrates the relationship between depression and the level of complexity in the job environment. The broken line illustrates the relationship between depression and the level of job complexity preferred by the person. Though there is a tendency for depression scores to decrease both for individuals with more complex job environments and for individuals who prefer higher job complexity, neither relationship reaches statistical significance.

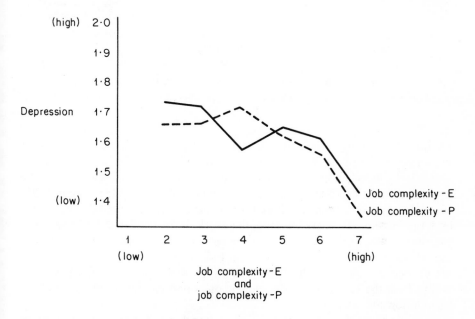

Figure 7.5 Relationships between scores on depression and scores on job complexity-E and job complexity-P. Etas = 0·14 (NS) and 0·19 (NS) respectively. $N = 318$ men from 23 occupations (from Caplan *et al.*, 1975, p. 90)

The person and environment scores on job complexity were combined into a person–environment fit score by subtracting the amount of complexity preferred by the individual from the amount of complexity on the job. The relationship between depression and person–environment fit on job complexity is presented in Figure 7.6. Depression is lowest for those with perfect fit and increases with either too little job complexity or too much job complexity. This

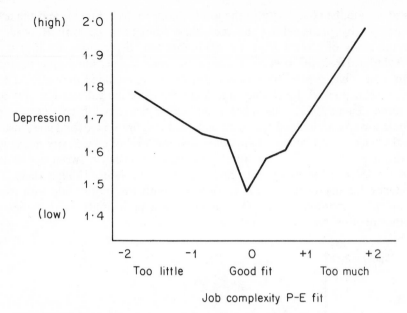

Figure 7.6 Relationship between job complexity P–E fit and depression. Eta $= 0.26$ ($p < .002$). $N = 318$ men from 23 occupations. (From Caplan *et al.*, 1975, p. 91)

relationship closely approximates the hypothetical U-shaped relationship presented in Figure 7.4. When the qualitative demands of the job are too great (P < E), the individual may be threatened with job loss, or at least loss of the esteem of others and a lowered sense of competence. Too little job complexity (P > E) may also prevent the individual from gaining a sense of competence and the esteem of others because the work lacks challenge and meaning. Harrison (1976) further analysed the same data to determine whether or not the relationship between depression and P–E fit on job complexity was found within occupations as well. The relationship was significant and U-shaped within 13 of the 16 occupations having enough participants to justify checking the relationship.

Analysis of the same data set shows that the relationships between P–E fit on work load and strains are more complex. Work load was a measure of the quantitative demands of the job and the multiple item index included items concerning the amount of work to be done, the amount of time to think and contemplate, and the time available to do the work. Harrison (1976) found that the shape of relationships between P–E fit on work load and strains varies by occupation. The relationship between P–E fit on work load and job dissatisfaction is presented separately for administration, assembly line workers, and policemen in Figure 7.7. Work overload (P < E) is rèlated to increased job dissatisfaction in all these occupations. However, the relationship between work underload (P > E) and job dissatisfaction changes from

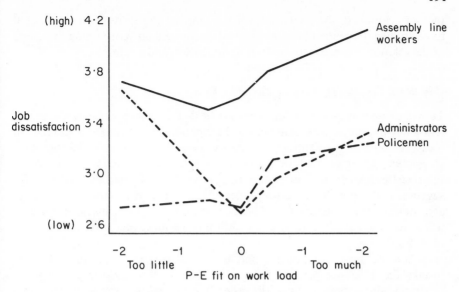

Figure 7.7 Relationships between job dissatisfaction and P–E fit on work load. For assembly line workers, $N = 102$, eta $= 0.31$, $p < .04$. For administrators, $N = 239$, eta $= 0.38, p < .001$. For Policemen, $N = 108$, eta $= 0.29, p = .05$

one occupation to another. Work underload seems to have little effect on the job dissatisfaction of assembly line workers and policemen.

Why should the effect of work underload vary across the occupations? House (1972) found that, on the average, white collar workers have been found to want a high level of intrinsic gratification in their jobs. Work underload can reduce the availability of intrinsic gratification and thus increase job dissatisfaction. Blue collar workers have been found, on the average, to be less concerned about intrinsic satisfaction in their jobs. Work underload would therefore not be expected to increase the job dissatisfaction of assembly line workers. House (1972) had no data concerning policemen. It is reasonable, however, to interpret somewhat differently the lack of relationship between underload and job dissatisfaction for them. For administrators and assemblers, the amount of work done is crucial to the job. For policemen, however, the availability to do work may be crucial. A large component of their job is performing routine duties while being available for emergency calls. When work underload is experienced, it may be viewed as a necessary part of the job and have less impact on the intrinsic gratification associated with the job.

The differing relationships between job dissatisfaction and P–E fit on work load support P–E fit theory in two ways. First, the predicted curvilinear relationships between P–E fit and strain are observed. Second, the interpretation of the P–E fit dimension in terms of its meaning for the motives and goals of the individual is emphasized. No specific relationship can automatically be assumed to exist between a particular P–E fit dimension and strain. One must consider the implications of the dimension for the motives and goals of the individual to be studied. Only then can specific predictions be made concerning the shape of the relationship between the P–E fit dimension and strain.

Additional variance in strain predicted by P–E fit

To what extent does the use of measures of P–E fit improve the prediction of strain beyond predictions made using the component environment and person measures separately? Considering the extensive literature using fit measures to predict outcomes, very little information has been presented concerning this question. A review of literature using measures of P–E fit by Kulka (1976) suggests that only three studies systematically deal with this issue. Before considering the findings of these studies, two statistical problems must be noted which are inherent in the question of additional variance predicted by a measure of P–E fit.

By far the most common method for calculating the score of P–E fit is to take the difference between the environmental score and the person score by simply subtracting one from the other. The fit score is a simple linear transformation of the component environment and person scores. Variance in strain which is linearly associated with P–E fit is therefore statistically indistinguishable from variance and strain which are linearly related to both the E and P components. Expanding upon this observation, Cronbach and Furby (1970) conclude that when only linear variance in outcomes is predicted, only the component scores need be used since the more complex discrepancy scores offer no empirical advantage. The equal or superior performances of the component scores over discrepancy scores in accounting for linear variance and strain also have implications for asymptotic relationships between P–E fit and strain. Though asymptotic relationships are non-linear, they are still monotonic. Nunnally (1967) points out that linear relationships will typically account for most of the variance in measures which are monotonically related. Asymptotic relationships between P–E fit and strain should therefore account for only marginal additional variance in strain beyond that accounted for by linear relationships with E and P components. When the relationship between P–E fit and strain has the non-monotonic U-shape, little variance in strain will be accounted for by linear relationships with the E and P components. In the case of U-shaped relationships between P–E fit and strain, therefore, P–E fit should account for substantial additional variance in strain over that accounted for by linear relationships with the E and P components.

A second statistical issue arises from the correlation typically found between the E and P measures. In field studies the level of a job characteristic is typically correlated with the level of that characteristic preferred by the individual. This positive correlation reflects the processes of job selection and job socialization. In selecting a job an individual tries to find one where the job characteristics match his preferences. Similarly, a factor used in hiring is selecting individuals whose abilities and preferences match the demands of the job. Once on the job, the fit between the individual and the job will tend to improve as the individual is socialized into the value system of the work group and as the individual's abilities to do the job improve with experience on the job. Statistical tests using a non-additive model (i.e. $E + P +$ interaction of E and P) typically assume that the E and P measures are uncorrelated. Violation of this assumption may artificially reduce or enhance the likelihood that the interaction term will account for additional variance in strain (cf. Althauser, 1971). Caution must therefore be used in interpreting the results for any one relationship between the strain and the P–E fit dimension. The overall pattern of results across several relationships between P–E fit dimensions and strains will still provide useful information concerning the general ability of predictions derived from P–E fit theory to account for additional variance in strain.

The most complete evidence concerning the ability of P–E fit measures to account for additional variances in strains is presented by Harrison (1976). Figures 7.5, 7.6, and 7.7, which were discussed above, are based on these data. Additional findings concerning the relationship between fit and job complexity and several psychological strains are presented in Table 7.1. Scatter plots and polynomial analyses were used to examine the shape of relationships between fit on job complexity and the strains. The six relationships in Table 7.1 were found to be U-shaped. The simple transformation of taking the absolute value of each fit score was used to make the relationships approximately linear. For example, fit scores of minus 1 and plus 1 would both be given a general misfit score of 1. (Cronbach, 1958, notes that the expression k ($|P-E|$) is equivalent to the expression c ($-PE$), where k and c are constants. The absolute value scores may therefore be regarded as a measure of interaction similar to a standard cross-product term.) The standard statistical techniques of correlation and multiple regression were used to quantify the relationship between the measure of misfit on job complexity and the strains.

The first three columns of Table 7.1 present the correlations between the

Table 7.1 Correlations and multiple correlations between strains and E, P, and misfit indices of job complexity

| | Correlations | | | Multiple correlations | |
Strains	Environment (E)	Person (P)	Misfit ($|E-P|$)	E and P	E and P with additional effects of misfit
Job dissat.	− 0·31	− 0·30	0·47	0·34	0·50*
Boredom	− 0·51	− 0·34	0·51	0·51	0·61*
Somat. cmplnts	NS	NS	0·16	NS	0·18*
Anxiety	NS	NS	0·21	NS	0·25*
Depression	NS	− 0·12	0·22	NS	0·23*
Irritation	NS	NS	0·15	NS	0·20*

Note $N = 318$ men from 23 occupations. For all correlations presented, $p < ·05$.
(From Harrison, 1976.)
*The addition of misfit increases the multiple correlation significantly.

strains in the left margin and the amount of job complexity in the environment, the amount preferred, and the amount of person–environment misfit, respectively. The fourth column presents the multiple correlation of both the environmental level and the preferred level of job complexity with the strains. These values represent the combined ability of the environmental measure and the person measure to predict the strains. The last column presents similar multiple correlations, except that the predictive ability of the misfit measure has also been included. The difference between these last two columns represents the variance accounted for by the misfit measure beyond that accounted for by the environment and person measures. The measure of misfit on job complexity accounts for significant additional variance in each of the six strains.

In addition to fit on job complexity, Harrison (1976) also examined the effects of fit between job characteristics and individual preferences on work load, responsibility for other people, and role ambiguity. Eighteen strains representing a variety of psychological, behavioural, and physiological responses were also measured. Either a deficiency (P > E) or an excess (P < E) on each of the four P–E fit dimensions was expected to reflect insufficient supplies for motives. Therefore, when a significant relationship was found between a P–E fit dimension and a particular strain, it was expected to be curvilinear in shape. Twenty-seven significant relationships were found between a strain and a measure of E, P, or P–E fit on a dimension. In 18 of these relationships, P–E fit measures accounted for variance beyond that accounted for by linear relationships between the strain and the E and P components together. Additional variance was accounted for in relationships between each of the four P–E fit dimensions and three or more strains. The additional variance in strain accounted for ranged from 1·5% to 14%, with a median increase of 3·3%. On the average, the increased variance in strain accounted for by the P–E fit measure equalled the amount of variance predicted by linear relationships with the E and P measures together.

House (1972) measured fit on several motive dimensions and reports data relating fit to job satisfaction in men from several occupations. Of the 18 fit dimensions in the study, 16 were significantly related to job satisfaction. Of the 16 fit dimensions, five were found to account for variance in job satisfaction beyond that accounted by the E and P components. The additional curvilinear variance in job satisfaction was small, however, ranging from 1·2% to 2·7%. This small increase in variance accounted for is understandable, however, since all five relationships were found to be asymptotic in shape.

Kulka (1976) measured P–E fit between high schools and high school students and its impact on several measures of strain (e.g. self-esteem, depression, the number of days school skipped). Of the 363 relationships between fit measures and strains, 260 were classified as linear, 46 were classified as asymptotic, and 57 were classified as U-shaped. The ability of P–E fit measures to account for variance in strain beyond that accounted for by the E and P components was examined in a subset of the data. Of 205 significant relationships between P–E fit dimensions and strains, P–E fit accounted for additional variance in 44 (about 20%) of the relationships. The amount of additional variance predicted in the strains ranged from 1% to 5%.

The findings reviewed above clearly demonstrate the existence of the curvilinear relationships between P–E fit dimensions and strain which are predicted by P–E fit theory. The findings demonstrate that measures of P–E fit can account for variance in strain which cannot be predicted by linear relationships with the E or P component measures, either singly or together. These findings demonstrate the usefulness of the theory and justify its continued use and development.

Contributions of E and P measures

The evidence that P–E fit can account for additional variance in strain does not necessarily mean that P–E fit measures can totally replace the component E and P measures in predicting strain. The theory of person–environment fit assumes that the E and P component measures have meaning primarily in relation to each other, i.e. the components have no independent effects on strain. Many examples can be found, however, where the E and/or P components of the fit measures have main effects on strain which are not accounted for by the fit measure. Table 7.1, which was presented earlier, presents an example in the relationship between job complexity and boredom. Together the E, P, and misfit measures account for 37% of the variance in reports of boredom ($R = 0.61$). The environment and persons scores together account for 26% of the variance in boredom ($R = 0.51$). Misfit on job complexity therefore accounts for an additional 11% of the variance in boredom. The table also shows, however, that misfit on job complexity by itself accounts for only 26% of the variance in boredom ($R = 0.51$) and the addition of the E and P measures accounts for an additional 11% of the variance in boredom. Some of the linear effects represented by the components are clearly independent of their relation to each other. Examples of component measures accounting for variance beyond that accounted for by P–E fit measures can be found in reviewing data reported by Harrison (1976), House (1972), and Kulka (1976). What implications do these independent relationships between the component measures and strains have for P–E fit theory?

Implications for theories of stress

The findings which have been reviewed demonstrate the usefulness of P–E fit theory in understanding how job stress results in health strain. The curvilinear relationships between measures of P–E fit and strains have not been predicted from theories which focus on the environment alone or on the person alone. Findings demonstrating independent effects of the measures of the environment and of the person raise doubts about the sufficiency of P–E fit theory to account for the total relationship between job stress and strain. Two interpretations of the findings are (1) that theories describing person–environment fit must be combined with theories describing the direct effects of characteristics of the environment and of the person, or (2) that the findings that characteristics of the person or the environment have independent effects on strain result from methodological problems and the theory of P–E fit is conceptually sufficient to account for the relationships.

The first interpretation takes the findings at face value. In addition to operating in relation to each other, characteristics of the environment and of the person can also operate independently. This conclusion suggests the need to develop theories describing the independent operation of the characteristics as they reflect job stress and result in health strain.

The second interpretation of the findings argues that the evidence has not tested the sufficiency of P–E fit theory, only its necessity. The data which are currently available have two major methodological limitations. One limitation results from systematic bias in the measures of the environment and the person. The individual's abilities can affect reports concerning the environment. For example, an individual's response to 'how much work load do you have' is likely to be affected by his perception of his ability to handle the work load. Similarly, the individual's environment can affect reports of his abilities and goals. The measures of the person and the environment are *contaminated* by each other so that each reflects to some extent the fit between the person and the environment. To the extent that measures of the environment and the person reflect P–E fit, the percentage of variance in strain accounted for by the components should be inflated. Furthermore, measures of P–E fit derived from contaminated E and P scores will underestimate the percentage of variance which should be accounted for by P–E fit (cf. French *et al.*, 1974; Harrison, 1976).

The second methodological limitation results from the *confounding* of measures on any one dimension with measures on other dimensions of P–E fit. For example, perfect fit will occur when an individual both has and prefers a job with a fixed routine or when an individual both has and prefers a job with a high level of complexity. More complex jobs, however, typically have higher pay, status, and other rewards than routine jobs have (Quinn and Shepard, 1974). The complexity of the job is therefore confounded with P–E fit on dimensions of pay, status, and other rewards. The measure of the actual complexity of the job will reflect supplies for these other dimensions. When these dimensions are related to strain, the confounding between these dimensions and the complexity of the job will result in a main effect being found between strain and the E component of job complexity. This explanation suggests that if all relevant dimensions were identified, P–E fit on the dimensions would account for relationships between strain and measures of either the person or the environment.

Additional research will be necessary to determine whether or not independent effects of measures of the person and environment can be explained as the result of the methodological problems of contamination and confounding. Measures and measurement methods must be developed which discriminate between environmental scores, personal preference scores, and P–E fit scores. Research is also needed to identify sets of dimensions which together encompass many, if not all, of the major interrelationships between a person and the environment.

For the present, the evidence is clear that researchers studying job stress should take advantage of the predictive power of measures of P–E fit and of the underlying P–E fit theory. At the same time, independent effects which the component measures of the person and the environment have on strain should also be studied. Such independent effects may be interpreted using P–E fit theory. The evidence does not, however, exclude the interpretation of these effects by theories describing the independent operation of characteristics of either person or environment (cf. Hope, 1975).

Implications for reducing job stress

The theory of person–environment fit provides the framework for conceptualizing many activities designed to reduce job stress. The theory emphasizes that job stress will not be reduced by general programmes which treat all individuals identically. The relationship between each worker's needs and values and the job environment must be considered. This relationship can be considered at one point in time, over the time the individual holds the job, and over the career of the individual. After discussing implications of the P–E fit theory from each of these perspectives, some practical limitations on improving P–E fit will be pointed out.

P–E fit at one point in time

The fit between the individual and the job should be carefully considered during the hiring process. Personnel psychology and personnel management have developed a vast array of instruments to measure individual abilities and their fit to the demands of specific jobs (e.g. the General Aptitude Test Battery and the Occupational Aptitude Patterns instruments of the US Training and Employment Service). By contrast, little attempt has been made to develop dimensions describing the supplies the job offers for the motives of the individual. How much appreciation and respect go with the job? What opportunities for achievement does the job offer? P–E fit theory emphasizes the fundamental role of misfit between job supplies and individual's motives in producing job stress. Measures of these types of dimensions need to be developed and the information be made available to both the employer and the potential employee when hiring decisions are made.

Once individuals are on the job, their fit with the job can be periodically reviewed. Measures of person–environment fit can be used to identify those individuals experiencing high levels of misfit. These individuals can then be the focus of special attempts to reduce stress through procedures such as counselling, training, and job transfer. If the misfit represents abilities and values for more challenging work, promotion may be considered. Again it must be emphasized that fit with respect to the individual's needs and values must be considered in addition to fit with respect to the individual's abilities.

P–E fit over the tenure in the job

While checking P–E fit at various points in time is important, it is also necessary to conceptualize processes occurring through time. By doing this the focus can shift from improving misfit to maintaining good fit.

Over a period of time, changes may occur both in the demands and supplies of the job and in the values and the abilities of the worker. How can good fit between worker and the job maintained? One approach would be to attempt to continually monitor the fit between the worker and the job. This has traditionally been a part of a supervisor's role. Another approach suggested by findings about participation and fit (French and Caplan, 1972) would place much of the responsibility for reducing stress on the individual worker. By increasing the control workers have over their jobs, they can modify the demands of their jobs themselves to bring about a better fit with their individual preferences.

This approach should not be confused with job enlargement or job enrichment. Proponents of job enlargement assume that all individuals want challenging and involving experiences at work. The evidence supporting person–environment fit theory suggests that enlarging an entire set of jobs may improve fit for some, but it will also worsen fit for others who prefer simpler job routines. Advocates of job enlargement programmes often propose giving people more participation in decisions affecting their jobs. They assume, however, that providing the worker with more control will meet the needs for challenge and involvement felt by all individuals. While person–environment fit theory also suggests that increasing worker participation is important, the theory suggests it is important because a more complex process can then occur. The increased control allows the worker to structure the job to better fit his abilities and values, whatever they may be. Those who want more complex and challenging jobs can take advantage of the opportunities opened up to them. Those individuals who prefer simpler jobs can choose to delegate decision making to others who want this job demand. Remaining tasks can be routinized in ways which minimize their demands on the worker.

The tremendous advantage of allowing some individualization of the job is the creation of a mechanism for the ongoing maintenance of good fit. As either personal preferences or job demands change, the individual can—without outside intervention—cope by making adjustments in the job to lessen stress and improve fit.

P–E fit over a working career

Considering an individual's entire working career provides a still broader perspective of the processes involved in obtaining and maintaining good fit between the individual and the job. This broader perspective highlights the distinctions between the individual's current fit with the job, the fit he expects to have at some future point in time, and the fit he actually experiences at that future time.

The preceding discussion has focused almost entirely on the degree of P–E fit which is currently experienced. Many job environments are selected for their anticipated effect in improving P–E fit in the future. For example, an individual will go through 4 years of postgraduate education and another year of internship to become a physician. Having decided that occupation will be a good fit with his needs and values, the individual begins to cope with the present lack of fit between himself and the job by acquiring the skills and abilities which are necessary. The effects of the misfit experienced during job training or on a particular 'step' of a 'career ladder' may be tolerated by the individual if they are perceived to be of relatively short duration and can be viewed as leading to the desired goal. The same level of misfit may have much more pronounced effects on strain if no improvement in P–E fit is anticipated.

The degree of P–E fit the individual actually experiences in the future may or may not match the individual's expectations. The P–E fit may be worse than expected if the individual misperceived the demands and supplies associated with the job, if the job environment changes, or if the individual's needs, values, or abilities change. The individual may cope with the resulting misfit by making a mid-career change to a job which then appears to offer a better fit. It is possible, however, that P–E fit will actually be better than would have been anticipated. For example, an individual may have originally seen a job as a temporary experience which was necessary for obtaining another position. Later the individual may find that his values and goals have changed as a result of socialization in the job. His P–E fit with the current job may become better than it would be were he to move to another position.

The present and future perspectives of P–E fit emphasize the need to understand more about the selection of careers, career paths, and changes in the individual's values and goals at various stages in a career. This information can then be used to provide more help in career counselling. Going beyond fit with a particular job, the individual can be helped in making long range plans which will enable the individual to match needs and values—in addition to abilities—with the appropriate job environments. This includes selecting jobs for the career paths associated with them, mid-career changes to jobs more suited to the individual's needs and values, and dealing with retirement when the individual's needs and values will no longer be met in the job environment. Planning to maximize good fit through all of these stages should minimize job stress at any given point in time and contribute to the individual's total personality growth by continually enhancing the individual's sense of self-worth.

Problems in improving person–environment fit

The inescapable conclusion of person–environment fit theory is that in order to reduce job stress for all persons, programmes must allow *individualized* treatment of a worker. It must be recognized, however, that this objective can conflict with the technology associated with the job, with organizational control structures, and with the system for allocating rewards.

Flexibility in meeting job demands may be severely limited by the technology of the job. The technology may determine the extent to which the job can be varied both in its content and in its work place. The cost of transforming the technology in an existing job is weighed against the potential benefits of redesigning the job to allow for better fit with the person over time. The development and use of technologies which give the worker more control over the work environment (e.g. team production rather than assembly line production) will allow for more individualized treatment of the worker.

Bureaucratic approaches to control require formal role descriptions. All individuals filling the same role are expected to perform the same jobs in a roughly equivalent manner. The control and co-ordination structure of the organization is based on the interlocking descriptions prescribed for the various work roles. As jobs are individualized, however, a greater variation in behaviour may occur across individuals holding the same jobs. New approaches for co-ordination between the individualized jobs will have to be developed. Suggestions for more flexible control structures include increasing individual participation, building worker teams, and improving co-ordination across work groups (e.g. Likert, 1967; Beckhard, 1972; Katz and Kahn, 1966).

The individualization of work also raises questions concerning the rewards— financial and otherwise—associated with the job. Pay systems have typically been built around sets of formal role descriptions with some individual variance for performance. With individualized jobs there is a greater variety in what individuals actually do. It becomes more difficult to distinguish one job classification from another. Modified systems for allocating pay and other rewards will have to be developed as jobs become more individualized (cf. Lawler, 1973).

Given the conflicts involved, it is probable that job stress cannot be totally eliminated. It can, however, be minimized to the extent that the benefit is worth the cost. Lawler (1976) points out that the true cost of job stress is gradually being realized. The costs to industry include decreased quality of work, increased absenteeism, increased turnover, and the increasing expense for group prepaid health insurance. Job stress can impair the psychological and physical well-being of the individual worker and thereby affect the well-being of the worker's family. On the societal level these effects can be manifest in increased welfare cost, increased socially disruptive behaviour such as alcoholism and drug abuse, and less involvement in the community. As the far reaching consequences of job stress are understood, more resources will be used to reduce it. To the extent that improving person–environment fit is found to reduce job stress and its consequences, greater emphasis will be placed on programmes which allow individualized treatment of the worker.

Future development of P–E fit theory

The usefulness of the theory of person–environment fit has been demonstrated by its ability to predict health strain and to suggest procedures which will reduce it. The benefits of the theory in its present form suggests that additional effort should be made to further develop the theory.

The types of dimensions used to measure P–E fit must be differentiated and their implications understood. One problem is identifying dimensions which are relevant both to the person and to the job. For example, French and Kahn (1962) point out that the dimension of 'love' better describes an individual's needs and values than the demands and supplies of the job. Graham (1976) has identified 120 dimensions which are generally recognized to be relevant both to the individual and to the environment. Even when a dimension has been identified, however, the precise meaning of P–E fit on it may still have to be specified. For example, Wanous and Lawler (1972) find that an individual will give different responses to questions asking how many units on the dimension are *wanted* and how many units *should there be*. Lawler (1973) suggests that the 'want' measure reflects the individual's aspirations for personal goals and that the 'should be' measure reflects an equity comparison or fairness measure. Another distinction to be considered is that between how many units on a dimension would be *ideal* or how many units would be *acceptable* (Miller, 1963). Since individuals can differentiate between these various questions, it is likely that they reflect different values and goals which are associated with the dimension being measured. Making one of the values or goals more relevant may shift the degree of P–E fit and its implications for strain.

A broader understanding of the meaning and impact of job stress will be obtained as P–E fit on the job is related to other domains of the person's life. For example, Cobb (1976) and Pinneau (1976) find that social support from wife and family may reduce job related strain. The process by which activities off the job affect job stress will be understood only as dimensions relevant both to the job and to the home are considered. An understanding of the relationship between the job and the individual requires research into the meaning of the job for the individual through the life cycle. The individual acquires a portion of the total self-identity from the job. This identity is affected by job change, job loss, and retirement. Other major life events, such as marriage and child rearing, must to some extent affect the individual's reactions to the job. To understand the impact of such events, dimensions of P–E fit must relate the various environments to each other and to the individual.

For any given individual, the most accurate predictions of strain will occur when P–E fit is measured on dimensions which reflect the values and goals of that individual. When P–E fit is measured on a particular dimension for a number of individuals, the dimension will predict strain only as it has the same meaning for each individual's values and goals. This observation suggests that any one list of dimensions may be limited in its ability to predict strain. Pervin (1976) presents an approach where the dimensions relevant to the interrelationships between the person and the environment are identified for each individual. The usefulness of this idiographic approach in defining dimensions of person–environment fit needs to be explored.

In the preceding discussion the assumption was made that stress was lowest when environmental demands and supplies perfectly matched the individual's motives and abilities. A modification of this assumption must be entertained. The reviews of Feather (1975) and Kulka (1976) summarize arguments of many authors pointing out that constant perfect fit may result in boredom and the lack of development. On some dimensions (e.g. those associated with achievement motives) small discrepancies may be experienced as being equally pleasant or more so than perfect fit. Of course, large discrepancies would still increase stress. Some instances of lowest strain scores occurring with small levels of misfit have been reported (e.g. Caplan, 1972). The motivation associated with small discrepancies may arise from the individual's time perspective. The individual may anticipate that successfully dealing with small discrepancies which are presently experienced will lead to better fit on important dimensions in the future. The experience of successfully dealing with the manageable discrepancy may also become in and of itself a goal of the individual. The theory of P–E fit must be developed to specify the various conditions under which either perfect fit or a small discrepancy will best represent the point of lowest stress.

Only a handful of studies have attempted to relate measures of person–environment fit to physiological outcomes. While some significant relationships have been demonstrated, the results have not been impressive (e.g. Caplan, 1972; Harrison, 1976). The weak findings may to some extent reflect the use of surveys rather than experimental studies. With more control over factors affecting physiological responses, experimental studies seem to have had more consistent success with physiological responses than have surveys. The weak relationships found in field studies suggest that relationships between P–E fit and physiological responses should be further examined in more controlled settings.

Many additional issues concerning the development and operationalization of P–E fit theory have been identified. Feather (1975) presents a detailed review of literature and theoretical issues dealing with the fit between the environment and the individual's values. Kulka (1976) reviews an extensive literature dealing with person–environment fit in many situations. Harrison (1976) reviews much of the literature relevant to person–environment fit and job stress. Both Harrison (1976) and Kulka (1976) consider many methodological issues raised by the use of P–E fit measures. Hope (1975) discusses theoretical and statistical relationships relevant to the prediction of strain from characteristics of the environment, the person, and discrepancies between the two.

The theory of person–environment fit emphasizes the interrelationship between the person and the environment and the complex processes which underlie this relationship. Much of the future work in developing the theory will involve the integration of theories covering limited domains: perception, coping and defence, self-identity, socialization, adaptation, and psychosomatic relationships. The model of person–environment fit presented in Figure 7.1 is an attempt to provide a framework within which a comprehensive theory describing various processes relating stress through health strain can eventually be described.

Note

The author expresses his appreciation to John R. P. French, Jr, for helpful comments on drafts of this chapter. Some of the material presented in this chapter was originally presented at the 1976 convention of the American Psychological Association. Much of the research reported in the chapter comes from a study supported by Contract SHM–99–72–61 and Grant 1 RO1 OH 00563–01 from the National Institute for Occupational Safety and Health, US Department of Health, Education, and Welfare.

References

Althauser, R. P. (1971) Multicollinearity and non-additive regression models. In Blalock, H. M., (ed.), *Causal Models in the Social Sciences.* Chicago. Aldine.

Appley, M. H., and Trumbull, R. (eds) (1967) *Psychological Stress.* New York. Appleton-Century-Crofts.

Atkinson, J. W. (1964) *An Introduction to Motivation.* Princeton. Van Nostrand, Reinhold.

Basowitz, H., Persky, H., Korchin, S. J., and Grinker, R. R. (1955) *Anxiety and Stress: an Interdisciplinary Study of a Life Situation.* New York. McGraw-Hill (Blakiston).

Becker, H. S. (1969) The self and adult socialization. In Norbeck, E. (ed.), *The Study of Personality.* New York. Holt, Rinehart, Winston.

Becker, M. H., Drachman, R. H., and Kirscht, J. P. (1974) A new approach to explaining sick-role behavior in low-income populations, *American Journal of Public Health,* **64**, 205–216.

Beckhard, R. (1972) Optimizing team-building efforts, *Journal of Contemporary Business,* **1**, 3, 23–32.

Binder, J., Mayman, M., and Doehrman, S. (1974) Self-ideal self discrepancy as a defensive style, *Comprehensive Psychiatry,* **15**, 335–343.

Campbell, D. B. (1974) *A Program to Reduce Coronary Heart Disease Risk by Altering Job Stresses.* Doctoral dissertation, The University of Michigan, 1973. *Dissertation Abstracts International,* **35**, 564–B (University Microfilms no. 74–15681).

Campbell, J. P., Dunnette, M. D., Lawler, E. E., III, and Weick, K. E., Jr (1970) *Managerial Behavior, Performance, and Effectiveness.* New York. McGraw-Hill.

Caplan, R. D. (1972) *Organizational Stress and Individual Strain: a Social-psychological Study of Risk Factors in Coronary Heart Disease Among Administrators, Engineers, and Scientists.* Doctoral at dissertation, The University of Michigan, 1971. *Dissertation Abstracts International,* **32**, 6706B–6707B (University Microfilms no. 72–14822).

Caplan, R. D., Cobb, S., French, J. R. P., Jr, Harrison, R. V., and Pinneau, S. R., Jr (1975) *Job Demands and Worker Health: Main Effects and Occupational Differences* (USGPO Catalog no. HE 20.7111: J57. USGPO Stock no. 1733–00083). Washington, DC. US Government Printing Office.

Caplan, R. D., Robinson, E. A. R., French, J. R. P., Jr, Caldwell, J. R., and Shinn, M. (1976) *Adhering to Medical Regimens: Pilot Experiments in Patient Education and Social Support.* Ann Arbor, Michigan. Institute for Social Research.

Caudill, W. (1958) Effects of social and cultural systems in reactions to stress, *Social Sciences Research Council Pamphlet No. 14,* June.

Cobb, S. (1976) Social support as a moderator of life stress, *Psychosomatic Medicine,* **38**, 300–312.

Coch, L., and French, J. R. P., Jr (1948) Overcoming resistance to change, *Human Relations,* **1**, 512–532.

Cronbach, L. J. (1958) Proposals leading to analytic treatment of social perception scores. In Tagiuri, R. and Petrullo, L. (eds), *Person Perception and Interpersonal Behaviour*. Stanford, Calif. Stanford University Press.

Cronbach, L. J., and Furby, L. (1970) How should we measure 'change'—or should we? *Psychological Bulletin*, **74**, 68–80.

Evans, M. G. (1969) Conceptual and operational problems in the measurement of various aspects of job satisfaction, *Journal of Applied Psychology*, **53**, 93–101.

Feather, N. T. (1975) *Values in Education and Society*. New York. The Free Press.

French, J. R. P., Jr (1971) Assessment of research on integration–disintegration. In Kaplan, B. H. (ed.), *Psychiatric Disorder and the Urban Environment: Report of the Cornell Social Science Seminar*. New York. Behavioural Publications.

French, J. R. P., and Kahn, R. L. (1962) A programmatic approach to studying the industrial environment and mental health, *Journal of Social Issues*, **18**, 3, 1–47.

French, J. R. P., Jr, and Caplan, R. D. (1972) Organizational stress and individual strain. In Marrow, A. J. (ed.), *The failure of success*. New York. AMACOM.

French, J. R. P., Jr, and Kahn, R. L. (1972) A programmatic approach to studying the industrial environment and mental health, *Journal of Social Issues*, **18**, 1–47.

French, J. R. P., Jr, Rogers, W., and Cobb, S. (1974) A model of person–environment fit. In Coelho, G. V. Hamburgh, D. A. and Adams, J. E. (eds), *Coping and adaptation*. New York. Basic Books.

Freud, A. (1966) *The Writings of Anna Freud*. Vol. II, 1936, *The Ego and Mechanisms of Defense*. New York. International University Press.

Graham, W. K. (1976) Commensurate characterization of persons, groups, and organizations: development of the Trait Ascription Questionnaire (TAQ), *Human Relations*, **29**, 607–622.

Hackman, J. R., and Lawler, E. E., III (1971) Employee reactions to job characteristics, *Journal of Applied Psychology*, **55**, 259–286.

Harrison, R. V. (1976) *Job Demands and Worker Health: Person–Environment Misfit*. Doctoral dissertation, The University of Michigan, 1976. *Dissertation Abstracts International*, **37**, 1035B (University Microfilms no. 76–19, 150).

Hope, K. (1975) Models of status inconsistency and social mobility effects, *American Sociological Review*, **40**, 322–343.

House, J. S. (1972) *The Relationship of Intrinsic and Extrinsic Work Motivations to Occupational Stress and Coronary Heart Disease Risk*. Doctoral dissertation, The University of Michigan, 1972. *Dissertation Abstracts International*, **33**, 2514–A (University Microfilms no. 72–29094).

Hulin, C. L., and Blood, M. R. (1968) Job enlargement, individual differences, and worker response, *Psychological Bulletin*, **69**, 41–55.

Katz, D., and Kahn, R. L. (1966) *The Social Psychology of Organizations*. New York. Wiley.

Katzell, R. A. (1964) Personal values, job satisfaction, and job behavior. In Borow, H. (ed.), *Man in a World of Work*. Boston. Houghton Mifflin.

Kroeler, T. C. (1963) The coping functions of ego mechanisms. In White, R. (ed.), *The Study of Lives*. New York. Atherton Press.

Kulka, R. A. (1976) *Person–Environment Fit in the High School: a Validation Study*. Doctoral dissertation, The University of Michigan, 1975. *Dissertation Abstracts International*, **36**, 5352B (University Microfilms no. 76–9438).

Lawler, E. E., III (1973) *Motivation in Work Organizations*. Belmont, Calif. Wadsworth Publishing Company.

Lawler, E. E., III (1976) Can the quality of work life be legislated?, *The Personnel Administrator*, **21**, 17–22.

Lazarus, R. S. (1966) *Psychological Stress and the Coping Process*. New York. McGraw-Hill.

Levinson, D. J. (1970) Role, personality, and social structure in the organization setting.

In Smelser, J. J. and Smelser, W. T. (eds), *Personality and Social System*. New York. Wiley.

Lewin, K. (1951) *Field Theory in Social Science*, ed. Cartwright, D. New York. Harper & Row.

Likert, R. (1967) *The Human Organization: Its Management and Value*. New York. McGraw-Hill.

Locke, E. A. (1969) What is job satisfaction?, *Organizational Behavior and Human Performance*, **4**, 309–336.

Lofquist, L. H., and Dawis, R. V. (1969) *Adjustment to Work*. New York. Appleton-Century-Crofts.

McDougall, W. (1908) *Introduction to Social Psychology*. London. Methuen.

Mason, J. W. (1975) A historical view of the stress field. Part I, *Journal of Human Stress*, **1**, 1, 6–12.

Mechanic, D. (1968) *Medical Sociology*. New York. The Free Press.

Miller, D. R. (1963) The study of interaction: situation, identity, and social relationship. In Koch, S. (ed.), *A Study of a Science*. New York. McGraw-Hill, vol. 5.

Miller, R. S., and Worchel, P. (1956) The effects of need achievement and self-ideal discrepancy on performance under stress, *Journal of Personality*, **25**, 176–190.

Morse, J. J. (1975) Person–job congruence and individual adjustment and development, *Human Relations*, **28**, 841–861.

Moss, G. E. (1973) *Illness, Immunity, and Social Interaction: the Dynamics of Biosocial Resonation*. New York. Wiley.

Murray, H. A. (1938) *Explorations in Personality*. New York. Oxford University Press.

Murray, H. A. (1959) Preparations for the scaffold of a comprehensive system. In Koch, S. (ed.), *Psychology: a Study of a Science*. vol. 3, *Formulations of the Person and the Social Context*. New York. McGraw-Hill.

Nunnally, J. C. (1967) *Psychometric Theory*. New York. McGraw-Hill.

Pervin, L. A. (1968) Performance and satisfaction as a function of individual–environment fit, *Psychological Bulletin*, **69**, 56–68.

Pervin, L. A. (1976) A free-response description approach to the analysis of person-situation interaction, *Journal of Personality and Social Psychology*, **34**, 465–474.

Pinneau, S. R., Jr (1976) *Effects of Social Support on Psychological and Physiological Strains*. Doctoral dissertation, The University of Michigan, 1975. *Dissertation Abstracts International*, **36**, 5359B (University Microfilms no. 76–9491).

Porter, L. W. (1961) A study of perceived need satisfactions in bottom and middle management jobs, *Journal of Applied Psychology*, **45**, 1–10.

Quinn, R. P., and Shepard, L. J. (1974) *The 1972–73 Quality of Employment Survey: Descriptive Statistics with Comparison Data from the 1969–70 Survey of Working Conditions*. Ann Arbor. Survey Research Center.

Ross, E. A. (1908) *Social Psychology*. New York. Macmillan.

Scott, R., and Howard, A. (1970) Models of stress. In Levine, S., and Scotch, N. A. (eds), *Social Stress*. Chicago, Ill. Aldine, pp. 257–278.

Slocum, J. W., Jr, and Strawser, R. H. (1973) Racial difference in job attitudes, *Journal of Applied Psychology*, **56**, 28–32.

Wall, T. D., and Payne, R. (1973) Are deficiency scores deficient?, *Journal of Applied Psychology*, **58**, 322–326.

Wanous, J. P., and Lawler, E. E. III (1972) Measurement and meaning of job satisfaction, *Journal of Applied Psychology*, **56**, 95–105.

White, R. W. (1963) Ego and reality in psychoanalytic theory. *Psychological Issues Monograph II*. New York. International Universities Press.

Wolff, H. G. (1953) *Stress and Disease*. Springfield, Ill. Charles C. Thomas.

Zung, W. W. K. (1965) A self-rating depression scale, *Archives of General Psychiatry*, **13**, 63–70.

PART V

Dealing with Stressors and Strains

Chapter 8
What People can do for Themselves to Cope with Stress

Albert Ellis

State University of New York

As the other chapters in this book ably demonstrate, many important kinds of stressors exist in today's world and significantly contribute to various harmful experiences and symptoms on the part of virtually all humans. Some of the main pernicious effects that seem rampant in modern society include acute and prolonged feelings of anxiety, depression, inadequacy, hostility, and low frustration tolerance. Moreover, people who react poorly to stressful conditions and acknowledge that they cannot bear such conditions or function effectively when they encounter them, frequently add still another harmful outcome to their already 'overburdened' lives: they berate and condemn themselves for their poor reactions to stress. They thereby make themselves anxious about feeling anxious, depressed about their depressions, and inadequate about their lack of adequacy. An enormous vicious circle of self-flagellation leading to further self-denigration thereby results.

What can such sufferers from stress do? Many different systems of psychotherapy, ranging from classical psychoanalysis to encounter groups and behaviour therapy, have tried to answer this question. Not content with their answers, I and my associates at the Institute for Rational Living and the Institute for Advanced Study in Rational Psychotherapy in New York City (and in various affiliated institutes throughout the world) have given much thought and experimentation to this matter and have come up with our own answers, incorporated in the theory and practice of rational–emotive therapy (RET). We have presented these in many publications—for example, Ellis, 1962, 1971, 1972, 1973, 1975, 1976, 1977a; Ellis and Harper, 1975; Ellis and Grieger, 1977; Hauck, 1974, 1976; Knaus, 1974; Kranzler, 1974; Lembo, 1974, 1976; Morris and Kanitz, 1975; Tosi, 1974; and Young, 1974. In addition, RET has made its appearance in the recent psychotherapeutic literature under several other names, including cognitive-behaviour modification, cognitive restructuring, rational behaviour therapy, decision therapy, multimodal therapy, and cognitive therapy. Some of the many important writings that have appeared under these headings include those by Beck (1976), Davison and Neale (1974), Goldfried and Davison (1976), Goodman and Maultsby (1974), Greenwald (1976), Lazarus (1971, 1976), Maultsby (1971, 1975),

Mahoney (1974), Meichenbaum (1974, 1977), and Rimm and Masters (1974).

What does rational–emotive therapy (RET) have to say about what people can do for themselves to cope with stress? A great many things, some of which other popular forms of therapy either ignore completely or deal with in a somewhat cursory manner. Let me outline the RET approach and show how almost any person, including one who lives in a highly 'stressful' set of conditions at home, at work, or socially can minimize unnecessary stress and can accept and successfully cope with 'stress' that he or she cannot eliminate.

Self-creation of stressful conditions and reactions to stress

A fundamental premise of RET (and many other forms of cognitive-behaviour therapy) states that stressful conditions do not exist in their own right but vary significantly in relation to the perceptions and cognitions of those who react to these conditions. This does not mean that *no* set of circumstances has intrinsically stressful predicaments attached to it; for a few almost unquestionably do. If, for example, a thousand humans, picked at random, suffer extreme loss of sleep, lack of nutrition, or physical torture for a sufficiently long period of time, it seems reasonable to conclude that just about all of them will experience 'too much' stress and will tend to crack under the strain. Some of them will literally die in fairly short order, and just about all the rest will 'live' quite a length of time—but with severe feelings of anxiety, anguish, depression, and suicidalness.

In such extreme circumstances, we may legitimately note that very stressful conditions directly 'cause' human fear and despair. Or, in rational–emotive terminology, a set of Activating Events or Activating Experiences (at point A) cause or create a subsequent set of emotional and behavioural Consequences (at point C). Strictly speaking, the Activating Experiences (A) really do not cause the behavioural Consequences (C)—between the stimulus (or Activating Events) and response (or Consequence) we invariably have the organism itself; and its particular biosocial make-up or predisposition to act in certain ways really makes it respond. Another organism—such as an amoeba, a rat, or an ape—would obviously respond quite differently to the same set of stressful conditions than would a human.

In any event, extremely stressful situations, such as prolonged lack of sleep or physical torture, rarely occur in human lives. Instead, much weaker stressors occur—such as loss of a job, rejection by a mate, or failure at school. And when these Activating Events happen, people clearly act quite individually. For example, out of every hundred successful business executives forced to retire by their companies because they have reached a certain age (such as 65 or 70), a certain number feel severely depressed, another group feel moderately sad and frustrated, and still another group feel content or happy. Obviously, the same 'stressor' leads to quite different results in these three groups of retirees.

In the case of ordinary or moderate 'stressful' situations, people choose, decide, or create their own feelings of anxiety, depression, and self-downing (which occur at point C) by picking a certain kind of Belief system (at point B) *about* the situations, or Activating Events, that happen to them (at point A). Their disturbed reactions—or emotional Consequences—at C follow directly from their Beliefs; and although what happens to them at A significantly *contributes to*, it hardly *causes*, C.

A specific example of this process? Fine. Let us take, again, a successful business executive who has to retire, say, at the age of 65, even though he does not want to do so, and would just as soon keep working until his seventies or even eighties. And let us take one who finds retirement exceptionally 'stressful' and consequently feels anxious and depressed after his firm lets him go. Economically, he easily has enough money to live on; physically, he has no diseases or disablements; emotionally, he gets along fine with his wife, his children, and his friends. So his only great 'stress' (or the Activating Experience that has newly occurred in his life at point A) consists of his forced retirement. And at C, his emotional Consequence, we find anxiety and depression.

If, as RET theory claims, this retired executive's Activating Experience (forced unemployment) does not directly cause his emotional Consequence (anxiety and depression), what does? Answer: B. And precisely what Beliefs does he have at B that make him experience panic and despair at C? Two main sets.

First, he has a set of rational Beliefs (rBs). These mainly consist of such ideas as: 'How annoying to have to retire so early in life! I wish my company didn't have this silly rule! I don't like retiring and I feel determined to do something about this unpleasant state of affairs. Damn it!'

What makes these particular Beliefs rational? Mainly, this executive's desires, wishes, preferences, values, or goals. His aim, if he had his druthers, involves working for several years more—perhaps until the day before his death. And since this seems a perfectly legitimate and theoretically achievable goal, and the conditions at point A bar him from accomplishing it, he sounds perfectly rational or sane if he notes his annoyance and displeasure about A and strives to do something about changing the Activating Events that have forced him to retire.

What would this executive feel if he rigorously stayed with these rational Beliefs (rBs)? Answer: sorry, disappointed, displeased, irritated, annoyed, frustrated.

Not depressed or anxious or angry? No: these inappropriate feelings would stem, if he felt them, from his irrational Beliefs (iBs) about A—which we shall consider in a minute. If he really stayed with *only* these rational Beliefs (rBs), he would feel appropriately sad and frustrated; and because he had such appropriate feelings, he would tend to act, in a determined manner, to change the Activating Events of his life, and replace them with other events: such as, finding another enjoyable job; devoting himself to some active avocational pursuit; or getting so busy with his friends, with travelling, or with something else, that he would no longer care that much about continuing to work.

'By rational Beliefs, then, you mean ideas or attitudes that help the individual adjust to an unwanted set of conditions or Activating Events? And by appropriate emotions (or emotional Consequences) you mean those feelings which again help this person to make his or her life more satisfactory when he or she finds it unsatisfying? Right?'

Yes: exactly right. In RET, we start with a basic value or goal—usually, the person's desire to survive and to live happily, in accordance with his or her own tastes; and once one chooses this value or goal (such as working until one reaches the seventies or eighties), rationality simply means aiding or abetting that purpose; and appropriate feeling means an emotion that helps one maximize one's basic values and to minimize one's disvalues.

By the same token, irrational Beliefs, in RET, consist of ideas, opinions, and attitudes that sabotage one's fundamental desires. And inappropriate or self-defeating emotions comprise feelings that help one, again, block or interfere with, rather than abet, one's chosen goals and purposes. Thus, in the illustration of the forcibly retired executive, if he made himself feel depressed, anxious, self-hating, or enraged (at point C) about what happened to him (at point A), we would consider these feelings inappropriate and self-sabotaging: because they would almost always hinder rather than help him solve his problem of working for the rest of his life or of feeling reasonably happy even if he could not work again.

What kind of irrational Beliefs (iBs) would we look for in the case of the executive who found retirement exceptionally 'stressful' and who reacted poorly to such an Activating Experience (A)? Usually, one basic irrational premise and three major foolish deductions from this premise. As for the irrational premise, that would almost always consist of some form of what I call *must*urbation—the devout and quite untenable belief in some absolutistic or dogmatic form of *should*, *ought*, or *must*. In the case of the forcibly retired executive, for example, I (as a rational–emotive therapist) would immediately look for irrational Beliefs like these:

'I *must* not get seriously blocked in the fulfilment of any of my basic desires, such as my desire to work productively and creatively until I reach a much older age than 65. The Board of Directors of my company, especially considering how long and how successfully I have worked for this company, *should* allow me to go on working just about as long as I wish to do so. I *have to* keep working and doing the fine kind of a job I have done for years, for only in this manner will I fulfil my destiny and prove that I exist as a worthwhile individual.'

Starting with these absolutistic and empirically invalidatable *musts*, this retired executive would most probably (I, as his rational–emotive therapist, would predict) have at least three major illegitimate and indefensible irrational Beliefs or conclusions. Namely:

(1) 'Since I *must* not get seriously blocked in the fulfilment of any of my basic desires, and the Board of Directors actually has banned me from continuing to work productively for my firm, I find it *awful* and *horrible* that this terrible state of affairs has come about.'

(2) 'Since the Board of Directors *should* allow me to go on working just about as long as I wish to do so, and it actually will not give me this right that I fully deserve, I *can't stand* it! How utterly *unbearable* my life remains as long as they stick with this criminal position!'

(3) 'Since I *have to* keep working and doing the fine kind of a job I have done for years in order to fulfil my destiny and prove my worth as an individual, and since my horribly unjust superiors won't let me do what I have to do, I can only find my entire life ruined and view my existence as utterly miserable and worthless.'

Rational–emotive therapy contends that these four major irrationalities (the basic *mus*turbatory premises and their three 'logical' illogical conclusions), and *not* the conditions of enforced retirement itself, truly (and certainly directly) 'cause' or 'create' the retired executive's emotional Consequences of anxiety, depression, self-hatred, or rage at his superiors. Even though conditions of real 'stress' (or deprivation) truly exist in his life; and even though he may not have brought about these conditions himself, but mainly gets victimized by them, these 'stressors' merely contribute to, but do not actually cause, his state of panic and depression. For he could—as we shall see later in this chapter—choose, at point B (his Belief system), other ways of reacting to the 'stressful' Activating Experiences (at point A). His *particular* choices, and the irrational Beliefs which constitute them (at point B, again), *really* create most of his 'stress'. And only if he acknowledges and forcefully works against these Beliefs will he be likely to cope better with, and possibly almost completely eradicate, his 'stress'.

To summarize what I have said thus far: although most systems of psycho-therapy and personality theory highlight the stimulus or environmental factors in people's 'stressful' reactions, RET does not neglect these factors but more importantly emphasizes the perceptual-cognitive factors. It holds that humans react 'stressfully' when they perceive a given situation as extremely 'difficult' or 'burdensome', and that they appropriately feel sorry or disappoin-ted about such 'difficulties' when they preferentially evaluate them as 'unlike-able' or 'unfortunate' or 'annoying'. But they inappropriately feel anxious, depressed, worthless, or angry about such 'burdens' when they absolutistically and exaggeratedly insist that they must not, should not exist and view them as 'awful', 'horrible', or 'unbearable' when they actually do.

The double whammy of 'stressful' reactions

Once people perceive a situation as very 'stressful' or 'burdensome', they almost always have another perceptual-cognitive reaction to it that tends to enormously increase their feelings of anxiety, anger, and despair. For humans (unlike practically all the 'lower' animals) not only can think but also think about their thinking; and they importantly perceive and cognize *about* their own reactions to 'stress'. Thus, if Joanne Smith sees her lover's or husband's rejection of her as extremely 'stressful' or 'terrible', she will most likely make herself feel anxious and depressed about this situation. But once she feels like a worm because of the way she chooses to react to this 'stress', she then will most likely observe her own reactivity and acknowledge that she feels downed or 'worthless'.

Joanne will consequently, in many if not all instances, upset herself about her anxiety, depression, and self-downing by telling herself something like this: 'I must not react anxiously or depressedly to the stressful conditions of my life, since not everyone would react in that self-defeating manner, and I really could behave otherwise. Because I over-react to stress the way I *shouldn't*, I find it *awful* that I act that way; I *can't stand* my own over-reactivity; and I am a pretty rotten person for behaving in that rotten manner!' By these kinds of irrational Beliefs (iBs) about her anxious reactions to stress, Joanne thereby makes herself anxious over her anxiety, depressed about her depression. Now she really has cooked herself!—and feels so extremely upset that she diminishes her ability to see exactly what she did to create her original anxiety and what she could do to uncreate it.

In other words: people not only partly create (or conceptualize) the original 'stressors' they experience, but they also bring about their over-reactions to these 'stressors'. Then, to crown their self-imposed inequity, they damn themselves for damning themselves—and thus immensely escalate their 'stress'. A vicious circle—or endless spiral, if you will—that seems to have no finish line!

Other *mus*turbatory attitudes that lead to over-reactions to stress

Can we outline the main *mus*turbatory or absolutizing attitudes that lead to people's over-reacting to stress and creating needless anxiety and despair, not to mention various behavioural and physiological symptoms? Fairly easily, if we use the rational–emotive approach. For RET hypothesizes that humans seem prone to invent three major absolutistic musts; and that practically all of their 'emotional' disturbance stems from devout belief in these three absolutes. They include:

(1) The dire need for success and approval

As Karen Horney (1965) noted a good many years ago, most of us run our lives by the 'tyranny of the shoulds'. And the worst should of the lot, probably, runs: 'I should (or must) succeed greatly or outstandingly at the goals I select and value and win utter and secure approval from everyone whom I consider significant for my achievements.' With this tyrannous should we almost inevitably make ourselves anxious, depressed, despairing, insecure, self-downing, and 'inadequate'. Even when relatively little stress or frustration abounds, and we have unusual competence and talent, we can easily disturb ourselves with this assumption by simply raising it a bit: 'I should (must) succeed *perfectly* and win every significant person's approval *constantly*.' Then, even with the genius of a Leonardo or a Beethoven, we really cook ourselves!

(2) The dire need for considerateness and justice

Whether or not we achieve outstandingly and win the unusual approval of others, we can easily upset ourselves with another unrealistic should: 'People *must* treat me kindly, considerately, and fairly, and when they don't they rate as horrible, wicked individuals who deserve severe blame, damnation, and ceaseless punishment for their terrible sins.' With this Utopian and crazy should we easily make ourselves angry, resentful, hating, vindictive, and depressed. For what chance do we have that people—yes, fallible humans—will consistently act the kindly and ethical way that they presumably should and must? Incredibly little!

(3) The dire need for immediate and constant gratification and ease

Few of us do not over-react to our own and others' failings and do not condemn ourselves and them for their human fallibilities. And even these few seem to endorse a third, and almost ubiquitous, foolish assumption: 'World conditions, and particularly those under which I personally live, must make things easy for me, give me practically everything I want immediately, and prevent me from undergoing any severe deprivations, pains, or hassles.' Whereupon, believing this utter rot, we quickly acquire intense feelings of low frustration tolerance, internal and external whining, and self-pity.

Given any one of these three major *must*urbatory ideas, people will take almost any 'stressful' situation and make it into a virtual holocaust. Given two or three of them simultaneously, almost certain emotional disaster—and continuous and intense disaster at that!—will occur. Let us take, for example, a fairly common 'stressful' occurrence: Joanne Smith's husband, John, discovers that she has begun to show a real interest in his best friend, Jim, and that Jim—of all things!—returns this interest and has had a few dates with Joanne behind John's back.

Naturally, we cannot expect John to wax enthusiastic about this 'stressful' state of affairs. We might well, instead, expect him to wonder at his own adequacy as a husband to Joanne ('Have I really treated her well recently? Have I satisfied her sexually and amatively?'). We might also surmise that he feels less than friendly towards Jim ('I don't mind his screwing around all he wants. But with *my* wife? And behind my back, when he frequently tells everyone he considers me his very best friend!'). And we might guess that he hardly feels good about the conditions surrounding Joanne's and Jim's betrayal ('Cripes!—just when I had to keep working overtime at the office, to meet the bills that Joanne and I had run up because of this goddamned inflation the country's having. And when my blasted back has started bothering me, during the past few weeks, so that I couldn't even take care of Joanne sexually if I wanted to. What crummy luck! Everything seems to work against me these days!').

But, in addition to his frustration and sorrow about his own inadequacies as a husband, about Joanne's and Jim's lying to him and betraying him behind his (aching) back, and about the poor economic and physical conditions he has to confront, we can also expect that John, if he feels immensely upset about these problems, will tell himself one, two, or three crazy shoulds. Such as: (1) 'I *should* have acted better to Joanne all along. What a dunce I amount to, for not treating her better for the last many months!' (2) 'Joanne and Jim *should not* have lied to me, as they obviously did. What bastards, for doing what they *shouldn't* have done!' (3) 'How awful that economic conditions and the state of my health have turned out so miserably! They *should not* exist that way; and I can't stand it when they gang up on me like that!'

John's anxious, hostile, and self-pitying reactions to the stress of his wife's dating his best friend, Jim, behind his back do not merely stem, therefore, from his strongly desiring less stressful conditions and intensely disliking the conditions he actually experienced. They also, and more importantly, stem from his demanding, insisting, and commanding that such conditions should, ought, and must not exist, and from his whining and wailing about the 'horror' and the 'awfulness' of their actuality. Without his own awfulizing and demandingness, he certainly would not feel very good about the 'stress' of his wife's and his best friend's behaviour; but neither would he feel horrified about it.

How to relieve and eliminate self-created over-reactions to stress

Suppose John Smith (or any other individual who over-reacts to 'stressful' conditions) comes to me about his feelings of anxiety, depression, rage, and self-pity. How can I, as a rational–emotive therapist, help him with his problem? Or, more to the point, how can I help him help himself to deal more sanely and satisfactorily with the 'stress' he experiences? Mainly, by showing him how to Dispute, at point D, the irrational Beliefs (iBs) that he keeps telling himself, at point B, about the Activating Events that he experiences at point A. I show him, in other words, that A does not really cause or create (though it may significantly contribute to) C; but that he, John, causes most of his own over-reactions to the 'stress' of A by irrationally viewing it, or telling himself nonsense about it, at B. And then I help him Dispute, at D, what he tells himself at B.

More specifically, I take each of John's irrational Beliefs (iBs) and actively–directively Dispute it, at D. I thus say to him, first, 'Why *should* you have acted better to Joanne all along? And how do you rate as a dunce for not treating her better for the last many months?'

'Because', John may well reply to me, 'if I had treated Joanne better, she might well have not got interested that much in Jim, and had those secret dates with him. And since I didn't, obviously, do what I should have done, I clearly acted stupidly—and therefore am a dunce!'

Whereupon I immediately start Disputing (at D) John's irrational Beliefs (iBs), in a dialogue that goes something along these lines:
THERAPIST: Why *should* you have treated Joanne better?
CLIENT: Because I would have got better results thereby. She probably

wouldn't have got involved with Jim had I shown more interest in her and satisfied her more sexually.

THERAPIST: Let's assume that—though we really don't know that it would have worked out that way. You still haven't answered my question. You've told me why *it would be better* if you had treated Joanne more considerately. But why *must* you do what would be better?

CLIENT: Because—uh, because only if I did would I get the results I want.

THERAPIST: But you're still only telling me that if you treated Joanne one way, you'd get good results and if you treated her another way, you'd get worse results. But you're still not telling me why you *should*, why you *have to* treat her so that you get good results. That's a *preference*, getting better results. But why is it a *necessity*?

CLIENT: Oh. I see what you mean now. I guess it isn't. I could exist with worse rather than better results. So I don't *have to* treat Joanne more considerately—even though it would probably be better if I did.

THERAPIST: Right! You really don't *have to* do anything, you know. If you want to live, then you have to do a few things: like eat, breathe, and defecate. But you don't *have to* live. You could always choose to not live, to die. So the belief 'I have to eat in order to live' is only a *contingent* necessity. It depends on your *choice* of surviving; and is not an *absolute* must. But your statement 'I *have to* treat Joanne considerately' is put forth as an absolute must. It means, 'Under all conditions, no matter what, I *must* treat her considerately.' But this, obviously, is nonsense. For if you *had to*, under all conditions, treat her considerately, you *would*. That would be a law of the universe. And you'd *have to* follow it. But is there any such universal law?

CLIENT: Uh, no. I guess there isn't.

THERAPIST: No, there isn't. You just set it up as John's law. And you don't exactly run the universe!

CLIENT: You seem to mean that it would be highly preferable if I treated Joanne considerately, assuming that I want to keep her as a loving wife and not let her run off with Jim. But I don't have to act preferably. And if I don't, I'll merely get unpreferable results—such as her waltzing off with Jim.

THERAPIST: Yes. And even if you treat her preferably, don't forget, you merely increase the *probability* of your getting what you want from her. She still, no matter how well you deal with her, can decide to waltz off with Jim, or with someone else. You still have no *certainty* that she will stay happily with you. And isn't that what you're really demanding: that you *must* treat Joanne better so that she *absolutely* and with *no doubt whatever* will stay with you?

CLIENT: Yes, now that you point it out to me, I see that you're right. I'm not merely *wanting* Joanne to stay with me and love only me. I'm *demanding* that she certainly do so. And I guess that, my certainty-seeking, is what's really making me anxious.

THERAPIST: Exactly! Most of the 'stress' that you're placing on yourself arises not from your desire for Joanne's love but from your *needing*, you're *absolutely insisting*, that you completely have it. Your anxiety, in the face of the 'stressful' condition that she has an interest in Jim and that you may lose her to him, largely arises from this need, this insistence of yours; and not from the undesirability of your losing her.

CLIENT: And does my hostility to Joanne and to Jim arise from this same kind of certainty-seeking, absolutistic thinking on my part?

THERAPIST: It definitely does. You keep demanding that 'Joanne and Jim *should not* have lied to me, as they obviously did. What bastards they are, for doing what they *shouldn't* have done!' But, of course, they *should have* lied to you; and they are not bastards. Do you see why?

CLIENT: Yes, I guess I do—or almost do. They should have lied to me because they *did*. However undesirable their lying may be, they should have done it because they actually did it. That's the way they acted; and I'd better accept their actions, even though I'll never like these acts. But if they lied, they lied!

THERAPIST: Yes, whatever they did, they did. And no matter how well you could prove that they were wrong for doing it, so they were wrong! And, of course, they *should* be wrong if they indubitably are wrong! That's the way fallible, screwed-up humans often are: wrong!

CLIENT: How about my belief that 'it's awful that economic conditions and the state of my health have turned out so miserably. They should not exist that way; and I can't stand it when they gang up on me like that'? I can see that there might be something foolish or irrational about those beliefs, too.

THERAPIST: There distinctly is something foolish or irrational about those beliefs, too. What do you think is irrational about them?

CLIENT: Well, for one thing, it doesn't seem to be *awful* but only *highly undesirable* that economic conditions and the state of my health turned out so miserably.

THERAPIST: Because?

CLIENT: Well, because *awful*, as I've read in RET writings, means more than undesirable—101% undesirable. And neither economic conditions nor the state of my health can be *that* undesirable. Nothing can very well be more than 100% bad; and my awfulizing makes it 200% or infinitely bad. How can it be *that* bad?

THERAPIST: Right! At worst, economic conditions and the state of your health can be 99.9% bad; and when you call them *awful* or *terrible* or *horrible* you really mean that they're more than 100% bad. And how can *anything*, as you're now seeing, be that bad? Fine. You're really beginning to see things within a realistic framework. And how about the idea that you *can't stand it* when things gang up on you like that?

CLIENT: Well, I don't think that I *can*! When things gang up on me all at once, I just feel so upset that I have to, well, practically go off the wall, or run away from the situation, or burst out in a fit of intense rage. My emotions seem to show that I can't stand it.

THERAPIST: Hogwash! Your emotions merely follow logically from the illogical *belief* that you can't stand it. If you think, for example, that if you lose at playing tennis a huge blue devil will run after you and stick a sharply pointed pitchfork up your rear end, how will you feel about playing tennis?

CLIENT: Uh, I guess I'll feel that I can't risk it, can't stand playing the game—and I'll do everything possible to avoid engaging in it.

THERAPIST: Right! Your *thought* about the blue devil—who, of course, has no existence whatsoever and is a pure fiction—will 'make you' unable to stand tennis. But really—*can* you stand the game?

CLIENT: I see what you mean. I really can. But I *think* I can't, and therefore I 'can't'.

THERAPIST: Yes, your thought creates your feelings about tennis; and your feelings create your actions or inactions about the game—your 'inability' to stand playing it. Actually, however, can't you stand just about anything you don't like—including the blue devil sticking the pitchfork up your rear end, assuming that could ever happen?

CLIENT: You mean, couldn't I truly bear it, if it occurred? Would I *die* of it? Couldn't I actually *take* it, no matter how painful it was?

THERAPIST: Yes, and even if you did die of it—highly unlikely, but it could theoretically occur!—couldn't you stand it, bear it *until* you died?

CLIENT: Oh, I never thought of it that way before. I see what you mean. Even if the blue devil finally killed me with the pitchfork, couldn't I stand being killed like that?

THERAPIST: Yes. Couldn't you, or anyone for that matter, stand just about anything that happens to you—until, perhaps, you die of it?

CLIENT: Mmm! You've got something there! I guess—I guess I could. And anyone could. Whatever occurs to us, we can certainly *stand*. No matter how we abhor it or what damage it does to us. We can stand it because—well, because 'stand' really means continue to exist and bear it, until, well, until, as you point out, we finally expire of it. But until we expire—

THERAPIST: —you can stand it! Any human can stand anything that occurs, even extreme torture, up until the point he or she dies of it. The phrase 'I can't stand it', 'I can't bear it', or any equivalent phrase, seems to be pure nonsense. For the one thing you can *always* do, whatever occurs in your life, is to stand it, to bear it. To like it or love it—no, of course not. Even to continue to live with it may be impossible—since, occasionally, the 'unstandable' thing, like torture, will actually kill you. But just as long as you do continue to live, why can't you stand or bear anything, yes anything, that occurs in your life?

CLIENT: Mm. Maybe I can. Come to think of it, I can! Never thought of that before. But I obviously can!

As a therapist, I continue along these lines, showing my stress-prone client that he, John, always upsets himself and is not upset by 'stressful' events. And that he, John, can always see, review what he tells himself to make himself anxious and depressed, and can invariably Dispute (at D) his own irrational Beliefs (iBs) until he gives them up. Then, even though the stressors of his life still definitely exist, he refuses to take them *too* seriously and stops upsetting himself about them.

Emotive and behavioural techniques of rational–emotive therapy

RET, as shown in the previous section of this chapter, largely consists of cognitive or philosophic methods of helping people under 'too much' stress see what they do to exacerbate the conditions of their lives and to over-react to them; and also to show them how to Dispute, as the therapist does with them, their own irrationalities until they give them up. But it also consists of a good many emotive and behavioural techniques that go right along with, and have an integral connection with, the rational methods of cognitive restructuring. For humans, as I showed in *Reason and Emotion in Psychotherapy* (Ellis, 1962), simultaneously think, emote, and behave in a dysfunctional (or, for that matter, functional) manner. And their thinking not only leads to disordered emotions and actions but also partially stems from such feelings and acts.

A good RET therapist, therefore, always uses 'non-cognitive' or 'semi-cognitive' methods to help clients under stress think and act less anxiously. In the case of John, for example, I would probably first give him what Carl Rogers (1961) calls 'unconditional positive regard' or what in RET we call 'full acceptance'. I would show him that I, his therapist, can completely accept him in spite of his stupid and self-defeating behaviour (e.g. his original poor behaviour with his wife and his later hostility towards her) and that though I may not like his *acts* or *performances*, I can easily accept *him*. By my giving him this unconditional kind of acceptance, and treating him as a fallible human (and not a 'louse' or a 'rat') I would have an easier time teaching him that he could do the same for himself.

I would quite probably also use dramatic role playing techniques with him, to show him that he could feel and behave more effectively. I would very vigorously and powerfully (not namby-pambily) show John that he *doesn't* have to perform beautifully with Joanne and that she *does* have the right to act wrongly. I might well give him some of the famous RET shame attacking exercises, whereby he deliberately does something foolish, asinine, or ridiculous in public, and sees that the 'shame' he feels when doing it comes from his own chosen thoughts and feelings and not from the 'humiliating' acts themselves. I would probably teach him, and get him to use on himself, rational emotive imagery, invented by Dr Maxie C. Maultsby, Jr. (Maultsby, 1975; Maultsby and Ellis, 1974), in the course of which he implosively lets himself feel downed or angry when imagining some of the worst possible things that might happen to him in connection with his wife and her extramarital interests, then changes his feelings to those of disappointment and regret instead of anxiety and depression, then sees what cognitions he uses to effect these changes, and then practises making himself feel only disappointed rather than depressed about her behaviour.

Behaviourally, I would also use a good many reliable methods of helping John to change his basic self-defeating philosophies about himself and others. Thus, I might employ *in vivo* homework assignments, getting him to take definite risks with Joanne that he might not otherwise let himself take (e.g. discussing with her and Jim his feelings about their relationship). I would give him the cognitive homework assignments of filling out the RET special homework forms, which particularly emphasize finding and steadily Disputing irrational Beliefs (Ellis, 1977b; Ellis and Harper, 1975). I might well use some form of B. F. Skinner's (1971) operant conditioning or self-management principles derived from Skinner (Goldfried and Merbaum, 1973; Goldfried and Davison, 1976). I might also employ, as we have used in RET for many years, assertion training or other skill training techniques, to help John cope better with some of the practical problems of his life, and to show him that he does have the ability to change himself in important respects (Lazarus, 1971, 1976; Meichenbaum, 1977).

Although RET, therefore, uniquely and vigorously emphasizes cognitive restructuring, and shows people like John who over-react to 'stressful' situations that they have almost complete responsibility for their own disordered reactions and that they can significantly change these emotional Consequences by modifying their ideas, attitudes, and philosophies about various kinds of stressors that occur in their lives, it consists of a multi-faceted, cognitive–emotive–behavioural attack on dysfunctional thinking and acting. And, perhaps more than almost any other therapeutic system today, it specifically teaches people how to treat themselves: how to take present and future 'stressful' conditions, unwhiningly accept the fact that they exist, cope with them as sensibly as possible, contribute significantly to changing them for the better, and gracefully lump (and even to some extent like the challenge of) their continued existence. RET thereby encourages a realistic attitude towards life (rather than a Pollyannaish or a pessimistic outlook) that some sage originally expounded thousands of years ago and that several outstanding thinkers have periodically endorsed since then. This attitude—as epitomized in the writings of Marcus Aurelius, St Francis, Reinhold Niebuhr and others—says: 'I feel determined to strive to use whatever power I have to change the unpleasant stresses of life that I can change, to dislike but realistically accept those that I cannot change, and to have the wisdom to know the difference between the two.' This kind of a philosophy will not eliminate all stress or our overreactions to it. But it will significantly help!

References

Items preceded by an asterisk may prove particularly helpful to readers interested in the rational–emotive approach to coping with stress. The Institute for Rational Living, Inc., 45 East 65th Street, New York, NY 10021, USA distributes these books.

*Beck, A. T. (1976) *Cognitive Therapy and the Emotional Disorders*. New York. International Universities Press.
Davison, G. C., and Neale, J. M. (1974) *Abnormal Psychology*. New York. Wiley.
*Ellis, A. (1962) *Reason and Emotion in Psychotherapy*. New York. Lyle Stuart.
*Ellis, A. (1971) *Growth Through Reason*. New York. Science and Behavior Books. Paperback edition: Wilshire Books, 1974.

222

*Ellis, A. (1972) *Executive Leadership: a Rational Approach.* New York. Citadel Books.
*Ellis, A. (1973) *Humanistic Psychotherapy: the Rational–Emotive Approach.* Julian Press. Paperback edition: McGraw-Hill Paperbacks, 1974.
*Ellis, A. (1975) *How to Live with a 'Neurotic',* New York. Crown, revised edition.
*Ellis, A. (1976) *Sex and the Liberated Man.* New York. Lyle Stuart.
*Ellis, A. (1977a) *How to Live With—and Without—Anger.* New York. Reader's Digest Press.
*Ellis, A. (1977b) *Homework Report.* New York. Institute for Rational Living.
*Ellis, A., and Grieger, R. (1977) *A Sourcebook of Rational–Emotive Therapy.* New York. Springer Publishing Company.
*Ellis, A., and Harper, R. A. (1975) *A New Guide to Rational Living.* Englewood Cliffs, NJ. Prentice-Hall.
Goldfried, M., and Davison, G. C. (1976) *Clinical Behavior Therapy.* New York. Holt, Rinehart, Winston.
Goldfried, M. R., and Merbaum, M. (eds) (1973) *Behavior Change Through Self-Control.* New York. Holt, Rinehart, Winston.
*Goodman, D., and Maultsby, M. C., Jr. (1974) *Emotional Well-Being Through Rational Behavior Training.* Springfield, Ill. Charles C. Thomas.
Greenwald, G. (1976) *Direct Decision Therapy.* San Diego, California. Edits.
*Hauck, P. A. (1973) *Overcoming Depression.* Philadelphia, Pa. Westminster Press.
*Hauck, P. A. (1977) *Overcoming Frustration and Anger.* Philadelphia, Pa. Westminster Press.
*Hauck, P. A. (1976) *Overcoming Worry and Fear.* Philadelphia, Pa. Westminster Press.
Horney, K. (1965) *Collected Works.* New York. W. W. Norton.
*Knaus, W. J. (1974) *Rational Emotive Education.* New York. Institute for Rational Living.
*Kranzler, G. (1974) *You can Change How You Feel.* New York. Kranzler.
Lazarus, A. A. (1971) *Behaviour Therapy and Beyond.* New York. McGraw-Hill.
*Lazarus, A. A. (1976) *Multimodel Therapy.* New York. Springer Publishing Company.
*Lembo, J. (1974) *Help Yourself.* West Los Angeles. Argus Communications.
*Lembo, J. (1976) *The Counseling Process: a Rational Behavioral Approach.* New York. Libra Publishers.
Mahoney, M. J. (1974) *Cognition and Behavior Modification.* Cambridge, Mass. Ballinger.
Maultsby, M. C., Jr. (1971) Systematic written homework in psychotherapy, *Rational Living,* **6**, 1, 16–23.
*Maultsby, M. C., Jr. (1975) *Help Yourself to Happiness.* New York. Institute for Rational Living.
*Maultsby, M. C., Jr., and Ellis, A. (1974) *Technique for Using Rational Emotive Imagery.* New York. Institute for Rational Living.
Meichenbaum, D. (1974) *Cognitive Behavior Modification.* Morristown, N. J. General Learning Press.
Meichenbaum, D. (1977) *Cognitive Behavior Modification.* New York. Plenum Publishing Company.
*Morris, K. T., and Kanitz, J. M. (1975) *Rational–Emotive Therapy.* Boston, Mass. Houghton Mifflin.
Rimm, D. C., and Masters, J. C. (1974) *Behavior Therapy.* New York. Academic Press.
Rogers, C. R. (1961) *On Becoming a Person.* Boston, Mass. Houghton Mifflin.
Skinner, B. F. (1971) *Beyond Freedom and Dignity.* New York. Knopf.
*Tosi, D. J. (1974) *Youth: Toward Personal Growth, a Rational–Emotive Approach.* Columbus, Ohio. Merril.
*Young, H. S. (1974) *A Rational Counseling Primer.* New York. Institute for Rational Living.

Chapter 9

Stress and Socio-technical Design: a New Ship Organization

Ragnar Johansen

Work Research Institute, Oslo

Introduction

Stress seems to develop when there is a substantial imbalance between the task an individual faces and his ability or means to complete it. Work and life at sea are marked by such a lack of balance, which most seafarers experience as stressful. Many technological and social duties on board a ship have, at an increasing rate, become more complicated. But, at the same time, a lot of simple manual but time consuming duties, like maintenance, are still unchanged. This has also made the duties far more diverse than earlier (e.g. special requirements for new skills and new types of job content).

The seafarers' ability to cope with this new situation has not yet developed sufficiently. This is especially the case with ship organization and shipboard competence and ability to make decisions. This has increasingly led to seafarers having to put aside 'developmental goals' to solve the new problems, at the same time that the consequences of 'not developing' are becoming greater. The developmental goals concern not only operations, but also the seamen's own social and psychological needs.

The goal of satisfactory ship operation has also gone through considerable change in the last few years. Running and safety concerns are, of course, still central. What is new is that social and psychological demands from seamen have steadily become stronger and more differentiated, while at the same time there is an increasing understanding within the shipping industry that a satisfying response to these demands is closely tied to the safe and effective running of a ship. The problem has become, at present, to find working and organizational systems for ships and their owners, which jointly optimize the shipboard technical and social systems.

The social and psychological requirements of seamen are roughly equivalent to the psychological job requirements formulated by Emery and Thorsrud (1976). These job requirements build on the fact that people also have intrinsic needs they want fulfilled in their work. Increasingly, seafarers are interested in safe working conditions, and protection against arbitrary dismissal. Seamen also need jobs that are intrinsically rewarding. The following list represents at least some of the general psychological requirements that pertain to the intrinsic content of a job:

(1) the need for the content of the job to be reasonably demanding (challenging) in terms other than sheer endurance, and yet providing some variety (not necessarily novelty);
(2) the need to be able to learn on the job and go on learning (which implies known and appropriate standards, and knowledge of results). Again it is a question of neither too much nor too little;
(3) the need for some decision making power and autonomy that the individual can call his own;
(4) the need for some minimal degree of helpfulness and recognition in the work place;
(5) the need to be able to relate what he does and what he produces to his social life;
(6) the need to feel that the job leads to some desirable future.

Experience in recent years strongly indicates that such general psychological requirements influence the relationship between tasks and the likelihood of fulfilling these tasks. This results from several factors: *partly* it comes from the content of the job assuming traditional tasks are seen from a different perspective; *partly* from the fact that the satisfaction of psychological job requirements ensures that a ship develops new technical and social tasks while at the same time eliminating some traditional duties, *partly* from the need for the accepted way of solving problems (e.g. the balance of power between the owners and the crew in allocating responsibilities) to be re-evaluated and better adjusted to these general psychological requirements. Individuals' psychological job requirements are, in other words, not only determined on the basis of an evaluation of job content, but are also a strong guide to co-ordinating the changes in tasks, and the possibility of meeting task obligations. Our hypothesis is that poorly fulfilled general psychological job requirements are closely linked with a fundamental lack of balance between tasks and methods used to complete them. This leads to a non-satisfying working and living situation, which is expressed in different stress symptoms, such as frequent psychosomatic illness, frequent injuries to people and materials, high turnover in the crew, low operational effectiveness, and conflict between persons and groups.

A programme for improving the quality of working life at sea

The Work Research Institute (WRI) in Oslo in early 1960 began a programme of 'action research' to test and develop more democratic forms of work in industry. This programme, initially co-sponsored by the Norwegian Federation of Trade Unions (LO) and the Norwegian Employees' Association (NAF), was eventually financed by the government (see Emery and Thorsrud, 1968; Herbst, 1974, 1976), and led to further field experiments in other areas [service organizations, banking, schools, the shipping industry—see Work Research

Institute (1975) for a complete description of WRI's first 10 years of projects and programmes].

Since 1966, a group of researchers from WRI has tried, guided by the six psychological job requirements and socio-technical design principles above, to create a better balance between seafarers and their social and technological surroundings by re-designing ships. We hoped this would lead to more meaningful and democratic working and living conditions, and at the same time Norway would get a more effective shipping industry, traditionally an important element in the Norwegian economy. After a pilot study on six Norwegian ships, the WRI team identified three different viewpoints from which organizational conditions in the shipping industry could be understood.

(1) The organization on the ship can be viewed as an 'open socio-technical system', i.e. tasks and the allocation of work are decided partly by technological and partly by human needs. The technical and the social systems on board cannot be viewed in isolation. In addition, the ship cannot be viewed in isolation from technical and human contacts on shore.

(2) Seamen's career paths also affect the ship, because the work and life on board is part of a career pattern with long traditions. But this pattern is being broken down both by new technology and by a new educational system. More people are getting more education and more freedom to choose their job, and to change jobs when they wish.

(3) The ship, as a 24-hour society, or 'total institution', must be carefully considered if one is to understand the organizational conditions at sea. The combination of the seaman's work situation and free time on board and his role in family and society on shore is very important.

WRI researchers started with practical experiments on board ships, owned by a suitable firm, and in co-operation with the unions and other organizations and institutions involved. Preparations for the first field experiment were started in 1968 in connection with the shipping company Leif Høegh & Co. A/S. The field experiments were built on the three main viewpoints listed above. Since 1969 this research has been co-ordinated by an advisory committee with representatives from the government, the seamen, and the ship-owners. Within the programme the experimental ships have made considerable progress in improving the quality of work and developing more democratic forms of organization in both work and leisure. Just how far the experimental ships differ will be clearer if we briefly describe the conventional organization of ships.

The traditional ship organization

The traditional ship organization is marked by highly compartmentalized departments (deck, engine-room, catering) and sharply differentiated jobs within the departments (i.e. greaser, motorman, repairman, third engineer, second engineer, first engineer, and chief engineer); splitting of work planning (senior officers), control (senior officers, junior officers, petty officers), and execution (crew); separate mess-rooms and day-rooms and substantial differences between the officers' and the crew's cabins.

This organization is characterized by an excessive fragmentation, a pronounced hierarchical structure, and a substitution of crew members according to the principle that individuals can be shifted about like parts in a machine, and that new replacements do not alter the effectiveness of the total organization. Often the departments function as independent hierarchies with long established and quite inpenetrable barriers between each other. We find equally strict barriers between officers and crew. For example, there are typically three different mess-rooms (one for the captain and senior officers, another for junior officers, and a third for the crew). Even today many ships are designed so that officers and crew never have to meet each other when not at work—they have completely different territories. This organization is strongly dominated by the roles that were originally connected with certain tasks. But task needs tend to be less determinative when the interpersonal/social relations are built into these roles in such a way that they have important but often unintended psychological characteristics. These characteristics support a strongly bureaucratic organizational structure. For example, the captain's role in a typical ship has almost a god-like character. On the other hand, crew members are not expected to be able to be responsible: 'they need someone to manage them'.

There are many indications that this bureaucratic and authoritarian ship's organization creates a number of undesired psychological, social, safety, and operational problems such as various psychosomatic illnesses, interpersonal and intergroup conflicts, high turnover, work related injuries, and physical damage. An excessively fragmented and hierarchical ship organization with high turnover impedes members of the ship's company from helping each other. This is particularly unfortunate since a ship is already an isolated work place, in which technical and social problems are becoming increasingly complex and demanding, but one which inhibits people from solving problems in ways they might be used to on shore. This is of great importance to the seamen, because they have far fewer opportunities than people ashore to compensate for a work situation which has no meaning and is stress creating. The work and social system which follows from the way work is organized is the main source of satisfying important needs. A meaningful and satisfying job can lessen the impact of stress because the circumstances under which the work must be carried out make the seaman's job especially stressful (social and physical isolation and limited action possibilities).

For many people the main difference between living conditions ashore and at sea is that seafarers cannot live a regular family life, or in other ways participate in the social life ashore. Even in his own family, a seaman is mostly a passive member. This *social isolation* is in addition to the fact that people on board are tied to a social system which often provides a relatively narrow social milieu. There are several reasons for this. In part it is narrow because of limited social resources—a small number of people, a male dominated society, and a relatively uniform social background. In part it is narrow because of its isolation, which creates quite restricted norms for acceptable behaviour. Finally, the on board social system is narrow because free time and work are more intimately linked than on shore. In short, seamen are not only *locked out* of a relatively diverse social system ashore, but also *locked in* to a relatively narrow social system. The consequences are that seamen must for the most part rely on their own resources to fulfil their social and technical duties even in critical situations where life and commerce may be threatened.

A ship's organization should complete routine technical and administrative tasks effectively and in such a manner that optimum job satisfaction is given to everybody on board, while at the same time it should fulfil a wide range of complicated and special social tasks which, among other things, are connected with the crew's social and physical isolation. The traditional ship's organization no longer seems to be able to do this satisfactorily. This is to be expected, since the dominant character of a ship's organization has not changed over the last 50 years. It is, as already pointed out, an organization characterized by:

(1) a strong fragmentation of the organization based on bureaucratic organizational principles;
(2) a marked hierarchic structure which leads, among other things, to a nonhomogeneous organization;
(3) a strong influence from the shipping office over task distribution and decisions on board.

The following technical and social changes on ships and ashore over the last 10 years have led to critical consequences for the industry and a need to change existing tasks on board:

(1) Many tasks are too complicated and change too fast, often because of decisions made outside the ship by, for example, technology or administrative systems.
(2) Some tasks are undesirable: for example, a heavy work load in maintenance and cleaning, or apparently unnecessary report writing.
(3) Tasks are generally badly divided, for example, between the ship and the shipping office or between different groups on board.
(4) More tasks are missed on board—often because of strong centralization in the ship-owning office.

In addition, the *seamen's competence* can generally be said to be unsatisfactorily adjusted to the new technological, administrative, and social tasks on board. This is in part, because of:

(1) strong specialization of jobs;
(2) low competence in certain fields; the traditional deck officer's education, for example, is not sufficient for many loading–unloading systems made for special ships (gas ships, chemical ships, etc.);
(3) higher competence of newer recruits in relation to tasks which are assigned

to certain positions. The lower level jobs in the organization have not been adjusted to increases in recent years in for example, general technical knowledge among new seamen recruits;

(4) an absence of competence amongst shipboard personnel in economic, and administrative tasks.

Such an evaluation provided the concrete rationale for research in socio-technical design of an alternative ship organization. New ways of organizing work and social life on board a ship seemed to be critically needed.

Socio-technical design

As Herbst (1974) has indicated, the socio-technical, analytical model assumes that the technological system determines the characteristics of the social system through the allocation of work roles and the technologically given dependence relation between tasks. Performance is a function of the joint operation of the social and technical systems. Dysfunctional consequences of the social system are not easily modified in so far as the social structure is based on the requirements of the technological system (Figure 9.1). Stress. as a dysfunctional

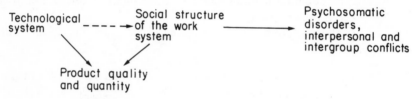

Figure 9.1 A socio-technical systems framework

consequence of the social system, will, according to this analytical model, be reduced by a joint optimization of the technical and social systems. One-sided changes of either the technical system (e.g. watch free engine-room) or the social system (sensitivity training) can lead to sub-optimal results, including stress, as a consequence. Implicit here is the proposition that if conflicts are built into the very organization of the ship, there is little to be gained by what is called 'human relations' training.

Joint optimization of a ship's social and technical systems demands, however, that we are able to specify certain minimum conditions to be satisfied by the ship's organization. WRI's shipping research programme has mostly been based on the following minimum conditions. The organization should:

(1) be adaptable to technological change;
(2) facilitate the effective use of leisure time;
(3) provide conditions for both autonomous and group based activities;
(4) be consistent with an exchangeable component structure; that is, it should not be too difficult to replace leavers and to integrate new crew members;

(5) be either an overlapping role structure or a multiple role structure;
(6) if possible, link 'mutual respect' relations to perceived and demonstrable competence;
(7) if possible, be consistent with and provide conditions for the development of collegial and friendship relationships;
(8) minimize the build-up of psychological tensions;
(9) provide effective control over interpersonal tensions;
(10) provide greater stability of crew membership.

Work roles should:

(1) provide a basis for technical or professional competence;
(2) facilitate both transition to and recruitment from shore with a minimum of retraining;
(3) be consistent with career advancement requirements.

The tasks and task elements developed on the ship should:

(1) be consistent with the requirements of the social system;
(2) consist as far as possible of complete task regions;
(3) provide to some extent conditions for operating towards a joint aim for the total crew.

The requirements have to be (1) feasible individually; (2) mutually consistent, and if possible mutually supportive.

An important relationship in the socio-technical planning of a new ship is the general direction that the Norwegian shipping industry has chosen for its development. The industry aims at technically advanced, capital intensive ships, which can offer an adaptable transportation service, supported by complex operating systems. All changes are in the direction of more automation, more effective computer systems and information transfer technologies. A special characteristic of this development is that changes occur at an increasing rate. The problem is, therefore, not to create a new shipping organization for a new technology, but an organization which can cope with a high rate of technological change. Since the development of a new ship organization takes far more time than technological changes, it is of great importance that a new ship, from its earliest organization, can cope with a continuous technological change process.

To achieve the desired level of adaptability, the organization must not be too well defined in the beginning. Initially, only a minimum of structure must be built into the organization. A ship's organization that is too highly structured can from the outset expect frequent and 'problem directed' restructuring.

The steadily increasing technological and operational changes, mean that the 'tasks for the crew' go through a similar change. An education for seamen that builds on a traditional task pattern will therefore be of less and less use. This means that the shipping industry will need people with higher education and interest for continued education—especially in technical subjects. Crews in the future will, in other words, be more homogeneous in relation to education and cultural background, which probably will lead to less isolation and fragmentation arising from status differentials.

The first shipboard action research efforts—the Høegh experiments (1970–1975)

The *Høegh Mistral* experiment began in Feburary 1970. (The ship is a car/bulk carrier on 24 000 d.w.—built in 1970.) The main objective for this experiment and the next—the *Høegh Multina* experiment—was to

(1) develop a more stimulating working situation on board and in the company, aiming at liberating the human resources. This will entail a development of the company's aim and policy in keeping up with society's changes in general and changes in ship technology in particular;
(2) influence and improve working conditions on board, specifically 'the ship's culture' and the training possibilities;
(3) create the foundation for the seafarers' profession, the company and the ship organization continually adapting to technological changes.

Our efforts in these two projects have for the most part gone in the direction of:

(1) increasing the autonomy of senior officers on board in relation to the shipping company;
(2) increasing the ratings' work autonomy;
(3) reducing status differences between officers and ratings both in work and free time;
(4) changing the roles of the deck and engine-room crews;
(5) improving the seafarers' conditions of appointment;
(6) stabilizing the ships' crew.

In the *Høegh Mistral* project these changes affected both senior officers (top management) and ratings (workers) more than junior officers (middle management). Although a genuine desire existed to do something about the junior officers' working situation, possibilities in this direction were limited—the junior officers were only indirectly affected by the change programme on board (see Roggema and Thorsrud, 1974).

One aim during the planning of the *Høegh Multina* experiment was to utilize some experiences from the *Høegh Mistral* concerning organization at the ratings' level. (The ship *Høegh Multina* is a fully refrigerated LPG/NH3 gas tanker with a cargo capacity of 52 000 m³. The ship—like the *Høegh Mistral*—has EO classification for the engine-room to be periodically watch free, and the alarm system, the automatic control loops, and the condition monitoring system are controlled by two computers.) But, in addition, the main aim was to carry out certain changes in organizational conditions at the junior officers' level, which would provide an opportunity to test a more

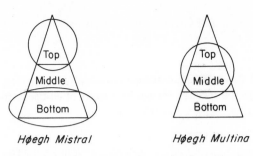

Figure 9.2 Relative focus of attention in two action
research projects

flexible organization form. This required that the junior officers had to some extent overlapping job competencies. Therefore, before *Høegh Multina* was launched, the mates received some technical–mechanical training, and the engineers and the electrician were trained in navigation (see Roggema and Hammarstrøm, 1975). The organizational changes in the *Høegh* projects led to a certain *horizontal integration*, i.e. people on the same level had more scope for shared work. This meant in practice that every individual in the crew got a variety of tasks to work on, which also gave him more contact with fellow crew members. This required more extensive training, and provided opportunities for being better qualified and more autonomous in his work. The result was, in other words, job enrichment and enlargement. This was also supported by other measures, e.g. eliminating the job of repairman *(Høegh Mistral)*. When it was discovered that not enough technical work was available for all the ratings, the repairman's position was abolished and the ratings were trained to do a number of the tasks usually done by the repairman. Raising the level of the crew's qualifications and autonomy also led to eliminating the boatswain's (i.e. foreman's) position, to extend the ratings' responsibility and independence. Horizontal integration led to the ships' organization being more homogeneous on all three levels (senior officers, junior officers, and ratings), and to decreased distance between the officers and the ratings. This was in harmony with the introduction of a joint day-room and mess-room for officers and ratings.

Integration of work on deck and engine-room, both by the ratings and junior officers, was dependent on joint 'work planning' for these two departments. This was, however, a problem the senior officers had to solve, even though the ratings were represented by one or two persons in the long range planning meetings (about one every month). The ratings' representation was, however, so little that it had practically no meaning. This was a main weakness in the *Høegh* projects. We did not manage to develop co-operative work planning successfully enough to significantly reduce the degree of bureaucratic ship organization. In short, *people planning their own work together seemed to be the main key to how successful the effort at vertical integration would be.* This became the keynote of the next experiment on board the M/S *Balao.*

The *Balao* project (from 1973); development of self-maintaining organizational learning through successive phases of co-operative work planning, training, and personal development

When the *Balao* project started in 1973, a special effort was made to develop and use work planning as a main tool to create a more meaningful and democratic ship organization (Johansen and Samuelsen, 1976). The M/S *Balao* was delivered to the Torvald Klaveness shipping company in Oslo in March 1973. At 27 000 d.w., it is a bulk carrier with two Kampnagel cranes (16–25 tons) that can be driven up or down or across the ship. The engine-room is fully automated (i.e. periodically watch free) with a main engine of the Sulzer type 6RND76 B.H.K. 12 000 rpm 122.

The superstructure of M/S *Balao* was quite different from superstructures of other Norwegian ships. In 1971 an *ad hoc* group (in which WRI participated) had in a very short time designed a new superstructure for the last four ships in a series of 13, which was delivered from Poland to the Bulk Carrier Group in Klaveness's Oslo office. The background for the change in these superstructures was that the ship-owners (and one in particular) felt that the future shipping environment would require a new form of shipboard social organization. However, the existing superstructure with its present physical layout reinforced the traditional social decisions and status differences within a ship.

Unfortunately, the design process itself limited the possibilities for such change. This led WRI to focus on the design process in new ship construction and on conditions for 'redesigning the design process' itself (see Rogne, 1974). We hoped that a new design process would lead to the construction of ships today that could function more effectively in 1990. For us, the problem was both in the technological and social design.

Balao has cabins of high quality and 'equality' for all on board. All cabins are placed high up in the superstructure which makes feasible large windows and good lighting in them. Further, each cabin has its own shower, toilet, and bedroom. On the main deck one enters a combination of lounge and coffee bar. This room is placed between the restaurant, swimming pool, and exercise room, with the intention of it being a 'contact point' where people can meet each other informally and relax over a cup of coffee. In the front of the superstructure on the poop-deck the ship's officers share a common office area, which provides facilities for continuous contact and collaboration in the ship's management. The ship's conference-room is here also.

The entire crew share in common all living-rooms: lounge, day-room with library, study-room, and restaurant. This was decided on at a conference in February 1973, where the whole crew participated, shortly before they took over the new ship. This 'crew conference' was very useful. The crew agreed on a programme for the experiment and at the same time they got to know each other under favourable conditions. This provided some experience of how we could work together on a more equal basis, and created the foundation for a good environment on board.

Plans for a joint restaurant—without assigned seating—and a common dayroom, lobby, and bar, were begun. This proved to be successful and contributed a great deal towards a good social atmosphere between all the different groups on board. The captain stated in a report after 3 months of operation: 'One can already assert that the shared restaurant on board is quite successful. I was in the beginning quite sceptical and anticipated a lot of problems. They were completely needless worries. We had no difficulties; on the contrary, it has been pleasant. And this goes for everyone, both ratings and officers, not to mention the undersigned.'

Work planning

For the first 5 months work planning was done by a group who met at least once a week. Here the captain took part, along with the chief engineer, chief mate, first engineer, the radio operator, the boatswain, and two representatives from the ratings. But, as with the *Høegh* projects, this was not satisfactory. Often in conjunction with these planning meetings there was a general meeting of officers and crew. The general meeting was a forum where the whole crew could participate in discussions and decisions about work planning and eventually other cases of common interest.

During that first summer in 1973, the crew agreed:

(1) to leave the weekly work planning to a semi-autonomous group, in which crew from deck and engine-room were represented;
(2) to intensify training so that the crew would be able to work together as an *integrated* group, with the whole ship as the work territory;
(3) to convert the boatswain's position into that of a manager of training;
(4) to work out a new combined training programme to support the further integration of deck and engine-room crews;
(5) to apply to the maritime authorities and branch organizations for approval of a suggestion from the ship to have a set monthly salary and an arrangement with flexible manning (i.e. the crew could vary somewhat during the year, around an agreed-upon average number of 23).

The next 3 months showed that the semi-autonomous group under certain circumstances could do the work planning. The main condition was systematic training of the crew, so that the majority could participate in planning, control, and carrying out regular work on deck *and* in the engine-room. However, it was clear this demanded lengthy development. Also, in the beginning, the new organization pattern was very vulnerable to changes in crew (men leaving for vacation or to work on other ships). This led to the chief mate and first engineer joining the planning meetings. The crew experienced this as a step backward in their autonomy, but it was accepted as necessary because of the low level of training and stability in the crew. During the summer of 1974 there was quite a big turnover in the crew. Therefore it was necessary to have a general meeting in August to summarize what had been attempted and learned to date, and to discuss and agree on further development efforts.

The crew agreed that:

(1) the six psychological work requirements would continue to be the guidelines for the developments on board;
(2) work planning was the key to further development;
(3) the training of the crew should follow the new programme developed for training of 'ship mechanics' (this programme was accepted by the Norwegian Co-ordinating Committee for Maritime Education in February 1974, as a means of giving full competence as both able seaman and motorman);
(4) it was very important to increase crew stability and recruit people who could fit the new training programme and the ship's new way of operating;
(5) all decisions in a general meeting would be valid until they were changed, if necessary, at a new general meeting.

Consistent with better training and higher stability in the crew, there was a positive change in the development of work planning. It was especially important that *planning of work and training were linked*. A point was made of dividing the work, so that the best possible training was available for everybody through the new training programme for ship mechanics. Integration of work and training made it easier to carry through the training in a systematic and controlled way. It also gave the individual more security in his job development and the senior officers more insight into what competence they had at all times available for the security and running of the ship.

To achieve greater effectiveness and co-operation in work planning, it was (in February 1975) decided to do some of the work planning in small groups. This especially applied to the question of *how* big and important jobs should be done. As more officers had become involved in the planning meetings over time it became important to ensure that the crew's point of view was given proper attention. It was felt that crew members would have better opportunities to communicate effectively in the smaller groups initiated at this point.

The weekly planning meetings were usually held on Saturdays. The ship's officers had their own meetings on Fridays to discuss their own matters. At these meetings, they worked out a preliminary list of *what* they thought should be the actual duties for the following week, based on the long term maintenance programme. The final work list was to be decided upon at the Saturday meeting with the participation of the full crew. The Saturday work planning meeting was therefore divided up between a plenary meeting (to make a work list and decide on *who* should do which jobs *when*), and small group work (for deciding on *how* a job should be done). This seemed to be an engaging, effective, and very informative way of planning.

These Saturday meetings gradually developed into a natural forum for cases normally taken up at general meetings, which no longer seemed so necessary. Senior officers gradually transferred things, which they had handled at their Friday meetings, to the Saturday meetings. In other words, the general meetings and Friday meetings were needed less and less. In the autumn of 1975, some adjustment in work planning was made. All duties for one week were now gathered into smaller groups of duties, which were then allocated to smaller groups of the crew. These smaller work groups had both officers and crew in them and changed their membership from week to week. The mate on duty (especially the first and second mates) were, however, prevented from participating in the planning meetings and in work groups because they had to stand watch, and there were still too few on board with navigation certificates.

Figure 9.3 shows the work planning procedure. This procedure was neces-

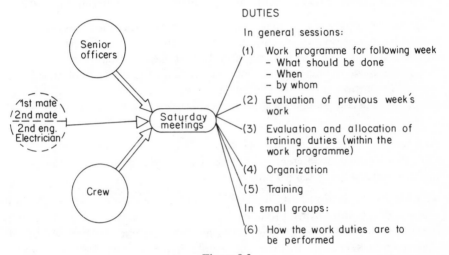

Figure 9.3

sary in order that partly autonomous groups could function as matrix organizations, where temporary work groups were created around particular types of tasks. Both tasks and groups might change from week to week. Work duties and functions were not divided according to deck and engine-room crews or between officers and crew, as is typical on conventional ships. Qualified members of the crew cover a variety of duties crossing the traditional functional and status dividing lines. The work load, training needs, and safety considerations were the critical factors in allocating specific tasks to specific people. This does not mean that everyone should be able to do everything on a certain level in the organization.

A matrix organization is built on the assumption that each person has his special duties which demand special qualifications, but he is also competent for duties overlapping other people's competence. As Herbst (1974) points out, every qualified crew member should then be able to be a manager, depending on the nature of the task, or work, as well as a member of a particular work group. This principle of a non-bureaucratic organization model is realized on *Balao* in that:

(1) the crew is integrated, i.e. former deck crew and engine-room crew now have the whole ship as a shared work area and a joint training programme;
(2) officers and crew together plan and control the training programme and the work itself;
(3) officers and crew together constitute a constantly shifting array of temporary, but still relatively autonomous, work groups, in a pattern that can best be described as a 'matrix organization' (Herbst, 1976);
(4) the whole crew has common dining and living facilities and similar individual cabins;
(5) the crew is permanently connected to the ship by fixed annual salaries, flexible manning requirements, and decentralized personnel administration.

At the very least it seems quite clear that the *Balao* experiment has been able, in part by relying on a combination of interdependencies around participation in work planning, special training, and decentralized personnel management, to achieve more than simply the job enlargement, job enrichment, and horizontal integration of earlier experiments. What has been achieved has the properties of a completely new type of organization.

Non-bureaucratic organization development—3 years of field experience show that learning on different levels leads to a new way of looking at things and new ways of living and working together

This ship organization rests on quite extensive changes of the crew's and officers' duties, duty distribution, co-operation, and living patterns. Essential ingredients of these changes were extensive training and the building up of diverse competences. In this way the people involved were able to determine *who* should do *what* work *when* and *how*—important elements in a democratic work organization. The conditions for increasing work democracy in ship organization seem to include:

(1) Common systematic training of the previously quite separate deck and engine-room crews (mostly by their participating in planning and managing their own work according to what needed to be done for the ship and for training purposes—this occurred through the weekly planning meetings).

(2) Constant discussions and 'experience exchanges' about the ship's organization—in planning meetings, general meetings, and in daily working and being together. In other words, the ship's operating policy is formed by continuous learning (Thorsrud, 1970) in which everyone is involved in successive phases of review, evaluation, and testing of new arrangements.

(3) A careful hiring of crew with technical training (e.g. 1 or 2 years of technical college).

(4) Taking care of the competence built up on board by encouraging a high

stability among the crew (e.g. by means of fixed annual salaries and flexible manning for the crew).

(5) Contact with other experimental ships, research centres, and trade unions, etc., for mutual learning and support (also through the network 'ship meets ship', see Johansen, 1975.)

Of all of these conditions, perhaps those having to do with the learning process are most central. The entire ship's community is strongly characterized by *learning* which seems to be occurring at three different levels simultaneously (Johansen, 1976).

(1) An extensive *individual learning* programme based on:

(a) More professional knowledge, both practical and theoretical, not only for more varied work and career development on ships, but also for more satisfying work on shore.
(b) How training and work can be planned, executed, and controlled as *integrated* activities.
(c) How this systematic training enables one to guide one's own occupational development. (In 1975 and 1976, four crew members were trained as ship mechanics on board *Balao*. The first two were also the first ship mechanics in the entire Norwegian Merchant Marine.)
(d) How these conditions (points a, b, and c) give meaning to, and security in, work and free time, which is shown in the exceptionally high stability among the crew, a significant decrease in the number of injuries and visits to a doctor, and a high level of job satisfaction expressed by crew members.

(2) A distinctive *organization learning* programme as seen in:

(a) Continuous surveying of problems by members of the ship's organization.
(b) A systematic search for alternative solutions to problems.
(c) A critical follow up and evaluation of self-initiated experiments.

This process has been expressed in a fundamentally different organizational structure and a clear understanding that:

(a) Work planning is the key to the goals of greater autonomy and meeting people's needs at work.
(b) Training is essential for the new organization structure to function satisfactorily.
(c) The ship's crew must have a strong influence on the personnel policy in order to recruit and hold well qualified crew members (decentralized personnel administration).
(d) Work planning, training, and personnel policy are closely linked.

(3) A far reaching social learning programme based on step-by-step changes of work and living patterns. This social learning is first of all expressed in the everyday routine among the crew. Today the social life on board is distinguished by a high degree of *mutual help and tolerance* among individuals and groups. The earlier situation, which is also typical of conventionally organized ships,

was characterized by people remaining aloof and apathetic, and by competition, for example, between deck and engine-room crews or between officers and crew. This new approach of relating to other people and having contact with them seems to decrease problems between them—or if problems occur they do not seem to develop into major traumas. It seems as if the crew has a greater ability than before to resolve these problems.

The relationships with people outside the ship, especially the family, also seem better. More persons claim to have a wider and more natural contact with their family. The social life on board seems to be more like social life within the family, which is also valued by society. The richer, more varied social life on board, based on extensive changes in the ship's organization, operation, and construction, has, in other words, developed a more friendly and tolerant view that *lessens the social isolation* many had previously experienced in relation to other crew members, the family, and others back home. This development of more communal and easy going social life and leisure seems to come quite naturally from a way of working and an organizational structure in which people get to know each other as part of their work. On board *Balao*, in contrast to conventionally organized ships, task sharing seems to lead to more meaningful, socially enriched leisure. In neither work nor leisure are people boxed up in relatively confined areas: task and living opportunities are equally available to all within the territory of the entire ship.

It might be easier to understand this development by looking at the changes beside the goals and values that we initially set out to attain: Joint mess-room and day-room facilities; similar cabins for all; a joint personal policy; participatory planning, control, and execution of work; cross-departmental training and more individuality in work (especially for the crew) are all measures supporting the belief that everybody on board has the same right to individually pursuing his work and free time activities. This individuality is mostly covered by the six requirements described above for psychologically fulfilling work.

The work planning and the ship mechanics' training are clearly in support of these psychological requirements. The way work is allocated has an important part to play in making sure that people get *meaning* and *variation* in their work and at the same time the chance to *learn* something. Participatory work planning in addition gives the individual a chance to have a say in *decisions* about the ship's maintenance and operation. It also gives room for more autonomy to individuals and groups in the control and execution of work. The combination of work and ship mechanics' training, for example, make the job more attractive for the future. What is important here is that when you are participating in organizing a productive activity (in this case the employees' work and free time), with special care taken concerning certain human needs, you are also creating your own relationships with other people and your view of yourself and others. You and the organization become closer to being one.

A summary and preliminary evaluation

A preliminary evaluation of results has been made by the ship itself and the company as well as by the Work Research Institute. The total crew has stated significant improvements on the six job criteria on which job redesign was based. Variation and learning on the job and increased participation in decision making improved most significantly among the rank and file, but such improvement was also evident at the middle and top levels of ship organization. For junior officers the improvements were least significant because of a close tie up with the routine watch system. The fourth criterion, social support and mutual help, again improved at all levels, but least so at the middle level. Improvements on the next criterion, the social impact of the job in the society outside, are shown in a number of ways, most significantly in the way all levels of the ship are involved in promoting their policies in other ships and shore organizations. The sixth criterion, the job as part of a desirable future, shows very clear improvements in three different ways: in terms of traditional promotion inside the company; in terms of more satisfying work through job redesign and horizontal as well as vertical job rotation; and last but not the least, the job prospects for sailors from this ship, if they want to take a job ashore, are much better than for sailors in the traditional system.

The ship also decided on a decentralized personnel policy and has gone a long way in this direction. Selection and replacement of crew at all levels, as well as the planning of periodic vacations, is taken over by the ship, with the central office personnel department acting in a service capacity. Training programmes for the whole crew are also worked out by the ship itself. The special problems of junior officers as mentioned above will be tackled when a new programme for integrated deck-engine officers' training is put into effect next year. Perhaps the most significant achievement in decentralized personnel policy is the system of variation of manning over different periods of the year. Manning goes up when work demands are high and when new people enter the ship for training. The average manning is still close to the minimum established by regulation.

How do these improvements on the six job criteria and in decentralized personnel policy show in actual behaviour? First, anyone visiting the ship will be struck by the continuous and highly effective learning activity on board. The Saturday work planning is at the moment the driving force for learning, but other arrangements have been used before and, if necessary, new ones will certainly be created and institutionalized. Second, the rate of turnover of personnel on this ship is far below the average for similar ships and the same applies to the number of accidents and sick leaves. Third, the ship has a very good record on its level of maintenance and its operational efficiency. The work planning system helps to keep the number of days—or even hours— of staying in port to a minimum. Fourth, one cost element increased during the first two years of operation, namely the cost of manning. The ship decided to analyse this problem in depth and one of its crew, the radio operator, spent 3 months at the Work Research Institute with all the cost data and specialist help made available to him from the shipping company. This year the personnel cost of the ship is probably turning out to be the same as that for similar ships. Perhaps more important is the fact that maintenance costs and days lost for

240

repairs, etc., are significantly below average.

The ship and the company clearly realized that effective, continuous evaluation of results can only be done by the ship itself. This is perhaps the most important point about evaluation and about the experiment itself.

References

Duckert, H., and Kevin, R. (1975) *Drift av skip* (Ship operations). Oslo. NR/SAF Felleskontoret.

Emery, F. E., and Thorsrud, E. (1968) *Form and Content in Industrial Democracy*. London. Tavistock.

Emery, F. E., and Thorsrud, E. (1976) *Democracy at Work*. Leiden. Martinus Nijhoff Social Sciences Division.

Herbst, P. G. (1969) Sosiotekniske og psykodynamiske variabler i planlegging av en ny skipsorganisasjon. (Socio-technical and psycho-dynamic variables in the planning of new ship organization), *Tidsskrift for samfunnsforskning*, nr. 3–4. (Also in English in Herbst, 1974.)

Herbst, P. G. (1974) *Socio-Technical Design*. London. Tavistock.

Herbst, P. G. (1976) *Alternatives to Hierarchies*. Leiden. Martinus Nijhoff Social Sciences Division.

Johansen, R. (1975) *Nettverk der skip møter skip* (Network: ship meets ship). Oslo. WRI.

Johansen, R. (1976) *Opplaering om bord M/S Balao* (Training on board the *Balao*). Oslo. WRI.

Johansen, R., and Samuelsen, E. (1976) *Planlegging av arbeid om bord M/S* Balao (Work planning on board the *Balao*). Oslo. WRI.

Roggema, J., and Hammarstrøm, N. K. (1975) *Nye organisasjonsformer til sjøs* (New Organizational Forms in Seafaring). Oslo. Tanum-Norili.

Roggema, J., and Thorsrud, E. (1974) *Et skip i utvikling* (A ship in development). Oslo. Tanum.

Rogne, K. (1974) Redesigning the design process: superstructures of ships, *Applied Ergonomics*, **5**, 4, 213–218.

Thorsrud, E. (1970) Policy making as a learning process. Invited paper, UNESCO Social Science Conference, Paris, 1970. (Also in Cherns, A. B., *et al.* (eds), *Social Science and Government, Policies and Problems*. London. Tavistock, 1972.)

Work Research Institute (1975) *Catalog of Programs and Projects 1965–1974*. Oslo. Work Research Institute.

Chapter **10**

The Increasing Relevance of Group Processes and Changing Values for Understanding and Coping with Stress at Work

Harold Bridger

Tavistock Institute of Human Relations

Le poisson ne sait qu'il vit dans l'eau que
quand il est déjà sur la rive.
(Old French saying)

We shall not cease from exploration
And the end of all our exploring
Will be to arrive where we started
And know the place for the first time.
(T. S. Eliot)

Introduction

It could be said that the development of the individual through earlier as well as adolescent years and young adulthood is also the development of the capacity to meet and withstand stress—internally and externally, physically and mentally. There is no best way, however, of passing through that sequence of different qualitative settings from conception onwards, with their appropriate degrees of protection and exposure. The richness of experience and the complexity of the forces and influences involved ensure that we are 'lucky' in some ways and dimensions and unlucky in others. It would appear that we are not all born with the same degree of what we might call the 'will to love' or 'zest for life' any more than we are born equal in intellectual, emotional or physical attributes. We can, however, make more or less of what we have so that some may fare better with fewer resources if these can be mobilized and deployed effectively, given the opportunity and making the effort. It is commonly known that putting the growing individual under inappropriate pressures before he is ready, or giving him too much and ill advised support when internal resources should be given more chance to become integrated, can make for a fragile boundary at certain points and for a 'thick skin' at others. Vulnerability, in stress terms, is therefore not just prevented by having strong defences, but rather by ensuring that an optimal balance of forces, situations, of inner strength and surrounding conditions, insight, integrity and capability for action have already developed by that time. In mentioning the positive aspect of these attributes it will be recognized that the 'optimal balance' also refers to 'managing' their other aspects. The effect of the death of a parent, for example, is almost always a painful and distressing experience, but to what extent, after mourning and adjustment, the loss becomes a trauma or catastrophe will depend on the way these other forces and dimensions can be realized. To use the 'language of organization' for organismic processes and events it could be said that the individual is encouraged to manage a succession of 'boundaries' and acquire strengths and capabilities to move on to the wider ones set by society and the culture in which the person is living. In these respects there is, in addition to the sequence of womb, mother, family, school, and so on, that other process of testing out and developing the capacity to internalize learning and experience. Winnicott (1971) gave the latter even more emphasis when he referred to the value of various means ('transitional objects', from earliest soft toys to later games and activities) in the developmental sequence as depending 'not so much on the object used as on the use of the object'.

The individual, group, organization and community

Coming to terms with or 'mastering' our individual environment and adapting it to our needs while developing and ordering our internal affairs thus begins at -9 months and proceeds throughout life. 'Managing' these personal 'boundaries' in thinking, feeling, deciding, and acting is then based on a complex of attributes and expectations; it is met not only by responses from others but from forces within oneself. These early beginnings in coping and 'managing' take on a wide range of strengths and a wide variety of directions as the individual, man or woman, internalizes and creates his or her own set of 'maps' of the external world and builds 'images' of the different social groupings he or she expects to meet or take part in.

The development of the individual through the roles he undertakes in groups and the experiences (achievement, love/hate satisfactions, triumphs, and humiliations . . .) he undergoes requires and becomes a process of learning, unlearning, and change. In the course of this development and maturation the individual is fulfilling new and growing capacities of resources while often reluctantly relinquishing skills, expertise, satisfactions, power, and authority associated with past roles and groups. This represents a continuous experience of problems and challenge for the individual. Arising from these experiences, the individual builds sets of values, standards, assumptions, stereotypes, and expectations in different situations. In groups and interpersonal contacts he tests out his 'maps' and risks his 'endeavours'. He may weigh up, consciously and unconsciously, the 'price tag' associated with different situations and different decisions or choices he makes—or, for example, he may avoid this 'managerial' balancing and optimizing, letting events or others decide for him. The entrepreneur, the professional manager, the trade union leader, the ward sister, the government minister, the team practice (of clergy, doctors or lawyers), the housewife, the autonomous work group, are in these respects 'brothers and sisters beneath the skin'.

Ultimately the life or death of any group depends on the capacity of its members to 'manage' not only themselves but the technological and structural systems employed while ensuring the achievement of its objectives. This 'leadership function' of the group may be 'organized' or carried out in a variety of forms but essentially it needs to be relevant to the tasks, activities, and goals of the group—for both the short and long term. The interdependence required today to cope with the balancing and optimizing of internal and external cultures and forces thus makes increasing demands on the quality and form of co-ordination and control in *every* kind of institution. In addition this interdependence has also to achieve a balance between conflicting objectives.

The group needs to provide a climate within which the member can try out his capabilities and grow, if the individual is to have the chance of contributing or withholding his own participation and commitment to common objectives. On the other hand, the group may also be experienced as a 'tyrant' forbidding certain 'freedoms' and even manipulating or invading personal privacy. Between these extremes lies the infinite variety of individual/group relationships with which organizations themselves have to cope.

Changing patterns of values and roles

Earlier patterns of community, family, and individual care no longer suffice in a world of accelerating technological, social, and economic change. There are far wider and deeper considerations which have created new dimensions in social living whereby the individual is faced with the need for continuous reappraisal of his relationships to the groups and institutions to which he belongs. In the recent past the individual, group, organization, and community had more distinct 'boundaries' in the wider society which gave them, in turn, clearer and more recognizable identities. These boundaries are now, for the most part, so 'open' to their various environments—and to the pressures, uncertainties, and complexities in them—that revised concepts of 'identity' are required. For example, the individual member of an organization is, in general, likely to have a 'career' which is far less related to that single institution and much more related to changes in role, function, and even in the career itself. The sum total of such changes in the quantity and quality of information (i), forces (f), and events (e) affecting a person, his family, work, and leisure— and influencing his decisions and actions—might be represented in a somewhat oversimplified way as in Figure 10.1. The changing position and nature of C, as portrayed in the sketch, plays an increasingly unsettling part in determining the behaviour and actions of 'ME' in his or her total life space. The

244

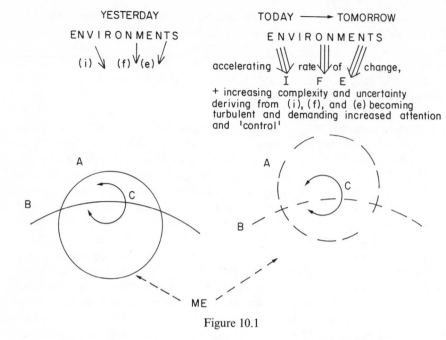

Figure 10.1

'ME'—my roles, relationships, and skills in family, work, and social interests
 —my values and standards acquired and patterned through development and experience
 —my aspirations, hopes, and fears
 —my 'identity'
 —etc.

A = my concern and preoccupation with exploring, testing, controlling (regulating), learning from, and contributing to the various environments
B = my boundary with other individuals, groups, institutions, and the environment generally
C = the part of 'me' which mediates the transaction of learning from and contributing to the environment

reduced effect of old established institutions and values, deriving from a more recognizable culture, have combined with an increased strain deriving from uncertainty and complexity, to make new demands on people.

It will be noted that to cope with the increasing complexity and rate of change, A has had to give increasingly more attention to the environments, with consequent implicit changes in the nature of C. A, therefore, has to become more 'open' to those environments and more involved with them. C's reciprocal relationship with those changes in the environments may be entirely neglected or rejected by 'ME'. If, however, they are indeed 'listened to', the individual will be adapting his own internal world by taking in new learning and developing a readiness for unlearning or relinquishing older established concepts, values, and behaviour acquired and patterned through his own development and experience.

When and how can stress be changed into useful experience?

Stress does not have to be a 'bad thing'. There is only one kind of person without conflicts—a dead one. What matters is the degree and quality of stress which the individual is undergoing in the particular *situation* he is in. An equally important factor is the balance of stress from within and the pressures from outside which that individual or group is having to cope with. For all sorts of reasons and despite the choice of transport we make, travelling in a train is likely to be less stressful than travelling by car or plane; working under difficult conditions or in danger with those we trust is less stressful than when that confidence is missing in others or ourselves. We are individually different as regards the circumstances which arouse stress or conflict within us. In turn, the capacity to tolerate it depends not only on the inner defences we have built in the course of our development and experience but on the chances we get to try out, or test out, our strengths and limitations in similar, less drastic or critical situations. If we trace our personal development from birth we see that much of our preparation for adulthood is based on quite stressful experiences, but ones which can be 'worked through' to give us that inner strength which comes from the feeling of 'having been there before' (even if we are not actually conscious of it). It was John Kennedy who applied this principle during the Cuban crisis, when he instituted a whole series of 'decisions' based on the different sets of circumstances as they occurred and in *possible* anticipated actions by the Russians. He did not have to implement any of those particular 'decisions' but when he had to respond to his opponent's initiative he was better able to produce a quicker and better quality decision than he would otherwise have done. However, the opportunity to learn from some earlier form of experience seldom if ever gives us the actual answers in advance. It is true that we often *expect* training or experience to give us the ability to find the actual 'right solution' in life, career, and work decisions. The Spartans took this idea to ridiculous lengths by exposing their babies to the unreasonable stress of the elements as a means of ensuring a future hardy race. When we fall into that trap we are forgetting the importance of finding conditions and a 'climate' which give an individual the chance to work things out at a rate and in circumstances which enable him to build that total experience into himself and make it part of him. Learning to swim may be achieved by 'being thrown into the deep end' but, as with the Spartans, we must consider the 'price tag' that goes with it. On the other hand the opposite extreme of providing conditions which do not allow the individual any or after him too little opportunity of trying himself out in appropriate ways, where he can *explore* the world around him and can match his resources to the demands made on him, will cause him to avoid or to be inadequate in equivalent situations of later life. Searching for ways of improving that *balance* not only differentiates humans from animals but also from the mechanistic and technological wonders man himself invents. When we only use drugs or even tranquillizers to cope with tension or stress states we must realize that we are not enabling a person to meet future situations in his life but are dealing with an immediate condition or symptom. Only by using the stress state to understand and work things out will the insight gained become the 'working capital' for future personal effectiveness. The 'understanding and working thing out' at times of tension are often hard and painful to face and we need those special conditions for learning (or therapy) which can enable us to earn that 'working capital' without retreating into facile rationalizations or erudite psychiatric labels. For those who do practise building this reality into themselves under favourable conditions there is no doubt that—as with the Kennedy experience—they have a better chance to meet what comes; it does not promise the 'right answer' but they can 'risk themselves' to greater effect. Perhaps the best examples of a transitional or temporary experience which enables us to learn under conditions of some degree of stress are natural ones like puberty and adolescence. Many of the experiences we undergo during those phases, both internally and externally, can be profitably exploited (in the best sense) if we have appropriate situations within which to make use of that temporary phase which 'nature' provides. Adolescence is itself also a 'second chance' to cope with unresolved problems of earlier years as well as a *temporary system* to build more 'working capital' for the future. The best kind of *temporary systems* therefore provide such opportunities for working things over again as well as for creating and innovating new ways of exploring and tackling the future.

The simplest kind of 'temporary systems' lend themselves to primitive solutions restricted to coping with the immediate situation. In emergencies this may be a 'good thing' to do but present expressions of tension and exacerbated stress often arise out of solutions to long past struggles or unresolved conflict. For example, current negotiating methods in trade union, management, and government relations can be regarded as crude and constraining attempts to use modes of handling problems based on attitudes and circumstances pertaining to early days of exploitation and understandable lack of trust. But trust is not built on repetitious negotiation.

Coping with stress

We vary as regards out capacity to tolerate uncertainty and anxiety according to the situation we happen to be in.

The threat may come from without and be real; in which case the way we react depends on the response it evokes in us—and this in turn can depend on past experience, the values and standards we have developed, etc., as well as on our capacity to understand the nature of the threat. Logical and intellectual understanding is seldom sufficient in itself to allay or prevent a reactive response if emotional tensions or conflicts are also aroused, unless some form of 'temporary system' is available to support the forces which are making for security in the individual or group—countering or preventing stress.

Stress can be *normal and appropriate*. For example,

(1) fearing that one has been deserted at various stages in early childhood and thus needing to test and find out (scream) that 'mother world' is still around one;
(2) trying oneself out in a new job or with promotion with the sense of being untried or deskilled.

Stress can be *inappropriate*. For example,

(3) when the threat of redundancy, whether real or imagined, affects the individual, his family or the organization carrying it out, in a variety of ways—leading to faulty thinking and decisions, distorted actions, etc.

'Temporary systems' to ameliorate or provide a basis for prevention of the stress (whether appropriate or inappropriate) may be created or 'invented' by ourselves or by others. The 'temporary system' itself can aggravate stress if it is inappropriate to the situation at the time, e.g. to give reassurance when a direct confrontation of the situation is required.

The following examples will illustrate both 'natural' and 'invented' experiences by which our personal resources are developed to cope with stress.

Natural development

(1) As well as all its other functions the family itself can be regarded as the means of coping with stress from the different members of the family and their relations with each other. It can, of course, act in the opposite direction and aggravate the stress as when it increases 'abrasion' between family members.

(2) In the earliest years we have the 'teddy bear', 'Linus' blanket' (see Charlie Brown in the Peanuts strip), and favourite toys.

(3) Games such as peep-bo can almost be regarded as *training experiences* for dealing with anxiety and stress situations since they provide learning experiences for testing out assumptions. Useful temporary systems usually have this quality, e.g. the apparent childish performance of the Vietcong and American representatives in Paris who spent 9 months deciding on the shape of the table to be used. Clearly other forms of test were being made under this guise however depressing it may be to realize that such devices have to be resorted to. But this is also an indicator of the *degree* of stress involved.

(4) The pet, with a life of its own, can be a 'temporary system' for the adult, the child or the family as a whole providing opportunities for developing care, affection, and responsibility, etc.—from both sides (Bridger, 1970; Bridger, 1976).

Intra-personal development

(5) We may try to provide our own *rationalization*, such as the dreams of

favourite meals and homely scenes experienced by soldiers of World War II in the desert. (These are provided by our own inner resources and relate to the comforting fantasies spontaneously evoked in earliest years.)

(6) Daydreams, hopes, and aspirations 'pained' with pictures. More creatively we produce poetry, music, and art in a variety of forms, materials, and dimensions. Artistic expression not only copes with stress but can be the medium for health and purpose.

Social and community development

(7) The Red Cross organization is an excellent example of an ameliorative 'temporary system' which is created to deal with national and international stress conditions. As a special case within this, the Red Cross parcels service for P.O.W. is a further example.

(8) There were the community schemes like Port Sunlight and Bournville which were relevant adaptive systems for the benevolent authoritarians of the early 1900s. Today they would aggravate by the 'music' they would communicate.

Structural and institutional development

(9) Lavatories and lift doors become the contrived as well as the spontaneous meeting places for all levels and functions in the hierarchy in modern office blocks.

In general community terms the shopping centre and volunteer (paid and unpaid) services need to exist. Without them the stress can become decisive and lead to ghost-town phenomena (Jacobs, 1972).

(10) High-rise buildings can be regarded as 'temporary systems' which can go desperately wrong. The 'self-contained' flat and the commuting population with jobs elsewhere than in the community often lead to isolation and loneliness of flat dwellers. The balance of independence and inter-dependence can be fruitful or destructive according to the forces and factors acting in the area. The tendency is for joint positive action to arise under conditions of common external threat to occupants rather than—as in more mature communities—towards common goals for the improvement of the joint good (the whole being greater than the sum of its parts).

(11) On the other hand the crowded House of Commons with its club atmosphere creates conditions which promote the warmth of humanity and recognition of rules for living together despite the cut and thrust of debate or the heat of conflicting ideas. In contrast the more clinical and legalistic chambers associated with other governing bodies tend to stress form and structure. This example is simply given to illustrate the effect which space and structure can *contribute*; it does not of course determine what will happen— the people themselves do that. But we can help or hinder matters with our use of such conditions and situations—as our town planners have discovered.

'Normal' stress and its value in building capacity for dealing with 'crisis' stress

In the normal course of development we experience natural situations which enable us to practise physical and behavioural skills to stand us in good stead. Much of our art and imaginative expression can help us create steps or 'platforms' from which to explore and adapt to new conditions and cope with changes in our personal and social environments.

Quite simple situations contribute to the building of this experience in coping with the more natural forms of 'stress'. We know the distinction which we learn from earliest times of 'being at home' in certain surroundings and not in others. The former conveys a sense of *comfort;* the other *discomfort.* For example,

(1) Looking around to see how to behave in situations to which we are not accustomed; picking up the right knife and fork; what dress to wear—customs and conventions which enable us to develop social 'maps' of living; rituals which help us to establish a 'recognition system' by which we can be 'at one' with others.

(2) This may have its obverse side—i.e. when we tend to make a virtue out of some of the 'prisons' into which our social situation may place us. The following are examples of 'temporary systems' of the past which outlive their usefulness and *break down* under changing social mores and educational development:

—the housewife who makes a virtue out of the 'kitchen sink'
   and 'washing machine'—a state which has already *broken down*
   in our current society as against the past;
—the manager or operative who makes a virtue out of the
   'assembly line', the commuter train journey, or long years in
   a dead-end job; these too have 'broken down' as has the
   notion of continuing with an unhappy marriage for the
   'sake of the children'.

(3) One particular and topical example of social and personal stress exists in the use of examinations, their style and purposes. Many of the changes taking place are directed towards people having to contribute greater attention to self-assessment and self-appraisal.

The Education Act of 1870 led to the spate of examinations not only as a method of judging educational standards but as a means of selection and rejection for jobs in our civil and local government services and so on. It is not often recognized that examinations originally served yet another purpose, i.e. of preventing nepotism—or at least as an attempt to guard against it. Such underlying reasons can, understandably, make it much more difficult to give up examinations even when the need for them becomes unnecessary or inappropriate with improved methods of selection and judgement. This is not an unusual form of resistance to change and which requires that the conditions and situations under which the established mechanism (the examination in this case) has to be considered alongside the other anxieties which are being allayed or excited.

(4) A telling example of a 'temporary system' for dealing with the stress of what might be called an 'ultimate examination' is the story of Scheherezade and the Caliph—the prelude to the 'Arabian Nights'. Most of us would say that Scheherezade kept the Caliph intrigued by telling him involved and continuous stories which had to be 'broken off' each night—and by which methods she kept her head when others had lost theirs in attempting to interest their lord and master.

In fact the original story describes a more valid 'temporary system' and one much more likely to cope with the stress of that situation: Scheherezade tells the stories to a boy in the presence of the Caliph, who 'listens in' to accounts which have to be broken into because the lad has to go to bed at a more reasonable hour.

It is only a step for us to recognize the wisdom of the BBC in putting on the kind of films (and stories) during children's viewing hours which adults can see and listen to 'and thus have some time and keep company with the children'. The adults can use the children's viewing times as a temporary system for looking at films they might not be prepared to see (yet might want to) if presented at 9 p.m. in case it was perceived as 'childish'.

(5) Some forms of stress which in the past have been treated as 'normal' are now more readily recognized as creating conditions for potential breakdown or for low tolerance of separation of personal responsibility later in life. The work of James and Joyce Robertson concerning mother/child separation in early years for a variety of reasons describes the circumstances and process by which the stress is increased or modified and the different kinds of 'mark' it may leave for the adult in his later life (Robertson, 1958). John Bowlby's (1969, 1973) work is a fundamental contribution to experiences of this kind.

Organizational stress under conditions of social and technological change

(1) Leadership and the working group
The changing character of leadership required to cope with current demand for 'identity' and work satisfaction has been sadly underestimated. The group task needs to provide its members with the real and not artificial feeling of *meaning* something—not just 'being wanted' but genuinely 'being somebody' and having 'a piece of the action'.

The lack of tolerance for double talk and double values has become a feature of the attitudes of the younger people. On the other hand the problem of increasing 'participation' has yet to be recognized as also entailing increased commitment and responsibility for the job—and *accountability* for it.

Thus, being a 'pair of hands', for the use of which the company gives some £s, is a relationship offering little more than 'strikes' and 'more pay' as a basis for dealing with stressful differences between management, trade unions,

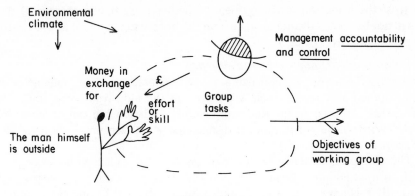

Figure 10.2

and their members, who are also members of the firm.

If, however, we find means for men and women to share in the realities we may find

(a) that some have not been accustomed, or want, to have those responsibilities
(b) that people can grow and find a variety of resources for particular aspects of the job—which not a few leaders, and supervision generally, may feel as a threat and have great difficulty in adapting to
(c) that learning to live with *interdependence* and a more 'crowded' sharing in the tasks and scope for ideas and trying them out, etc. This may mean reviewing the *whole task* as well as the way of working. Such new forms of work organization (Klein, 1976) require different concepts of leadership and control.

The relationship of 'authority' to 'member' changes in character since the member accepts some authority for the job. But, in so doing, he must be able

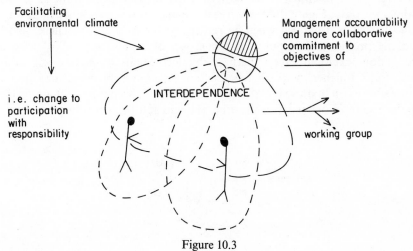

Figure 10.3

252

to trust the leadership ('management', whether of company or union!) that it will not be taken advantage of, i.e. that the 'rate' will not be cut as production or results improve (Bridger, 1971).

(2) Problems of multiple group membership
While the common, complementary, and diverse arms of 'management' and 'unions' now range much wider than in the industrial scene alone, the stress that can arise in the leadership/member relationship can occur within each. (Witness the not infrequent disagreement between union/shop steward or shop steward/member.)

The 'temporary system' used for resolving stressful conflict within or between such groups and interests is usually that known as 'negotiation' or 'bargaining'. Basically this appears as a crude and primitive method having early cultural origins, but, as with examinations mentioned earlier, satisfying anxieties about the state of distrust and other considerations such as conflicting values and norms. Of course this is not to say that in the hands of experienced exponents this primitive method does not also become 'a fine art', but the search for 'solutions' can only be conducted within a very limited kind of 'temporary system'.

Essentially the regression to this primitive approach includes the fears of having to face one's own group (managers or union members) with the recognition and awareness of

(a) the consideration and implications of issues ranging far outside the 'nitty-gritty' conflict under negotiation;
(b) the problems and concerns of the 'other side'.

Generally, therefore, the 'temporary system' of bargaining and negotiation is based on fight and win/lose. The system is bound to be repetitive.

But we could draw the situation as shown in Figure 10.4. And if we have government represented, which so frequently occurs in one form or another today, we have Figure 10.5, each participant with a ⌐⌐ (ghost) in front of him of what will happen when he returns to his own group. These 'ghosts' and the problems they pose for the group of representatives or delegates are seldom explored except perhaps by individuals in private—or in the 'corridors'. Further, working together on a common problem may become impossible when to do so is experienced as betrayal, becoming 'soft' or yielding up the 'rights' of one party or the other (Higgin and Bridger, 1964).

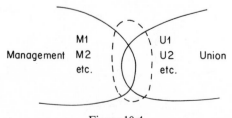

Figure 10.4

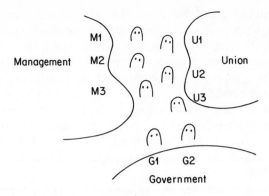

Figure 10.5

When management and unions can find it possible to work on *common tasks* actually affecting the company and the unions—and take up problems associated with the 'ghosts'—we may be nearer 'temporary systems' more appropriate to the situation. In fact where more mature relations exist it will be found that joint working on common tasks and exorcizing the 'ghosts' by bringing them out into the open is always a feature.

(3) Role differentiation and group integration
The conflictual element of community, family or organizational life usually referred to as 'personality clash' is seldom one of 'personality' alone. The roles, the jobs, the structure or the situation in which the people happen to be placed will frequently be an important determinant of the real position. Whether in superior/subordinate, colleague or other type of relationship, what the other person would think or act upon in future circumstances becomes an assumption on which to base decision and action. It is, unfortunately, all too common for people who might otherwise be quite good friends to be in roles, functions or in an organizational structure which makes them 'enemies'. Those who are in production, marketing, and accounting functions for example know how frequently the roles can introduce competitive feelings of status, competence, etc., instead of confronting the problem of optimizing in the face of the common task (Bridger and White, 1972).

Research, training, and action to deal with stress conditions

It has been a striking feature of the contemporary scene that it is the industrial organization rather than academic institutions which has engaged in research and development to resolve its own problems. Increasingly there is a growing recognition of the organization as an organismic, dynamic structure of roles, values, etc., to be kept under review and adapted to change in the light of the social needs of the wider society as well as towards the objectives of the organization itself. In some cases, the step has been taken to build 'internal institutions' whose function it is to collaborate with external professional social scientists in continuing and deepening the value of such work. It is perhaps not, after all, so surprising when one realizes the accelerating rate of change in the many facets of society today where people, in their roles and organizations, are endeavouring to control (regulate) the increasing complexity and uncertainty created by a 'turbulent' environment (Emery and Trist, 1965).

There is a corresponding necessity to identify the critical characteristics of that turbulence (e.g. information overload, accelerating technological innovation and obsolescence, etc.) so as to build and maintain optimum interdependence of resources and commitment. These conditions demand a shift in capabilities towards developing and managing new forms of work organization (Klein, 1976).

When groups, communities and organizations regard themselves as *relatively* independent of each other and of their environments in general, they lend themselves more readily to the simpler hierarchical/bureaucratic structural forms and control. Such relatively 'closed systems' come under stress, however, when socio-economic pressures and other environmental conditions force members of the system to review and cope with the reciprocal implications created internally—whether materially or through changes in membership outlooks and expectations. When the family, group or institution becomes more of an 'open system' it demands more continuous consideration of its structure and of its ways (processes) of working (Emery and Trist, 1960).

Learning to develop the capacity for self-review and appraisal individually and as a group or institution often runs counter to the traditional notion that introspection is 'unhealthy'. Certainly, this idea was more common in 'closed system' contexts but the problem of changing from one kind of living system to the other does occasion stress for many individuals and groups. The process of unlearning and relearning can be painful in developmental terms—to a much greater degree than in the direction of acquiring or re-orienting one's knowledge or skill (Bridger *et al.*, 1963).

In recent years many efforts have been developed to enable people and organizations to develop insights and capabilities which will facilitate the double task of

(1) fulfilling roles and responsibilities relating to the activities and tasks upon which working groups are engaged in the short and long term;
(2) exploring the group and institutional processes, within and outside those groups, and relating the insights gained to the former one.

The earlier tendency was to concentrate on (2) and then expect that (1) would follow. Such learning models, T-groups, encounter groups, and so on, inferred that if people could change their behaviour, working patterns would alter also—and stress would be reduced. In certain respects this was likely to happen just as personal therapy could help a person to be better able to face reality and social situations.

More effective designs have now been evolved which enable the actual working situation—as well as just training events—to be both the organization for achieving stated objectives and being the 'learning institution' in itself. In this connection the double task referred to earlier becomes the practice and endeavour of the organization itself. In one important sense we also see this happening not only in organizations but in families, in schools, and in public life generally. The change process is not unaccompanied by reactive forces—dropping out, violence, backlash, and many milder forms of resistance to change. Stresses can be externalized and projected into social and environmental settings in an attempt to deny or avoid their comprehension and the essence of changed conditions. On the other hand, the efforts to understand their nature must be encouraged and developed if stress and conflictual forces are to be regulated and 'managed' (Bridger, 1972).

Whatever changes in theory or technique may arise in future, therefore, it will be essential that the focus of attention in dealing with inappropriate stress conditions should lie in

(1) the study of the various internal and external forces which might affect our relationships, our roles and institutions in their various contexts;
(2) the application of this understanding to balancing and optimizing the interdependencies and divergences of interest within and between groups and institutions;
(3) the consultative relationship as an increasingly significant feature in leadership and membership competence, not least when dealing with participative forms of shared responsibility.

References

Bowlby, J. (1969) *Attachment and Loss*. vol. I, *Attachment*. London. Hogarth Press.
Bowlby, J. (1973) *Attachment and Loss*. vol. 2, *Separation: Anxiety and Anger*. London. Hogarth Press.
Bridger, H. (1970) Companionship with humans. Paper presented to the Health Congress of the Royal Society of Health, Eastbourne, 1970.
Bridger, H. (1971) A viewpoint on organisational behaviour. Proceedings of CIBA Foundation Symposium 'Teamwork for World Health'.
Bridger, H. (1972) Course designs and methods within the organisation. In Berger, M. L., and Berger, P. J. (eds), *Group Training Techniques Cases, Applications and Research*. Epping. Gower Press, pp. 34–48.
Bridger, H. (1976) The changing role of pets in society, *J. small Anim. Pract.*, **17**, 1–8.
Bridger, H., Miller, E. J., and O'Dwyer, J. J. (1963) *The Doctor and Sister in Industry. A Study of Change*. London. Macmillan (Journals) Ltd. Reprinted from *Occup. Health*, 1963, **15**.
Bridger, H., and White, S. F. T. (1972) Towards a policy for health of the manager. In Hacon, R. (ed.), *Personal and Organizational Effectiveness*. New York. McGraw-Hill, pp. 240–255.
Emery, F. E., and Trist, E. L. (1960) Socio-technical systems. In Churchman, C. W., and Verhulst, M. (eds), *Management Sciences, Models and Techniques*, vol. 2. Oxford. Pergamon Press, pp. 83–97. Reprinted in Emery, F. E. (ed.), *Systems Thinking*. Harmondsworth. Penguin, 1969, pp. 281–296, and Frank, H. E. (ed.), *Organization Structuring*. London. McGraw-Hill, 1971, pp. 41–53.
Emery, F. E., and Trist, E. L. (1965) The causal texture of organizational environments, *Human Relations*, **18**, 21–32.

Higgin, G., and Bridger, H. (1964) The psychodynamics of an inter-group experience, *Human Relations*, **17**, 391–446. Reprinted as Tavistock Pamphlet no. 10, 1965.

Jacobs, J. (1972) *Death and Life of Great American Cities*. Harmondsworth. Penguin.

Klein, L. (1976) *New Forms of Work Organisation*. Cambridge University Press.

Robertson, J. (1958) *Young Children in Hospital*. London. Tavistock. American ed. New York. Basic Books, 1959.

Winnicott, D. W. (1971) *Playing and Reality*. London. Tavistock. Also: Harmondsworth. Penguin, 1974.

PART VI

Issues in Research on Stress at Work

Chapter **11**
Epistemology and the Study of Stress at Work

Roy Payne

University of Sheffield

Most research in the field of stress has been carried out within the philosophical framework of an epistemology rooted in the experience of science and most conveniently summarized as positivism. This is a doctrine that has been much under attack in recent years and the attacks raise the possibility that more adequate intellectual frameworks exist for solving the problems of research in this field. With this possibility, and hope, in mind I shall summarize the epistemological writings of Stephen Pepper (1942). I refer only to him since I have argued elsewhere (Payne, 1975) that he raises the main issues and incorporates ideas from writers whose views are in conflict such as Popper, Kuhn, and Toulmin.

Stephen Pepper's *World Hypotheses*

Burtt (1943) commenced a review of Pepper's book with these words: 'A volume has recently appeared which, should the times prove ready for it, may well inaugurate a new era in the writing of systematic philosophy' (p. 590). Although current writers on epistemology refer to Pepper's work on values (Pepper, 1958) they seldom refer to *World Hypotheses* so it would seem that its potential was either unfulfilled or found inadequate. Whichever is true, it seems to me to provide enlightenment. Pepper is concerned with the processes by which knowledge increases or becomes 'refined'. Before describing the mechanisms of evidence and corroboration he demolishes the arguments for taking either a sceptical or a dogmatic stance towards epistemological questions. Scepticism is rejected on the grounds that the sceptic must ultimately produce reasons for his scepticism. And if his reasons are held dogmatically the sceptic can then be criticized for holding the dogmatist position. If the theory justifying the sceptical attitude is held undogmatically, then the theory must necessarily be a world hypothesis. That is, the theory is a theory about the world which is unrestricted in its scope. All knowledge can be fitted within it. The theory of evolution is not an unrestricted theory, for example, since it would exclude mathematics or physics. Dogmatism fails to be a world hypothesis since the cognitive criteria to which the dogmatist appeals turn out to be unsound.

The grounds for the dogmatist's position are:

(1) the dogma of infallible authority;
(2) the dogma of self-evident principles;
(3) the dogma of indubitable fact.

The dogma of *infallible authority* proves wanting as an ultimate criterion of knowledge because (a) supposedly infallible authorities often conflict, (b) the competence of authorities is often seriously questioned in terms of other criteria, and (c) such appeals to other criteria are often successful. The three reasons for rejecting *self-evidence* of facts as adequate grounds for knowledge are very similar: (a) claims to self-evidence or certainty often conflict, (b) claims to certainty are often questioned in terms of other cognitive criteria, and (c) such claims against other criteria are often successful. English empiricism is founded on the belief that the *facts are indubitable*. Pepper's rejection of this claim is, first, that facts conflict with each other; second, that descriptions of facts conflict with hypothetical descriptions of facts which can be supported by corroborative evidence; and, third, when doubt is cast upon a fact, there is no corroborative evidence, and this recourse is so often successful in establishing the fact, that its indubitability as fact *qua* fact, is in doubt. At one point in all three arguments Pepper makes the point, that once the grounds of the dogma have been refuted in one fair case, how can the criterion ever be trusted again?

Pepper's intention in criticizing the cognitive attitudes of scepticism and dogmatism is to

show that these extremities, in their efforts to avoid the uncertainties of theory, actually lay themselves open more widely to theory and to unjustifiable interpretations and assumptions than the moderate middle course of partial scepticism which we shall pursue. The term world hypothesis connotes this middle course. It signifies that these objects we are about to study [world hypotheses] are not final products of knowledge and yet that they do contain knowledge. ... and shall undertake to show that there is nothing cognitively legitimate in the claims (of dogmatism and scepticism) which is not accepted also by our attitude of partial scepticism. (Pepper, 1942, p. 3)

Having dealt with scepticism and dogmatism Pepper can now provide his resolution to the dilemmas they imply. It is this exposition of the nature of evidence and the process of corroboration of evidence that deals most effectively, in my opinion, with some of the problems raised by Phillips (1973) in his book *Abandoning Method*.

If there is no certain evidence or knowledge, then where does knowledge begin? Pepper's comment on this question is, 'The pathos of the question betrays the assumption behind it. For why should knowledge begin with certainties?' (Pepper, 1942, p. 39). Pepper's thesis is that the growth of knowledge is a process of refinement, where knowledge moves from being 'uncriticized' to 'criticized' or highly refined evidence. Uncriticized evidence can also be called common sense, and because it is uncriticized common sense must always be doubted. The name Pepper gives to common-sense knowledge is *dubitandum*; something to be doubted. Common-sense facts must be doubted because they remain uncriticized and as soon as they become criticized they are no longer common-sense facts. However, although every item of common sense is highly dubitable and subject to criticism and generally greatly altered by cognitive refinement, the total body of common-sense evidences is not highly dubitable.

While common-sense knowledge is insecure in the sense referred to above, it is completely secure in another. As Pepper graphically puts it, 'Water somehow and tomato in some way will always be waiting to receive the weary cogniser, however discouraged he may be in his search for perfect cognition' (Pepper, 1942, p. 43). Cognition cannot sink lower than common sense. Its knowledge is not reflected upon, it is just accepted. The problem is that common-sense knowledge often contradicts itself. It is what Pepper calls 'irritable'. Indeed, to the serious cognizer common-sense knowledge is a nightmare.

The paradox is that highly refined knowledge is eventually found to be wanting. It is ultimately based on refined pointer readings as in physics, or arbitrary definitions as in mathematics or tentative hypotheses as in philosophy. When knowledge is highly criticized and highly refined it becomes so only because it commits itself to very little. So, ultimately the critical cognizer is driven back to common-sense knowledge: 'After filling its empty definitions and pointer readings and hypotheses with meanings out of the rich confusion of common sense, it generally turns its head away, shuts its eyes to what it has been doing and affirms dogmatically the self-evidence and certainty of the common sense significance it has drawn into its concepts' (p. 45). As the errors of such dogmatism have already been exposed, critical knowledge is left with no alternative but to acknowledge the source of its significance and security in the uncriticized knowledge of common sense. In Pepper's words, 'The tension between common sense and expert knowledge, between cognitive security without responsibility and cognitive responsibility without full security, is the interior dynamics of the knowledge situation' (p. 42).

The goal of our 'rational enterprises' (Toulmin, 1972) then is to increase the stock of refined knowledge, but the ultimate criterion against which our refined knowledge is tested is common sense. And the tension between common-sense and highly criticized knowledge will remain until all common-sense knowledge is refined: a state of no ignorance.

Accepting the current state of knowledge as containing considerable ignorance, Pepper proceeds to consider the sorts of ways in which knowledge can be refined. Since it would be dogmatic to claim something is known self-evidently, knowledge becomes refined by a process of corroboration. Corroboration can be of two kinds: corroboration of man by man, and corroboration of fact with fact. The first sort of corroboration Pepper calls 'multiplicative corroboration', and the products of the process are *data*.

Corroboration of fact with fact is given the name 'structural corroboration' and its products are known as *danda*.

Multiplicative corroboration occurs when a number of men agree on the facts, or the results of their observations. Thus our knowledge about the strength of a chair could be refined by asking a number of men to sit on it, and if it did not break we could then draw the conclusion that the chair was strong enough to support a man's weight. The alternative strategy would be to hypothesize that, for the purpose of bearing a man's weight, the chair would need to be of certain sorts of wood, the wood being of certain sorts of dimensions, and being fixed together by screws and glue at various points of the structure. If all these separate facts apply then there is a structure of evidence which points to the validity of the fact at issue: structural corroboration.

Each of the components of structural corroboration rely ultimately on multiplicative corroboration, and in this sense data might appear to take priority over danda. There is, however, fluctuating tension between the two sorts of evidence. The problem with highly refined data is that it has been refined to such an extent that it commits itself to very little. In Karl Popper's terms it has a very low probability of being falsified, but as a result has a very low information content (Magee, 1973, p. 36). Furthermore, a refined datum would most likely be interpreted also as part of a more encompassing structural hypothesis. Returning to the strength of our chair: if the evidence suggests the chair is weak, but someone actually sat on the chair without breaking it, would one be inclined to assume the hypothesis was wrong, or would one interpret this datum in the light of the structural hypothesis? That is, assume the person was too light to break the chair, or he did not put all his weight on it. Unless such an event occurred many times the evidence would be interpreted in terms of the structural hypothesis, or the dandum. As Pepper puts it, 'The question is one of proportion and it appears that structural evidence does not give way to multiplicative evidence, unless the latter is based on very considerable agreement among many observers and unless it cannot be interpreted to fit the hypothesis which organized the structural evidence' (Pepper, 1942, p. 51). The conjecture would have been refuted, and as Popper (1963) has taken pains to point out even this does not lead to a victory for data, but to another opportunity for a better conjecture. The tension between data and danda reappears.

To someone obsessed with not being dogmatic it is important for Pepper to ensure that he is not accused of suggesting the existence of only two kinds of data or danda: refined and unrefined. There is a whole range, but Pepper is content to label just one intermediate point, to which he gives the beautiful names 'rough data' and 'rough danda'. Much of our knowledge falls into these categories, of course. Highly refined data of the sort provided by pointer readings and other sophisticated measuring devices is defined as 'empirical data': data which are invariant. These data are distinguished from 'logical data'. 'Logical data are the evidence for the validity of logical and mathematical transitions and for those organizations of such transitions which are called logical and mathematical systems' (Pepper, 1942, p. 57). They are data because their corroboration depends on the agreement of multiple men that the transitions are legitimate.

The belief that knowledge consists of empirical data, supported by logical data, is the one held by the positivists. They would exclude danda as a form of knowledge, taking the view that multiplicative corroboration is the only reliable ground for cognition. Pepper questions this on the grounds that the area of knowledge where such criteria actually work are very limited: physics and chemistry. And even there the data are frequently 'rough data', which ultimately rely on common sense for their security. A second counter-argument is more complex, but ends in demonstrating that the person wishing to propose that data are the only reliable form of knowledge must have a hypothesis as to why his position is held. The grounds for any such argument could not be based on data, but on some hypothesis about the world. That is on a dandum, the very sort of corroboration the positivist wishes to avoid. Thus a world hypothesis is one claiming knowledge about the structure of the world the evidence for which is based on structural corroboration (Pepper, 1942, p. 74). Since world hypotheses seem inevitable outcomes of attempts to systematize our beliefs about the world, Pepper argues we need to understand them, and the implications they have for the growth of knowledge.

The four main world hypotheses

Pepper admits there could be hundreds of world hypotheses, but in his view only four can be regarded as relatively adequate ones. Figure 11.1 presents Pepper's outline of the various paths to knowledge, which include the four world hypotheses as four types of danda. None of these four is superior to the others, and there is much discussion in the book about the criteria by which such a judgement is made. Simply, the criteria are precision and scope. A precise hypothesis fits all the facts exactly, and one adequate in scope covers all known facts. A hypothesis which does not cover all the facts is not a world hypothesis, and probably can be subsumed by one of the four relatively adequate world hypotheses: these are formism, mechanism, contextualism, and organicism.

Pepper is able to reduce the multitude of possible world hypotheses by constructing a theory of the origin of world hypotheses which he calls the root metaphor theory. Burtt (1943) describes it this way:

the philosophic imagination has drawn from experiences of common sense only a very few fundamental clues to world interpretation. Each of the main schools of philosophy has cognitively refined one of these basic clues, that is, has codified the implications of that chosen idea into a set of categories that hang together and claim power or corroboration by all evidence of every kind. That clue is its 'root metaphor'. (p. 592)

Pepper uses analogy as a synonym for metaphor, and the analogies turn out to be surprisingly unprepossessing. The root metaphor of formism is similarity.

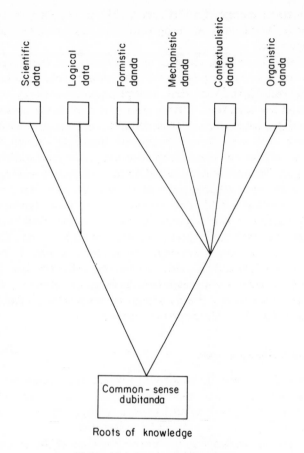

Figure 11.1 A tree of knowledge

Objects and phenomena are often very similar and thus can be classified into categories or types. The truth theory of formism is the correspondence theory: things are truer as a result of the degree of similarity which a description has to its object of reference. Maps and pictures are examples of close correspondences though ultimately the correspondence can be expressed in symbolic form as in a mathematical equation. Formism is better known philosophically by the terms 'realism' and 'Platonic idealism' and its best known exponents (dogmatic exponents at that, as is true of all exponents of the world theories) are Plato and Aristotle.

The alternative names for mechanism are naturalism and materialism and its major champions are Hobbes, Locke, and Hume. The root metaphor of mechanism is the machine, and cognitive refinement is obtained by interpreting the world as if it were a machine. Put oversimply, this involves three steps: first, the machine consists of a configuration of parts and it is necessary to define the precise *locations* of those parts. Treating a lever as a simple machine, this would involve stating precisely the length of the lever and the distance of one end of the lever from the fulcrum. The second step involves identifying the *primary qualities* of the machine. In the case of the lever this would be the weight exerted to work the lever. The actual weight could be a load of bricks or a tree stump but when working with the machine analogy one merely wants the weight or force applied, so as to describe the quantities necessary for the efficient functioning of the machine. Third, mechanism requires the statement of a *law* of the interrelationships among the parts of the machine. In the case of the lever this would entail an equation stating the required weights for balancing a lever with a given fulcrum length. The truth theory of mechanism is whether the machine works. Pepper uses the term 'workability' or the phrase 'causal adjustment', but it comes down to whether or not one's knowledge allows one to predict the outcomes of any causal adjustments made in the system.

On the face of it workability sounds a very pragmatic criterion, but pragmatism as philosophy has contextualism as its world hypothesis, and its root metaphor is the historic event: that is, the event alive in its present; or the act in its context. On page 232, Pepper says that only verbs should be used in the language of contextualism—doing, enduring, enjoying, etc. Weick (1974) refers to Bateson (1972) who has sounded the more evocative clarion call, 'stamp out nouns' (p. 334), but his reasons imply a contextualist's view of understanding the world. One of the major derivatives of such a philosophical stance is that change is endemic. The context will change and thus knowledge will need to change also. Consequently the truth theory of contextualism is 'qualitative confirmation' or verification, though such verification demands a thorough exploration of the context and texture of any event. Strictly speaking, it is not the event but a hypothesis about the event that is verified, so hypotheses, not events, are regarded as being true or false. Nevertheless, 'A true hypothesis, does in its texture and quality give some insight into the texture and quality of the event it refers to for verification' (p. 277). William James, C. S. Peirce, and G. H. Mead are the founding fathers of pragmatism.

The main originators of the organicist cognitive attitude were Hegel and Royce. Its alternative philosophical name is absolute idealism, which is sometimes called objective idealism. Burtt (1943, p. 593) describes its root metaphor as 'harmonious unity'. It, too, is concerned with understanding the historical event, but it differs from contextualism in that time is regarded as unimportant. It is the integration in the process rather than the duration of the process that concerns the organicist. His ultimate aim is to describe the enduring structure that the processes realize. Its truth theory is called the coherence theory of truth. The criteria of the coherence theory are 'the categorial features of the organic whole—inclusiveness, determinateness and organicity—and the ideal of truth is the absolute itself' (p. 310). Organicism thus proposes the existence of degrees of truth dependent on the amount of facts known and when all facts are known, as in principle they can be, then absolute truth has been obtained. This is a very different conclusion from the contextualists who will always believe that change is just around the corner, so that 'truth' may turn out to be false, and thus there is no absolute truth.

Pepper is always careful to refer to the four world hypotheses as only 'relatively' adequate. The differences between contextualism and organicism have already been mentioned and there are qualitative differences among all four theories. Some of the major strengths and weaknesses of the four are revealed in Figure 11.2 which is revision of a diagram of Pepper's (1942, p. 146) plus information from the text.

	Analytical theories	Synthetic theories	
Dispersive theories	FORMISM	CONTEXTUALISM	Indeterminate world: theories lack precision
Integrative theories	MECHANISM	ORGANICISM	Determinate world: theories lack scope

Figure 11.2 The scheme of world hypotheses

Formism and mechanism are analytical theories. The former concerned to allocate facts to categories on the basis of similarity, the possibility always being that a more precise analysis will establish another category. Mechanism is concerned to analyse the world into the component parts of the machine. Contextualism and organicism are synthetic. Organicism is searching for explanations in terms of organic wholes, and contextualism for a complete understanding of the event as it occurs in the specious present.

Contextualism and formism however are dispersive theories each taking the view that any structure in the world tends to be imposed upon the world by other parts of the world, but ultimately the world is unpredictable due to 'an inherent cosmic resistance to determinate order' (p. 143). Thus contextualists have no trouble in allowing any fact about the world, which is what gives contextualism its wide scope. Its inadequacy arises from the number of ways in which the same fact can be interpreted which is why contextualist theories have inadequate precision.

The integrative theories of mechanism and organicism have the problem of tending to reject facts. Mechanism proposes that there is a finite set of natural laws and consequently rejects facts that do not fit the current state of knowledge about those natural laws. Organicism rejects facts which jar with its search for harmony and unity.

By wishing perhaps too hard to get everything into one determinate order, they have to deny the reality of a good many things. Nevertheless, . . . it is amazing how much they are able to get into their order. And it is possible on their own showing that actually the entire universe is in a determinate order, and that the dispersive theories are only profiting on human ignorance. To which, of course, the dispersive theories reply that the integrative theories are only profiting on human propensities to rationalisation and sublimation. (p. 145)

The obvious question arises as to why it is not possible to be eclectic and take the best from each theory to make one world hypothesis. Pepper's detailed answer lies in the maxims he derives from his root metaphor theory, but a major problem is that once the theories are put together their categories compete for domination and nothing is gained. Contextualism and organicism both start with the historical event and in many ways are similar theories, but the fact that contextualism concentrates on the event in the present and organicism on the structure of the event regardless of time, is more than enough to make the two theories incompatible. On the other hand, since all four theories make a unique contribution to cognition, each should be pursued so as to increase the total stock of refined knowledge. These recommendations are reflected in the following quotation, which is included because it sums up the conclusions and the spirit of the whole book:

We wish in matters of serious discussion to have the benefit of all the available evidence and modes of corroboration. In practice, therefore, we shall want to be not rational but reasonable, and to seek, on the matter in question, the judgment supplied from each of these relatively adequate world theories. If there is some difference of judgment, we shall wish to make our decision with all these modes of evidence in mind, just as we should make any other decision where the evidence is conflicting. In this way we should be judging in the most reasonable way possible—not dogmatically following only one line of evidence, not perversely ignoring evidence, but sensibly acting on all the evidence available. (p. 331)

Has Pepper helped?

In his lengthy prelude to the recommendation to 'abandon method' Phillips (1973) makes the following points and provides some pointers as to how we may decide whether Pepper has helped:

What Kuhn does not point out, however, is that scientists must also decide what to regard as relevant techniques for deciding what is acceptable, they must decide what to regard as facts as well as what to consider as new facts, they must decide what to regard as excess empirical content, they must decide what constitutes corroboration, and they must decide what length shall be considered the 'long run' in determining whether a research program is to be considered progressive or degenerating. I do not mean that such decisions are made at the whim of the individual scientist, but rather that he must rely on common-sense understandings that he and his colleagues assume are taken for granted by all competent members of the particular scientific community to which he belongs. (p. 111)

The problems are how to decide what are facts and what corroborates them as facts, and whether particular lines of research are worth continuing.

In talking about facts Phillips was concerned about facts as things (X weighs Y lb) and facts as propositions (interaction increases liking). In drawing out the distinction between multiplicative and structural corroboration, data and danda, Pepper has clarified the difference between facts as things (data) and facts as propositions (danda). Although he does not use the same language as Pepper, Stephen Toulmin (1972, p. 173) states the different, but related functions of data and danda, rather well: 'Meaning in science is shown by the character of an explanatory procedure (danda); truth by men's success in finding applications for that procedure (data).' The exposition of the four world hypotheses also emphasises that cognitive refinement depends heavily on structural corroboration. The introduction of the idea that both multiplicative and structural corroboration are always in a state of development themselves, rough data and rough danda, also reminds us that even empirical data and logical data vary in the degree to which they approach the truth. The more that multiplicative and structural corroboration occurs the more one can believe that knowledge has approached the truth, though truth itself can never be known absolutely (Popper, 1972). The existence of dimensions of facts, from dubitanda to highly refined data, and danda, frees us from the insistences of the positivists for more data as the only adequate route to knowledge. It does not free us from the responsibility for deciding what might be termed 'working criteria' for both data and danda. Or put more vividly, how rough are we prepared to allow our data and danda to be? By what criteria can data and danda be judged?

Criteria for data: multiplicative corroboration

Since the basis of multiplicative corroboration is agreement among men the reliability of the observations and the instruments used to make them are important factors. This makes test–retest reliability particularly pertinent since the whole concept of test–retest reliability assumes that the observations are reliable over time and over different observers. The employment of standard procedures in the use of instruments is an attempt to ensure they remain reliable over observers, though instruments are not always thoroughly tested in this way and several studies have shown that instruments do appear to have different reliabilities and validities when used by different experimenters (e.g. Jung, 1971). It would appear that there is much room for improvement in the standards of multiplicative corroboration. In general there seems much scope for increasing the standards of inter-observer agreement on the classification of interview material and observational data. Internal reliability is also a criterion for data since it is based on the assumption that many people could see that the scores on the items vary according to some dimension and that people who score correctly on the even items are just as likely to score correctly on the odd items. Split–half correlation and item–whole correlation are merely short-hand ways of demonstrating this.

The commonly accepted distinctions about validity appear to be a mixture of data and danda. Face validity is clearly based on multiplicative corroboration since it is assumed that all or most men would agree that the item or test is a measure of the particular property in question. Similarly factorial validity is a more sophisticated way of demonstrating that the items or tests are part of the same construct (or factor). Given the results of a factor analysis many men could agree that the items always correlate in much the same way. Most other forms of validity are in the nature of danda. Convergent or discriminant validity is based on the hypothesis that if the measure is valid it will correlate with certain measures and not correlate with others. Similarly, criterion or predictive validity involves structural corroboration following from the expectation that the measure will predict some other quality or performance.

Validity and reliability are two of the six criteria listed by Zetterberg (1966), and of the other four the only one that seems a relevant criterion for data is the representativeness of the sample and the scope of the population. This is multiplicative corroboration in that it assumes that observations will be repeatable across the population. That is, there are lots of other examples to be seen should the observers wish to go and look at them.

Criteria for danda: structural corroboration

We have already listed two structural criteria in considering reliability and validity as criteria for data. They are construct (convergent and discriminant) validity as well as criterion validity. The latter is similar to Zetterberg's third criterion that there is a fit between the data trend and the theory. As Phillips (1973) points out this can be tested by assessing the percentage of predictable variance and by the application of the usual level of significance criteria. There are socially accepted conventions for the latter (the 5% and 1% levels of confidence) but none for the former, yet the size of the relationship might seem to be the more important of the two. In terms of predicting a criterion with more than one test predictive validity takes precedence over reliability (Guilford, 1954, p. 471). That is, a test which may be not too reliable is worth retaining if it has predictive validity, but just how much predictive validity it must have is unclear. The normal procedure is to test whether it adds significantly following the usual conventions. What the criteria are for adding practically, or usefully, or meaningfully is a lot less clear. Application of the index of forecasting efficiency is one way of estimating practicality, but ultimately the value must be judged in the light of the particular circumstances. Increasing the forecasts of the efficiency of a steel manufacturing plant by 6% might be very useful indeed, but the same margin of improvement in the prediction of graduate performance may not be worth the cost of collecting the necessary data.

Such remarks are related to another of the main criteria for structural corroboration quoted by Pepper, and that is the precision of the hypotheses. When one can account for 100% of the variance then the hypothesis is precise. Pepper's other criterion is scope, and this is similar to Zetterberg's last criterion which is that the proposition tested should be related as well as possible to a broader and well established theory. The more this applies the higher the level of structural corroboration. A way of ensuring this issue is adequately explored involves the use of Zetterberg's fourth criterion: that alternative propositions have been controlled. This is what experiments are designed to achieve, of course, but this condition is hardly met at all in the correlational designs typically employed in studies of organizational structure and organizational stress. This can still be achieved at the interpretive level but the practice of supplying more than one explanation for a set of data is not widespread. Such alternatives can then be tested by further studies of samples which test the differences. If the sample is *very* large some control can be obtained by multivariate statistical analyses. Multiple explanation tends to occur when the results are out of line with the original explanation, and the consequent learning is not to be devalued for that, but our search for structural corroboration may be advanced by greater prior speculation, since it might result in better designs and more comprehensive research. Popper insists that science is a matter of testing competing hypotheses, but it is indeed rare to see such competition made explicit. The criteria for data and danda may be summarized as in Table 11.1.

Table 11.1 Criteria for evidence

Data	Danda
(1) Test–retest reliability	(1) Concurrent validity
(2) Internal reliability	(2) Predictive or criterion validity
(3) Face validity	(3) Precision of hypothesis
(4) Factorial validity	(4) Degree to which proposition is embedded in a wider theory (scope)
(5) Representativeness of sample	(5) Control for alternative explanations

The data and danda of stress at work

Examination of the data on stress at work involves consideration of measures of stressors, symptoms of strain, predisposing personality factors such as anxiety, self-esteem or A type traits, and outcome variables of a behavioural and a physiological disease nature.

Data on stressors occur in four major ways. One is by comparing groups which have been exposed to very different conditions such as combat versus non-combat roles, or a major organizational change versus no change. These are relatively good data in the sense most men would agree there has been a difference in demands. The majority of studies have depended on taking a sample of people in different jobs and getting them to rate subjectively the degrees of stress in their work environment. Measures of role conflict, role ambiguity, and so on are indirect measures of such stressors. In terms of the criteria for data most of these measures have good face validity and 'acceptable' internal reliability. That is reliability coefficients around 0·7–0·8 (e.g. House and Rizzo, 1972) and test–retest reliabilities of a somewhat lower order, perhaps 0·6–0·7 (e.g. Buck, 1972). Hackman and Oldham (1975) quote reliability indices for job dimensions which range from 0·59 to 0·78. They also compared the views of the job holders with those of trained observers and the median correlation was 0·63. Reliabilities for observer's ratings were not quoted but with training these usually become quite good (Bales, 1950; Turner and Lawrence, 1965).

Such independent observers describe the nature of the environment (using measures for physical properties such as noise, heat) by recording the actual number of messages received, the phone calls answered, the decisions made in a given time, etc. These 'objective' assessments are usually done for a given type of job, of course, so that all people doing the same job are classified as being under the same degree of stress. This is different from the studies using subjective measures of stressors where each individual may perceive the situation quite differently. Buck (1972) used perceptual measures of stressors, self-report personality measures, and self-report felt-job-pressure. These intercorrelated very highly so that over 80% of the variance in job pressure was accounted for by the other variables though perceived stressors correlated so highly with the personality variables that adding the stressor variables only accounted for a little more of the variance (9% for managers and 17% for workers). Such confounding of the variables does of course make it difficult to assess the explanatory value of this study.

The fourth way stressors are assessed is by experimental manipulation, and the quality of these data depends on the subtlety of the experiment and the strength of the manipulation. The psychological component in stress shows its importance again here for Sales (1969) manipulated the degree of role over-load in an experiment and found a correlation of just over 0·4 between perceived role overload and objective role overload.

While most of these measures of stressors are potentially applicable to most work situations it could not be claimed that they have been applied to a representative sample of jobs, though a wide variety of jobs has been studied. The point is that any one of the above has been used in a much more limited way.

More justifiably perhaps most measures of *strain* are self-report measures. Measures are sometimes developed from projective tests or from observer ratings, peer reports, etc., but the vast majority are self-reports and this includes measures of stable traits such as anxiety and more passing states such as recent symptoms, job pressure or tension. These have reliabilities of a similar order to the stressors. The reliability ratings for the five dimensions of the Hopkin's Symptom Checklist (Derogatis *et al.*, 1974) range from 0·64 to 0·77. House and Rizzo quote reliability coefficients of 0·83, 0·76, and 0·72 for measures of job induced anxiety, somatic tension, and general fatigue respectively. Measures of job satisfaction and both state and trait anxiety (Spielberger, 1975) have similar orders of reliability. Once again very few measures in this area have been used on samples adequately representative of the general population though the different measures have been given to most segments of the population and they seem acceptable. While these data can not be described as highly refined they are not so rough as to be rejected out of hand.

Measures of outcome variables such as *behaviour* and *disease* are probably the most variable in terms of quality. It is easy enough to know a man drinks or smokes but much more difficult to know just how much. Similarly, one knows a man is absent from work, but just why he is absent is much more problematic.

As Clare points out in his book *Psychiatry in Dissent* (Clare, 1976) the unreliability of all but the most general psychiatric classifications is notorious, but diagnosis of physical illnesses is also much more dubious than the critics of psychiatry allow. Stomach troubles, back ache, dyspepsia, etc., may, or may not, have a real organic basis and it is often the case that they are genuine psychosomatic complaints and nobody is sure whether the psychological or the somatic component came first, is the main cause, and so on. As far as classifications of coping strategies in terms of what the person is doing to cope with (a) himself and (b) his environment are concerned then few exist and information on their reliability, etc., is virtually non-existent. The literature on defence mechanisms and on relaxation and meditation techniques provides some ways of looking at adjustment/self-cure strategies. Reichard *et al.* (1963) describe five patterns of adjustment in retirement, and Ackoff and Emery (1972) produce an interesting theoretical framework for classifying coping strategies but no data about their efficacy. Physiological indicators can of course be measured with great reliability, but they require base rates to be established for persons, are inconvenient to administer over lengthy time periods, and their validity as indicators of the presence of strain is still controversial. The data on the outcome variables, then, is possibly the 'roughest' of all, though much more variable than measures of stressors and strains. In *structural corroboration* these different measures are related to each other to test the structural hypotheses, so it is not surprising that these relatively 'rough' data produce, in combination, even rougher danda.

We saw on page 270 that the criteria for danda are concurrent and predictive validity and embeddedness in other structural propositions. Apart from well established measures of general traits such as anxiety it is hard to find good evidence of concurrent validity for measures of strain, stressors or outcome variables. This is partly because few measures have been seriously explored in these terms, but it is also due to the very complex relationships that exist among variables. Some stressors do combine to increase stress, but two stressors can combine to reduce stress. Or, while a stressor may be present in two situations it might be combined with high demands and constraints in one and low demands and constraints in the other. There is a tendency for low participation to go with certain supervisory styles, and certain forms of centralized control. But Payne and Pugh (1976) have reviewed the relationship between organizational structure and aspects of the climate such as support, pressure, etc., and found rather small relationships. Many studies in this area use the average of the ratings of a group of people and there is often not high consensus in the group as to just what is stressful about the environment. This is related to the validity of the measure and is a source of error too. Thus complex interactions of variables in the real world, and 'rough' measures combine to make the attainment of concurrent validity difficult.

Measures of strain do better, partly because they are usually all from the same person, and unless suffering from schizophrenia most people are relatively consistent in reporting that they feel tense about work, feel under pressure, and therefore do not like their jobs (Caplan *et al.*, 1975). Buck's study, to which we have already referred, produced relationships much higher than those of Caplan *et al.* but is another example of the greater consistency one achieves among self-report variables of this nature.

The distinction between concurrent validity and predictive validity begins to become a little vague since one can relate stressors to strains and strains to outcome variables and describe them as concurrent variables or dependent variables one is trying to predict. The fact is that measures of physiological responses such as heart rate, cholesterol, and diastolic blood pressure correlate with each other about 0·2. They then correlate with behavioural variables such as smoking and drinking coffee at about 0·15, and with stressor variables such as hours of work and perceived role ambiguity at about—0·10 (Caplan *et al.*, 1975). Kagan and Levi (1974) review the literature on the relationship between psychosocial factors and disease for four of the major psychosomatic diseases: coronary heart disease, thyrotoxicosis, hypertension, and gastro-intestinal disorders. For every one they conclude that there are good grounds for suspicion that psychosocial stimuli play a role in causing (and alleviating) these diseases, but while there is suspicion there is no proof of a causal relation-ship. The small correlations quoted above indicate that they may play a role, but that there are so many interacting variables at play that no one variable shows a strong, dominating effect. If we add these numerous small relation-ships together into a multivariate model then we can improve our ability to predict strain and disease. The multiple correlations of such studies vary between about 0·3 and 0·5. The question arises as to how useful such findings are. Else-where I have explored this question (Payne, 1976) which is a complex one, but my conclusions are conveyed by the quotation from Campbell's review of psychometric theory as it relates to industrial and organizational psychology (Campbell, 1976):

We can only hope that when a firm set of (psychometric) guidelines is finally mapped out they are not so complex as to be unusable .... For now, appropriate behaviour on the part of an applied psychologist would be to avoid developing empirical prediction rules on anything but very large samples and to double cross-validate in those instances. A single cross-validated estimate is never appropriate. (p. 216)

I know of no study of stress at work which meets these conditions. The issue is whether research in this tradition can attain these conditions and, if not, what alternative approaches are available. Pepper's world hypotheses present the most obvious framework for examining this.

It is my contention that the kind of research I have drawn on, and that most of the authors in this book have drawn on, has been carried out in the positivistic tradition for which mechanism is the root metaphor.

Mechanism

Mechanism has probably been the dominant metaphor during this century, and it has certainly influenced research in all areas of the social sciences. It has come under increasing criticism recently from all the social sciences and we have already seen that its proponents have not produced results which have been either theoretically inspiring or practically of great utility. It is such a powerful metaphor however that it seems there must be scope for its application. Without perhaps conceiving of it in Pepper's terms, Herbert's criticisms and conclusions seem the best evidence for the application of the mechanistic model to behavioural problems (Herbst, 1970).

Having concluded it is only possible to produce physical laws from postulates designed to deal with physical problems, Herbst (1970, p. 4) proceeds to examine the sorts of laws that might exist and to see which of these are in principle applicable to behaviour. Three laws are suggested, and they are labelled A, B, and C.

Type A

Both the functional form of the relationship and parametric values are universal constants.

The gas law is quoted as an example:

$$\frac{\text{pressure} \times \text{volume}}{\text{absolute temperature}} = R \text{ the gas constant}$$

The existence of such a law is discoverable by examining a large number of gases since it could be shown to apply to all the gases. In regard to the behavioural sciences Herbst feels very pessimistic about the possibility that such laws exist about behaviour due to the fact that 50 years of population studies have failed to even suggest one.

Type B

The functional form of the relationship is a constant but parameters are specific.

The rate of expansion of a metal rod with temperature is an example of a physical law of this kind. The formula would be $L = cT$, where L equals length, $T =$ absolute temperature, and c is a constant. The parameter c is specific for each metal but the relationship is the same for all metals. Herbst thinks it is possible that laws of behaviour could have this form where the parameters differed for each individual or each group. He points out that population studies would not reveal such a law because the law-like behaviour occurs within each individual, so that only the study of individual cases will reveal such laws.

Type C

Both the functional relationship and parameters are specific, but the generating rules for possible functional relationships are a universal constant. This law would fall outside the laws of physics.

It implies that each person and each group constitutes a behavioural universe which operates on the basis of its own laws. ... but also every person operates on his own measurement scales in terms of which he experiences and responds to both what he takes to belong to and be part of himself and what he regards as relevant aspects of his environment. We can in this case speak of laws only if we can find a set of generating rules for the possible range of behaviour principles that can come into operation. (p. 8)

Once again only the study of single cases is relevant, and this is the crux of Herbst's case: that every individual and every group is a behavioural universe with its own laws and measurement scales. Since behaviours do not possess the invariance properties (of functions and measures) that exist in the physical world the search for law-like properties needs to be of a different kind. What is required according to Herbst (p. 22) is 'to look for invariance properties at a more fundamental level. What we will arrive at is not a universal set of behaviour principles but a set of postulates which are able to generate the possible behavioural universes that can evolve and to exlude those that cannot come into being'.

Herbst illustrates the application of these ideas to individuals and groups and describes a number of study designs which can be used on the study of single cases—longitudinal time independent; cross-sectional where the individual carries out a cross-section of tasks; longitudinal phase transition technique where the development of an interpersonal relationship over time is shown to consist of a number of phases each of which achieves steady state conditions. In the preface to the book Herbst claims that all the longitudinal studies show that the process of structural development is not continuous, but that persons and groups go through phases which have steady state characteristics and the transition from one steady state to another is relatively abrupt. This is an important point since the limitation of Herbst's model to situations where steady state conditions exist seems at first sight to be very restricting and to limit severely the range of behaviours left to study. The fact that structures appear relatively quickly indicates that their scope is quite extensive. Nevertheless mechanism is seen as unsuitable for the study of populations such as has been attempted in stress research. It is the individuality of each case, of course, which leads to the small predictive correlations described in a previous section. Any prediction about a single individual from these studies of groups has such a large margin of error that it is of very little practical value. As we shall see, formism appears lacking for not dissimilar reasons.

Formism

A formistic study of stress would involve an increasingly sophisticated taxonomy of stressors, strains, diseases, and behaviours, so as to be able to decide in what ways different situations, persons, diseases, and coping behaviours were similar. In this way it would eventually be possible to 'draw a map' of the person most likely to do well or badly in a particular set of circumstances. This achievement would imply the existence of a law, but that is quite possible in formism since a law is itself 'a form' (Pepper, 1942, p. 177) which connects one set of basic particulars to another set. From a scientific point of view the search for the forms of laws is what increasing knowledge is really about, and the descriptions of the qualities of particulars are only building blocks in the edifice of knowledge. An analogy which illustrates such an approach is to be found in biology where it would be possible to make a good guess at the kind of animal or plant that might survive a given ecological circumstance. In industry and commerce personnel selection attempts this very problem using a formistic root metaphor by drawing up job and man specifications and trying to find the person who best fits the categories. Some of the reasons why selection systems are less successful than was once hoped are that the taxonomies of jobs, people, and performance criteria are inadequately developed and somewhat unreliable in use. As we have seen, this comment applies equally, if not more forcefully, to the study of stress at work.

This potential unreliability emphasizes the importance of multiplicative corroboration within this structural metaphor. People must be able to agree what the appropriate categories are and it must be possible for many people to reliably place particular examples in the correct categories. The ability to classify persons, diseases, and coping behaviours is not well enough advanced (see Clare, 1976). Thus reliability, construct validity, and adequate sampling are the more important criteria for formism.

One cannot help but feel that in a field which lacks adequate taxonomies of independent, dependent, and intervening variables, much progress could be made by further attempts in the formistic mould. The prognosis does not seem good, however, particularly when one has to rely on the reports of human subjects whether they be given in interview or on questionnaire. Epidemiological investigations presently come closest to following the formistic metaphor in that they rely on placing people or situations into categories and finding some correspondences between categories and people and diseases. Birtchnell (1974) reviews the field of epidemiological studies of family factors in mental illness and in his abstract of the paper comments: 'It is concluded that at the present stage of research into families greater stress should be laid upon the verbal descriptive type of study and the researcher should beware of the temptation to seek false security in presenting his findings in numerical terms.' If the taxonomies can be considerably improved then this criticism might become invalid, but the attempts to improve psychiatric diagnoses and classifications have proven very resistant to progress of a significant kind as is reported in the symposium on the definition and measurement of mental health sponsored by the US Department of Statistics (Sells, 1968). Whether priority should be given to work within the formistic tradition then seems highly debatable.

Mechanism and formism are both analytic theories and this is partly why they have similar deficiencies. Contextualism and organicism are synthetic theories and also have similar faults and virtues. These two are possibly more similar to each other than mechanism and formism. Both are concerned with the event in its context, and both are concerned with the wholeness or quality surrounding the event. The major difference is that organicism assumes the existence of absolute truth in a determinate world, while contextualism assumes the possibility of continuous change. Apart from indicating a broader historical examination of the events, the two world theories would lead the researcher to do similar things in practice. Given this, and other arguments about the likelihood of there being absolute truth (Popper, 1974), I shall save time by concentrating on the relevance of contextualism for the study of stress, though I have argued elsewhere (Payne, 1975) it is the most relevant for social science at this time. It would be dogmatic and wrong to argue it was the only one.

Contextualism

The calls for more studies of organizational processes (Weick 1969), the injunction to include change within our theoretical frameworks (Argyris, 1972), and the plea to consider more subjective methods of data collection (Poole, 1972 and ethnomethodologists such as Garfinkel, 1967) all indicate that the contextualistic root metaphor is presently regarded as a most appropriate one for the behavioural sciences. Since this is so the implications of the metaphor will be considered in greater detail.

The root metaphor of contextualism is the act in and with its setting: 'These acts or events are intrinsically complex, composed of interconnected activities with continuously changing patterns. They are like incidents in the plot of a novel or drama. They are literally the incidents of life' (Pepper, 1942, p. 233). The stress on 'continuously changing patterns' is what distinguishes contextualism from the other world theories, for if there are unchangeable structures in the world such as the forms of formism, or the space–time structures of mechanism, then contextualism would be a restricted hypothesis, and hence a false world hypothesis.

The basic, fundamental categories of contextualism are quality and texture, and although it is conceivable that some future states may not contain these two categories in the world as we know it, it is quality and texture that provide the structure the world does have.

Pepper says that it is impossible to understand quality and texture separately, but they can be contrasted. The quality of a given event is its intuited wholeness or total character; the texture is the details and relations which make up that character or quality. The quality of contextualism itself is its root metaphor— the historic event. The texture is the categories of quality and texture. The quality of a performance of a ballet is the total effect it produces—the actual dancers, props, and orchestra are the texture of the event. As the gestalt psychologists would argue, we see the whole (quality) and it is only in later analysis that we see the parts (texture). Quality has three sub-categories: spread, change, and fusion.

Spread

The contextualists believe that an event can only be understood qualitatively by assuming the event is located both in the past and the future, as well as the present. They do not accept the primacy of linear time as the mechanists do. They accept linear or schematic time is useful, but for them qualitative time is more useful. Indeed schematic time is regarded as a derivative of it. In an actual event the present is the whole texture which directly contributes to the quality of the event (Pepper, 1942, p. 242).

Change

This refers to changes in the quality of events. Even as events occur each part of an event extends forwards and backwards in the specious present. As the event unfolds the quality of the event may change. Permanent structures may appear to exist but these are interpreted as historical continuities which are not changeless. While fundamental to the contextualistic position change itself appears like a backdrop—it is there, but the event is still interpretable.

Fusion

The quality of an event is determined by the degree of fusion in the details of its texture. This idea is well illustrated by some of the visual illusions used in the psychology of perception. The vase figure which is also the outline of a face shows a higher degree of fusion than the three rows of dots formed into a square. The former is always seen as a vase or a face, whereas many people may just see three vertical or three horizontal lines of dots rather than a square. A team of players who co-ordinate their play are more fused than a team of equally skilful individuals who are not 'getting together'. It is this degree of fusion which determines the unity of an event. In other world theories fusion is interpreted as vagueness, failure to discriminate, but it is a central feature of contextualism, since the contextualists believe that even the simplest things are fusions of details.

In practice its centrality is somewhat ignored since 'the analysis and practical control of events goes on in terms of the categories of texture. . . . But, without qualities, textures would be as empty as sentences the words of which had no meaning' (Pepper, 1942, p. 246). This interdependence is not confined to quality and texture. Pepper also takes the stance that the first two categories of texture, strands and context, are so interlocked with the notion of texture itself that all three must be considered together.

The categories are indeed complexly interlocked as the following quotation illustrates.

A texture is made up of strands and it lies in a context. There is, moreover, no very sharp line between strands and context, because it is the connections of the strands which determine the context, and in large proportion the context determines the qualities of the strands. But by way of definition we may say that whatever directly contributes to the quality of a texture may be regarded as a strand, whereas whatever indirectly contributes to it will be regarded as context. (p. 246)

Taking the decision making activity of a group of senior executives as an event, it might be said that the executives themselves are the strands of the event. But they are based in a context represented by their departments and in a wider context represented by their professional reference groups. These contexts of the strands obviously bring something of their quality into the texture of the event. Therefore, each of these strands can be reconceived as an event or a quality which will have its own texture and strands, etc. This interdependence is so clear to the contextualist that he ridicules the idea of analysing things into their elements since elemental analysis so easily distorts the real quality of the event. It is thus 'pragmatic' or practical to limit analysis to the degree to which it reveals the quality of the particular unity being studied. This pragmatic choice as to where the event ends is akin to having to decide where the boundary of a system lies when following a systems theory model. Both are, in an absolute sense, arbitrary decisions. It is perfectly legitimate for the contextualist to 'intuit' where the wholeness lies.

The third category of texture is references of the strands: these are a detailed specification of strands and there are four of them—linear, convergent, blocked, and instrumental.

(1) A linear reference has a point of *initiation*, a transitive *direction*, and achieves an ending or a *satisfaction*. The direction is forwards and backwards being consistent with the 'spread' of the event. Returning to our group of executives, the chairman's activities to keep to the agenda exemplify a linear reference. They start from the agenda, and as the group proceeds the agenda moves them forwards and backwards both directly and indirectly through its relation to past events. Finally, the meeting ends and the satisfaction of that particular linear reference is achieved.

(2) A convergent reference describes a situation where several linear references converge on one satisfaction. It is a contextualist's version of a form since the convergence implies some similarity. A consensus decision would be an example. The executives only have this similarity on this one issue, and become dissimilar, non-convergent, on others.

(3) Blocking refers to the blocking of a linear or a convergent reference. Strands do not always run smoothly from their initiation to their satisfaction. When they do we have order, and it is blocking that creates novelty or disorder. Usually the blocking is due to another strand conflicting with the strand. It is therefore likely that investigation of the blocking strand will show how the two strands arrived in conflict. It is thus not absolutely new or novel and is called 'intrusive novelty'. Most novelty is of this kind, but the contextualist allows the possibility of an absolutely inexplicable blocking which would be called an 'emergent novelty'.

(4) Instrumental references are secondary acts which remove the blocking reference or, if not remove it, circumvent it. Once again this can become

very complicated if instrumental references build one upon another, but what retains the integration is the original linear reference which was seeking satisfaction when the blocking occurred. In a sense, any instrumental reference is a texture in its own right with its own satisfaction, but it is guided by the terminal action it is serving and also by the blocking action it is trying to neutralize. This pattern can become so interlocked that what was originally a blocking can become like an articulated linear reference itself, giving the appearance of a total quality. Because of this what appeared to be discrete textures can become fused so that they far outreach the contextualistic present. This is how contextualism extends beyond the present event even though its categories are all derived from the present event.

The original truth theory of contextualism was known as *operationalism*. This is because it was regarded as a purely empirical examination of what men did when they called something true. That is, what happens when a strand is blocked? If the action taken to remove the block works then that is a truthful solution: 'Truth is the result of an instrumental texture which removes a blocking and integrates a terminal texture' (Pepper, 1942, p. 269). This view of the truth theory is also called 'successful working'.

The critics of contextualism have found this a very naïve view of truth on somewhat similar grounds to the criticisms of relativism. A major part of their criticism is that there is a hypothesis about which instrumental act will remove the blocking but it is the act, not the hypothesis which is regarded as true. The truth theory was accordingly modified to what Pepper calls the 'verified hypothesis' theory (1942, p. 272). This simply means that it is the hypothesis, not the act, which is true or false, and when there is no hypothesis there is no test of truth or falsehood, there is only successful or unsuccessful working. This is an important change since it makes it possible to consider the truth of a hypothesis which has not yet been verified.

Despite this improvement, proponents of the rival world theories still criticize the 'verified hypothesis'. They do so on the grounds that there is no link to the actual qualities of nature. It does not mirror nature directly such as the forms of formism do. Pepper's reaction to this is that it is over-harsh and that the spirit of contexualism itself can overcome it by what he calls 'qualitative confirmation'. That is, if the hypothesis is treated as a linear reference that achieves satisfaction then the examination of the strands of that hypothesis will inevitably extend to textures which are present in the event itself. In this way a hypothesis can lead to insight into the quality of nature itself. The notion of 'qualitative confirmation' seems particularly apposite to human stress research.

Some implications of contextualism in the study of stress

The most fundamental re-orientation would arise from the necessity to research events, and that means actual cases of people under stress. Most work has been epidemiological or correlational and there have been few studies involving the study of cases directly. Such studies raise practical problems of access to the cases for anyone who is not a physician. Since few physicians possess much social psychological knowledge and experience of organizations this almost certainly implies the need for multidisciplinary teams. One of the few studies that could be described as in the spirit of contextualism actually operated in this way. Weiner *et al.* (1973) set out to reduce the amount of lost time due to mental illness among workers in the New York garment industry. They involved the insurers, the trade unions, the managers, mental health professionals in special clinics as well as hospital staffs in neighbouring areas. Jointly these groups worked out a programme to encourage all concerned to identify, advise, and support people with symptoms of mental illness. Shop stewards, for example, referred 103 of the 718 cases seen in the clinic. The early diagnosis and support enabled many 'ill' people to continue work, so that work itself acted as a therapeutic agent. The essence of the programme's pragmatism is illustrated here: 'the professional saw himself as mediator, helping the individual negotiate the work system and helping the work setting change those patterns which proved dysfunctional to the particular worker' (Weiner *et al.*, 1973, p. 147).

I have great admiration for this work, but I would suggest that it might have been even more fruitful had it systematically followed the contextualist model. They had events identified in that persons were stopping work, or being ineffective. They had set a common linear strand—to return them to effective working. For each case they could have explored blocking strands (boss, family, skills, attitudes, and values, etc.?) and what might be instrumental in removing them (medical help, support from boss, support from wife, etc.?). A concern for the quality of the context of the event might have highlighted more fundamental questions about the kind of work done. It is true this might lead to the identification of political issues which might be against raising such questions. But these can be seen as blocking strands and faced, or the pragmatic decision might be made that the quality is acceptable given the constraints. Contextualism, if correctly pursued, forces examination of such issues, but in itself imposes no constraints on what is acceptable since the context itself must define that. What the categories of contextualism offer is a systematic guide to the exploration of events. It is a more reliable way of refining data, and identifying and testing danda.

Since contextualism involves finding the way to satisfy linear strands it is more likely to lead to action, since the hypothesis about what is blocking satisfaction cannot be verified unless one acts to achieve satisfaction. This surely places the researcher in a much healthier psychological contract with the researched than that which exists in the traditional, mechanistic research relationship where the researcher strives to avoid 'contaminating' the situation.

Contamination was avoided in mechanism, of course, so that results were not biased by the situation and were therefore generalizable. Is contextualist knowledge generalizable? In the sense that hypotheses that have worked in one context are the best bets for trying in another context which is similar

282

the answer is clearly 'yes'. But the additional bonus is the contextualist call, 'Beware, the situation may not be the same, so test it!'

This emphasis on verifying hypotheses ought to be enough to demonstrate that contextualism is not anti-experimental. An experiment is a way of creating an event. It might lead the experimenter to be more careful about assuming that the behaviour of the control group is only different because of the experimental manipulation and he might be encouraged to understand that event too. Since some researchers in human affairs claim there is no such thing as a control group but only different experimental groups then this might not be a retrograde step.

What is probably clear is that contextualism involves much more detailed work, and that means smaller studies. Since we have demonstrated that the large scale cross-sectional study has not been very helpful in predicting individual reactions to stressors then this cannot be counted too negatively. In-depth, clinical, and processual studies of the kind implied by pragmatism stand at least a chance of helping the individual case. Good and lasting solutions to such individual problems will surely have a reasonable chance of working in similar contexts.

When the famous neurophysiologist, Sir John Eccles, first read Popper on refutation in science its psycho-logic, rather than its logic, affected him. Instead of being depressed about an unsupported theory he was now called on to feel elated about the challenge to produce a better theory. And the same applies to contextualism. The standards for evidence, the use of experimentation and measurement are not lost in contextualism, but for the study of human affairs the stress on looking at contexts, on expecting change and on looking for wholeness and quality, psychologically have the right appeal. In the language of contextualism this chapter is itself a linear strand added to those of many others calling for a change in our philosophy of how to understand human behaviour (e.g. Chein, 1972; McGuire 1973). I only hope that not too many blocking strands (old attitudes, time, habits) will converge to prevent it achieving satisfaction.

References

Ackoff, R. L., and Emery, F. E. (1972) *On Purposeful Systems*. London. Tavistock.
Argyris, C. (1972) *The Applicability of Organizational Sociology*. London. Cambridge University Press.
Bales, R. F. (1950) *Interaction Process Analysis*. Reading, Mass. Addison-Wesley.
Bateson, G. (1972) *Steps to an Ecology of Mind*. New York. Ballantine.
Birtchnell, J. (1974) Is there a scientifically acceptable alternative to the epidemiological study of familial factors in mental illness?, *Social Science and Medicine*, **8**, 335–350.
Buck, V. E. (1972) *Working Under Pressure*. London. Staples Press.
Burtt, E. A. (1943) The status of 'world hypotheses', *Philosophical Review*, **52**, 590–601.
Campbell, J. P. (1976) Psychometric theory. In Dunnette, M. D. (ed.), *Handbook of Industrial and Organizational Psychology*. Chicago. Rand McNally.
Caplan, R. D., Cobb, S., French, J. R. P., Jr, Harrison, R. V., Pinneau, S. R., Jr (1975) *Job Demands and Workers Health*. National Institute of Occupational Safety and Health, US Government Printing Office, Washington DC.

283

Chein, I. (1972) *The Science of Behaviour and the Image of Man*. London. Tavistock.

Clare, A. (1976) *Psychiatry in Dissent*. London. Tavistock.

Derogatis, L. R., Lipman, R. S., Rickels, K., Uhlenhuth, E. H., Covi, L. (1974) Psychological measurements in psychopharmacology, *Mod. Probl. Pharmacopsychiat.*, **7**, 79–110.

Garfinkel, H. (1967) *Studies in Ethnomethodology*. Englewood Cliffs, NJ. Prentice-Hall.

Guilford, J. P. (1954) *Fundamental Statistics in Psychology and Education*. New York. McGraw-Hill.

Hackman, J. R., and Oldham, G. R. (1975) Development of the job diagnostic survey, *Journal of Applied Psychology*, **60**, 159–170.

Herbst, P. G. (1970) *Behavioural Worlds; the Study of Single Cases*. London. Tavistock.

House, R. J., and Rizzo, J. R. (1972) Role conflict and ambiguity as critical variables in a model of organizational behaviour, *Organizational Behaviour and Human Performance*, **7**, 3, 467–505.

Jung, J. (1971) *The Experimenter's Dilemma*. New York. Harper Row.

Kagan, A., and Levi, L. (1974) Health and environment-psychosocial stimuli: a review, *Social Science and Medicine*, **8**, 225–241.

McGuire, W. J. (1973) The yin and yang of progress in social psychology; seven koan, *Jnl Personality and Social Psychology*, **26**, 3, 446–456.

Magee, B. (1973) *Popper*. London. Fontana.

Payne, R. L. (1975) *Epistemology and the Study of Behaviour in Organizations*. Memo no. 68, MRC Social and Applied Psychology Unit, Sheffield University.

Payne, R. L. (1976) Truisms in Organizational Behaviour. *Interpersonal Development*, **6**, 203–220.

Payne, R. L., and Pugh, D. S. (1976) Organizational structure and climate. In Dunnette, M. D. (ed.), *Handbook of Industrial and Organizational Psychology*. Chicago. Rand McNally.

Pepper, S. (1942) *World Hypotheses*. Berkeley, Calif. University of California Press.

Pepper, S. (1958) *Forces of Values*. London. Cambridge University Press.

Phillips, D. (1973) *Abandoning Method*. San Francisco. Jossey-Bass.

Poole, R. (1972) *Towards Deep Subjectivity*. London. Allan Lane.

Popper, K. (1963) *Conjectures and Refutations*. London. Routledge Kegan Paul.

Popper, K. (1972) *Objective Knowledge; an Evolutionary Approach*. Oxford University Press.

Popper, K. (1974) Replies to my critics. In Schilpp, P. A. (ed.), *The Philosophy of Karl Popper*. La Salle, Ill. Open Court.

Reichard, S., Livson, F., Peterson, P. G. (1963) *Ageing and Personality: a Study of 87 Older Men*. New York. Wiley.

Sales, S. M. (1969) Organizational role as a risk factor in coronary heart disease, *Administrative Science Quarterly*, **14**, 325–336.

Sells, S. B. (1968) *The Definition and Measurement of Mental Health*, US Department of Health, Education, and Welfare, US Government Printing Office, Washington, DC.

Spielberger, C. D. (1975) Anxiety: state-trait-process. In Spielberger, C. D., *Stress and Anxiety*, vol. 1. Washington. Hemisphere/Wiley.

Toulmin, S. (1972) *Human Understanding*. Oxford. Oxford University Press.

Turner, A. N., and Lawrence, P. R. (1965) *Industrial Jobs and the Worker*. Boston, Mass. Harvard University Press.

Weick, K. (1969) *The Social Psychology of Organizing*. Reading, Mass. Addison-Wesley.

Weick, K. (1974) Middle range theories of social systems, *Behavioural Science*, **18**, 6, 357–367.

Weiner, H. J., Akabas, S. H., and Sommer, J. J. (1973) *Mental Health Care in the World of Work*. New York. Association Press.

Zetterberg, H. (1966) *On Theory and Verification in Sociology*. Totowa, NJ. Bedminster Press.

Concluding Remarks

In the introduction to this book we suggested that facts based on scientific study were perhaps stranger than fiction and certainly more complex. The reader was made well aware of this complexity in Kasl's chapter when he commented, 'I should like to close this section by reminding the reader that no matter how bewildered he or she is by this array of findings, the picture can only get worse were one to also consider other issues of a methodological or substantive nature.' This self-critical characteristic of science and scholarship is always a prerequisite, but it seems to have come to the fore unusually strongly in these essays. This suggests a time of reappraisal in this field of study. Kasl is totally objective about the poor methodological nature of past work as well as about the strength of those relationships in which we can have some degree of confidence. McMichael, too, is critical of much past work and, even in a volume about stress at work, reminds us that psychological and physical strains seem so idiosyncratic to the individual that he, rather than work, might be the appropriate focus of attention. This is not to say that McMichael does not recognize the interactive relationship between the man and his environment but only that factors within the individual appear to account for most of the variance; or would do if we could succeed in measuring them adequately. Beech, too, is cautious about translating behavioural techniques to work problems and reminds us of the need to properly evaluate them when they are used so as to increase our understanding of their relevance, positive qualities, and limitations.

As editors we feel this is as it should be. We set out to tell people what is known about stress at work, what is not known, and where further information can be found. We feel satisfied that we have done this. In doing this the authors have also proposed views about how the study of stress should continue in the future. This is the main focus of Payne's chapter, but all the chapters make some reference to this as it applies to the particular areas in which they have concentrated. The main suggestions are that there should be fewer cross-sectional studies; that too many studies have operationalized both dependent and independent variables from the subjective reports of the individual, and that such studies are of little scientific use even though strain is a subjective phenomenon; that there should be more longitudinal studies; that we should take all opportunities to use 'natural' experiments as sources of further knowledge; that interventions to improve work situations from the point of view of psychological and physical health should be properly evaluated and treated like a natural experiment; that research should not stop at the factory gate; since strain is an idiographic phenomenon, that more idiographic studies (pragmatic) should be carried out. An indication of pragmatism among researchers seems present in these chapters since there is no strong emphasis on defining and agreeing the use of terms. While it would seem desirable, there is no strong contender for this arena and fruitful, if frustrating, work seems possible without too much soul searching.

Another editorial aim was to provide some information about what to do about stress at work. Figure 1 summarizes some of the techniques that have been used to combat stress. The figure follows the philosophy of the book in considering the individual and the environment. The environment is classified

Figure 1
STRATEGIES FOR ACTION

| | ROLE OF PERSON | |
	INITIATOR	RESPONDENT
Organizational environment	PHYSICAL: He (and colleagues) design own environ-ment TECHNOLOGY: Designs own work methods (e.g. autonomous work groups) STRUCTURE: Designs own roles, duties, or negotiates	'Experts' design environment Time and work study design tasks Consultants or managers design 'best' structure
Interpersonal environment	Uses role-set models or other models of interpersonal relations to diagnose and treat interpersonal issues Initiates role negotiations, confrontation, problem solving meetings	Techniques applied: T-groups; role negotiation; inter-team confrontation; restructuring of roles, communication, authority; manipulate rewards
Person him/herself	Personal growth labs; will power training (self-help); acquires new skills, capacities; tries 'new' situations; meditation; yoga; karate; co-counselling	Counselling; psychotherapy; vocational guidance; medical care (drugs, hospital); rehabilitation; training and education

broadly into the interpersonal environment which includes relations with bosses, subordinates and the family, and the organizational which distinguishes between the physical environment, the technological environment, and the structure of the organization. In all cases the system in focus (the individual, the interpersonal, or the organizational) is considered as an initiator or as a respondent. This simply means the system can do things for itself or it can have things done to it, though these are usually with its agreement. The chapters in this volume deal with aspects of all six cells. The concentration tends to be in the respondent cells though Bridger's chapter directs our attention for systems at all levels to take an initiating role towards their situations. Beech and Ellis focus largely on the respondent cell at the individual level but the ideas of both are recommended for use in the initiator role. Handy's scheme provides a framework which could be used to analyse the family from either perspective. The chapter by Cooper and Marshall makes suggestions which cover all six cells in Figure 1, while Johansen's chapter stresses the importance of the relationship between the technology and the social structure as they affect individual jobs and interpersonal relationships. The chapter by Poulton provides a rich catalogue of how to improve the physical environment of jobs. Harrison's chapter also stresses the relationships among the cells since its emphasis is on the fit between the person and his environment. This frame-work offers rich suggestions as to what is, and is not, relevant to obtaining better fit. It appears particularly useful for consultants operating in the respondent cells.

Some of the possible actions at the individual level are not really dealt with in this book, such as meditation, karate, and co-counselling. Not a lot of research exists on these in the work place, but meditation, physical fitness programmes, and counsellors in the work setting are all on the increase and suggest areas of development for both research and practice.

Given the relatively pessimistic view of research in this book it is encouraging to find the applied field increasing and vigorous. There is almost a paradox in the sense that we do not appear to be able to claim we know much so, how can we recommend action? Well the answer is that we might not know exactly how A affects B but we have some good ideas of what variables are important even when we cannot measure them. Applied work is also by its nature more pragmatic and looking for things that solve the problem at hand. The applied researcher may bother less about why particular approaches work. But this suggests an unreal distinction between research and practice as roads to knowledge. We have already seen in the criticisms of past research that future studies must concentrate also on natural experiments and action research. The confidence placed in proposals for action in this volume, then, is based on evidence that many of the approaches tried work and that the same and other approaches will lead to better knowledge if the chance is taken to study such action properly.

One study illustrates the possibilities. Weiner et al. (1973) report an attempt to improve the mental health of employees in the New York clothing industry. The stress in this project was getting people to work or keeping them at work when they might have gone absent. It involved a community approach. There were researchers, medical staff who manned a clinic, the trade union, the managers, the insurer, and the community hospitals. It was very much a colla-borative approach where all groups were encouraged to aid in the diagnosis and care of the people who were ill. Data showed that this approach was very successful in that referrals came from all groups in substantial numbers. It was also successful in that work became a form of therapy in itself. But most of all it worked to show what was possible in research terms in a project which had a very practical orientation. This study signposts the future in several ways: first, that studies must take place over several years; second, that research is multi-disciplinary; and, third, that work is one of the few places where large numbers of people can be educated about mental illness, its recognition, its treatment, and its future prevention. For the community in general, and the research community in particular, the costs of mounting and funding such studies must surely be considerably less than the practical and theoretical benefits likely to accrue. Despite its difficulties, the study of stress at work is here to stay.

Reference

Weiner, H. J., Akabas, S. H., and Sommer, J. J. (1973) *Mental Health Care in the World of Work*, Association Press, New York.

Index

292